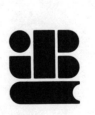

*A publication of the*
Association of American Medical Colleges

# Teaching
# Quality Assurance
# and Cost Containment
# in Health Care

*A Faculty Guide*

# John W. Williamson, M.D. and Associates

Daniel M. Barr, M.D.
Elizabeth Fee, Ph.D.
Mohan L. Garg, Sc.D.
James I. Hudson, M.D.
Mary Lee Ingbar, Ph.D.
William F. Jessee, M.D.
Donald R. Korst, M.D.
Madeline M. Nevins, Ph.D.
Jay Noren, M.D.
Frank T. Stritter, Ph.D.
Renate Wilson

# Teaching Quality Assurance and Cost Containment in Health Care

 Jossey-Bass Publishers

San Francisco • Washington • London • 1982

TEACHING QUALITY ASSURANCE AND COST CONTAINMENT IN HEALTH CARE
*A Faculty Guide*
by John W. Williamson and Associates

Copyright © 1982 by:   Association of American
Medical Colleges
One Dupont Circle, Suite 200
Washington, D.C. 20036

Jossey-Bass Inc., Publishers
433 California Street
San Francisco, California 94104

Jossey-Bass Limited
28 Banner Street
London EC1Y 8QE

**Library of Congress Cataloging in Publication Data**
Main entry under title:

Teaching quality assurance and cost containment in health
  care.

  Bibliography: p. 312
  Includes index.
  1. Medical care—Quality control—Study and
Teaching.  2. Medical care—Cost control—Study and
teaching.  3. Medical education.  4. Medicine—Study and
teaching (Graduate)  I. Williamson, John W.
RA399.A1T4  1982   362.1   82-48071
ISBN 0-87589-530-1

Manufactured in the United States of America

The paper in this book meets the guidelines for
permanence and durability of the Committee on
Production Guidelines for Book Longevity of the
Council on Library Resources.

FIRST EDITION

*Code 8223*

*The Jossey-Bass Series
in Higher Education*

# Contents

## ⚡⚡⚡⚡⚡⚡⚡⚡⚡⚡⚡⚡⚡⚡⚡⚡⚡⚡⚡⚡⚡⚡⚡

## Part Three: State-of-the-Art of Quality Assurance and Cost Containment Education

     Cost Containment Programs                       231
     *Mohan L. Garg*

12.  Future Trend and Needs                          258
     *John W. Williamson, James I. Hudson,
     and Jay Noren*

     Appendix A: A Historical Perspective on Quality
     Assurance and Cost Containment                  278
     *Elizabeth Fee*

     Appendix B: Efficacy of Selected Common
     Interventions for Coronary Artery Disease        297
     *Daniel M. Barr*

     References                                      312

     Index                                           337

# Foreword

This book serves as a resource and guide for modifying the education and training of physicians and other health professionals to include concepts of quality assurance and cost containment. In recognition of the diversity of approaches used at each educational level, it does not present a "model" curriculum. It does, however, describe educational experiences that will prepare future health professionals to continue monitoring the quality of care they provide throughout their professional lives.

It is clear that the rapid rate of growth in resources devoted to health care characteristic of the past will not continue into the future. Several segments of society, particularly the federal government, are already raising objections to the proportion of the Gross National Product expended on medical services. Proposals have been made to introduce more price competition and more regulation into the system as ways of reducing escalating costs. In light of this activity, the continuation of gains made in the care of the poor and the aged is threatened. Restriction of funding in the face of the increasing costs of new complex and expensive technology requires that greater attention be paid to the costs of medical care. At the same time, more effort must be made to assure that the highest priority of care is provided under the restrictions imposed. This book will help prepare physicians and other health professionals in meeting this critical challenge.

The Association of American Medical Colleges has undertaken a number of programs over the past decade in response to growing concerns about the quality and rapidly escalating costs of medical care. Among these were regional workshops to interest the faculties and to assist in incorporating these important subjects into undergraduate medical education and residency training. Based on these workshops, this volume and its companion, *Principles of Quality Assurance and Cost Containment: A Guide for Medical Students, Residents, and Other Health Professionals,* have been prepared by a group of experts to provide a resource and to extend this assistance to a larger group of educators.

The Association is pleased that these two important works on quality assurance and cost containment in medical care initiate its Series on Academic Medicine—one that will address important issues in the administration and conduct of medical education.

*July 1982*                                    John A.D. Cooper, M.D., Ph.D.
                                               *President, Association*
                                               *of American Medical Colleges*

# Preface

The codes established by all health care professions commit members to the highest quality of care and to professional excellence. Implicit in these standards is a responsibility of health care professionals to assess and improve the quality of care on a continuing basis. Until recently, however, few attempts were made to develop an extrinsic, systematic approach to monitor and improve care. This situation has changed within the past decade. Professional organizations such as the Joint Commission on Accreditation of Hospitals (JCAH) now require systematic quality assurance programs for hospitals and affiliated ambulatory care programs. Professional Standards Review Organizations (PSROs), established by the Social Security Amendments of 1972 to review quality of care and use of inpatient hospital services delivered to Medicare and

Medicaid patients, have expanded the scope of their review and are currently developing criteria for use in ambulatory settings and long-term care facilities. An implicit concern with quality and excellence has become explicit, and systematic assessment of care is now an integral part of medical services in the United States.

Concurrent with the increasing interest in quality assurance has been a growing concern with containing the costs of health care. The increase in federal expenditures for medical services and the rapid escalation of hospital costs are two of many factors that have led economists, government officials, and leaders of labor and industry to examine how to curb health care costs.

Both these trends imply that future physicians will be practicing in an environment that differs from that of their predecessors. In recognition of these changes, medical school faculties have undertaken to introduce formal training in quality assurance and cost containment into medical school curricula and residency programs. Their efforts have been impeded by the lack of published materials that present a broad-based approach to teaching these issues. This book provides a framework for integrating quality assurance and cost containment concepts and methods into medical school curricula and residency programs so that future physicians will be trained both to participate in existing programs and to develop their own approach to monitoring and assessing the care provided in their own practices.

The authors acknowledge that teaching quality assurance and cost containment is not an easy task. Definitions of quality assurance and cost containment vary, methodologies differ, and potential and actual sites for quality assurance and cost containment studies range from the large academic medical center to the office of the individual practitioner. Moreover, the state of the art is in flux, with changes in policy and procedures advocated frequently. This text proposes an approach that can be applied despite these difficulties. It offers suggestions for planning the curriculum, defines and explains key concepts that form the basis of quality assurance and cost containment efforts, and provides a description of the stages that constitute a successful quality assurance program.

## The Concept of Quality Assurance

As used in this text, *quality assurance* refers to a health care discipline that provides the theoretical framework and practical resources required for assessing and improving the effectiveness and efficiency of health care delivery in actual practice. In defining quality assurance in terms of both effectiveness *and* efficiency, it is recognized that quality assurance encompasses both the traditional concept of quality (that is, a high degree of effectiveness in providing care) and cost containment as commonly understood (that is, an efficient use of resources). Whenever the term *cost containment* is used, it refers to this second dimension of quality assurance— namely, assessment and improvement of the efficiency with which resources are used; it does not mean only a reduction in charges.

The purpose of assessing and improving health care effectiveness and efficiency, which is the purpose of quality assurance, is to effect a positive change in the health status of patient populations, in the satisfaction experienced by both patient and provider, and in the utilization of health care resources. Improving care, then, has as its ultimate goal improvements in one, several, or all of the outcomes of care. Quality assurance is the means by which this goal is attained at all levels of health services organization. It can be applied to delivery of care at the level of the individual patient/ physician encounter and at institutional, community, state, and national levels.

Regardless of the level of application, quality assurance involves understanding certain basic concepts and using systematic procedures. The problem-oriented approach on which the material in this text is based follows five basic steps: (1) identifying problems in health care delivery and selecting those that warrant investigation; (2) verifying selected problems; (3) identifying underlying factors that can be corrected; (4) implementing a plan that can effect improvement; and (5) reassessing health care delivery to determine the impact of the previous stages.

Several interrelated factors must be recognized and assessed in the quality assurance process: importance of the health problem; efficacy, effectiveness, and efficiency of interventions; and potential for achieving improvement. Importance is determined by examining the frequency with which a given health problem occurs within an identified population, the degree of actual or potential health loss associated with it, and the direct and indirect economic costs of both treatment and the health problem itself. Efficacy is established by estimating the degree of benefit to a defined population that can be obtained by particular health care interventions under ideal conditions of use. Effectiveness is evaluated by the extent to which the achievable benefit of interventions (established through efficacy studies) is actually achieved under ordinary conditions of care—that is, in day-to-day practice. Efficiency is measured as the extent to which the resources expended to achieve a given benefit have been utilized with minimum waste. The potential for improvement is gauged by comparing benefits that could be achieved with those that are actually being achieved and ascertaining the feasibility of effecting change with a more cost-effective expenditure of time and resources. All these factors are important in identifying and setting priorities for investigation, the first stage of quality assurance; all must be considered in the remaining stages of quality assurance as well.

### Content and Structure of This Book

The theory and stages of quality assurance, described briefly above, will be amplified and explained within the context of the primary purpose of this book: to facilitate the teaching of quality assurance and cost containment in medical schools and residency programs. The examples, drawn from quality assurance applied at the institutional level, use the aggregate of patients and providers within a given institution (for example, group practice, hospital) as the subject of the assessment and improvement study. Information on health care costs is presented primarily to illustrate how this information should be used as part of the assessment of health problem importance and health care efficiency.

The book has been designed as a faculty teaching resource to accompany a brief companion volume for students. As a teaching resource, it not only identifies and explains information to be covered in the teaching of quality assurance but also discusses ways in which the curriculum can be planned and implemented. We have tried to present a practical approach to the teaching of quality assurance and cost containment. The first part of the book, therefore, deals with planning, implementation, and evaluation of the curriculum itself; the second, and major, portion of the book contains the theoretical and practical information to be included in the curriculum; the final section describes past and present approaches to teaching quality assurance and cost containment and also discusses possible future trends in quality assurance that may affect the teaching of this important topic.

In Part One, "Integrating Quality Assurance and Cost Containment into Current Curriculum," basic curriculum planning theory is applied to the process of designing such a program (Chapter One); medical school courses and residency programs are examined and points where quality assurance and cost containment could be incorporated are identified (Chapter Two); and approaches are suggested for evaluating the components of the quality assurance curriculum (Chapter Three). The decision to place the discussion of curriculum development at the beginning of this book reflects the assumption that faculty members are seeking ways of teaching quality assurance and cost containment but, to date, have had few materials to assist in developing their programs. Without singling out any specific approach, these chapters attempt to provide a rationale and an implementation strategy applicable to development of curricula in a wide variety of situations; they offer curriculum goals and objectives that can be adapted to a comprehensive approach to teaching quality assurance and cost containment.

Part Two, "Incorporating Principles of Quality Assurance and Cost Containment into Curriculum Content," identifies and explains concepts to be addressed at various points in the curriculum and delineates the stages of the quality assurance process. Five chapters present basic information on core concepts of quality assurance: health problems as the framework for quality assurance studies, the importance of health problems as determined by their frequency and associated health and economic costs, the efficacy of interventions used to manage health problems, effectiveness and efficiency of health services provided under ordinary conditions of care, and improvement potential.

More specifically, Chapter Four discusses health problems as a framework for establishing quality assurance priorities. Chapter Five identifies the three major indexes of the importance of a health problem and provides information on health problems most frequently seen in ambulatory care and hospital practice and methods for determining their relative economic and social costs. The importance of using such frequency and cost information in setting priorities for quality assurance activities and for identifying appropriate areas for assessing health care effectiveness and efficiency is discussed. The material on health problem frequency is often incorporated into courses in epidemiology or public and community health, and the information on health loss and economic costs could be used in a course on health economics, thus making it possible to integrate quality assurance teaching at various points in the curriculum.

Chapter Six addresses two issues essential to quality assurance: how the efficacy of health care interventions is determined by research studies on a defined population under optimum conditions of care and how documented evidence of efficacy can be obtained for quality assurance purposes. Chapter Seven provides an overview of various methods currently used to measure the quality of care (that is, its effectiveness) and the cost-effective use of health care resources. Use of effectiveness and efficiency measurements to estimate the potential for improving care is explained. The material in Chapters Six and Seven can also be integrated into existing courses or programs. For example, the discussions of efficacy of health care interventions and of effectiveness and efficiency measurements, in conjunction with the material in Appendixes B and C, could well be incorporated into a course on research design.

Information on behavioral and cognitive approaches and on strategies for organizational, behavioral, and institutional change is presented in Chapter Eight. Chapter Nine provides detailed information on a systematic, five-stage approach to conducting a quality assurance study, including theoretical considerations and methods, and Chapter Ten reports a series of illustrative case studies conducted in different practice settings. The material in these three chapters is adaptable for inclusion in lectures, seminars, and discussion sessions specifically directed to quality assurance. It can also be learned through direct involvement in implementation of the concepts—for example, on rounds, in special research projects, or through participation on quality assurance committees. Learning of the material presented in Part Two can also be reinforced by including information on these concepts in discussions of individual cases during clinical clerkships or residency programs. Practical exercises and projects at the ends of chapters could be assigned to students or residents after the chapter content has been presented.

Two appendixes contain useful supplements to the teaching material in Part Two. Appendix A reviews the history of quality assurance and cost containment in medical practice. Factors that have contributed to present and proposed legislation on quality and cost review are presented, as are the broad outlines of the various federal laws. This information could easily be included in preclinical medical school courses that present an overview of the changing role of the physician in society, such as "Introduction to Medicine," "Introduction to Health Care," "Perspectives in Medicine," "Ethics in Medicine," or "History and Philosophy of Medicine." Appendix B illustrates in detail aspects of efficacy of selected common interventions for coronary artery disease.

The final portion of the text, "State-of-the-Art of Quality Assurance and Cost Containment Education," is again addressed to the faculty curriculum planner. Chapter Eleven reviews past and present quality assurance programs at academic medical centers, highlighting their strengths and weaknesses. Chapter Twelve offers a prognosis on quality assurance and cost containment methodologies that may become the assessment and improvement tools of the future. The information on the successes and failures of past and current teaching programs may serve as a guide for what is likely to work in teaching quality and cost to medical students and residents today. The discussion of future trends in quality assessment may prove useful for those upgrading existing programs as well as those starting new teaching programs in this area.

   In conclusion, it should be noted that this faculty resource is intended to be used in conjunction with a guide for medical students and other health professionals on conducting quality assurance studies. The guide differs from the faculty resource in two ways: (1) it is built around a case that illustrates the principles of quality assurance study, with each step of the five-step process explained in relation to the actual case presented, and (2) the material on importance, efficacy, effectiveness, efficiency, and improvement potential is greatly simplified. We hope that the use of these two companion volumes will facilitate the teaching of quality assurance and cost containment in the nation's academic medical centers.

*Boston, Massachusetts*                                    John W. Williamson
*August 1982*

# Acknowledgments

The preparation of this text was made possible by a grant from the Health Care Financing Administration (Grant No. 18-P-97124/3-01) to the Department of Health Services of the Association of American Medical Colleges and the School of Hygiene and Public Health of the Johns Hopkins University. The content of this text was adapted for use in *Principles of Quality Assurance and Cost Containment in Health Care: A Guide for Medical Students, Residents, and Health Professionals*, the companion volume to this book. The approach, as well as the fundamental principles of quality assurance on which this text is based, is the work of John Williamson, the principal author. The information on efficacy and its application to quality assurance was contributed by Daniel M. Barr. Some of the research on which Chapter Five was based was supported by the

National Fund for Medical Education through Grant No. 45/78A
sponsored by the American Hospital Supply Corporation. Jay
Noren contributed much of the material on effectiveness and efficiency; and William F. Jessee is responsible for the information on
achieving improvement. Material on curriculum development,
evaluation, and history was prepared by Mohan L. Garg, Donald R.
Korst, and Frank T. Stritter. The historical background of quality
assurance was developed by Elizabeth Fee and the prognosis for
future teaching of quality assurance was written by John W.
Williamson and James I. Hudson.

        The authors and project staff are particularly grateful to the
medical school students, residents, and faculty who participated in
the field testing of the original manuscript and whose recommendations led to the development of a separate text for students and
residents. It would be impossible to name all faculty and students
who participated in the field testing of this book. However, special
thanks are due to the following faculty who acted as coordinators at
the field test sites: C. M. G. Buttery, associate professor of community medicine, Department of Family Medicine, Eastern Virginia
Medical School; Herbert Lukashok, associate professor and acting
chairman, Department of Community Health, Albert Einstein College of Medicine, Yeshiva University; Kathleen Morton, deputy
director of Ambulatory Services, Montefiore Hospital and Medical
Center; Joseph Gonnella, associate dean and director of Academic
Programs, and Carter Zeleznik, associate director of the Offices of
Medical Education, Jefferson Medical College, Thomas Jefferson
University; William M. Marine, director of the Department of
Preventive Medicine and Comprehensive Health Care, University
of Colorado School of Medicine; Michael J. Garland, assistant pro-
fessor, Department of Public Health, University of Oregon Health
Science Center; Louise Ball, special assistant to the dean, and
Samuel C. Matheny, Division of Family Medicine, University of
Southern California School of Medicine; Charles Begley, assistant
professor, Department of Medical Humanities, Southern Illinois
University School of Medicine; and Herman S. Wigodsky, clinical
professor, Department of Pathology, University of Texas Health
Science Center at San Antonio.

A final word of thanks is extended to Dian Nelson and Katherine Hubscher, project secretaries in the Department of Health Services at the Association of American Medical Colleges, and to Bernice F. Culp, secretary to the Department of Health Services Administration at the Johns Hopkins University.

# The Authors

Daniel M. Barr is chairman, Department of Family Medicine, Illinois Masonic Medical Center, and associate professor, Department of Family Medicine, Abraham Lincoln School of Medicine, University of Illinois.

Elizabeth Fee is assistant professor, Department of Health Services Administration, School of Hygiene and Public Health, Johns Hopkins University.

Mohan L. Garg is professor, Department of Medicine, Medical College of Ohio.

James I. Hudson is staff associate, National Organization for Quality Assessment in Hospitals, Utrecht, The Netherlands.

Mary Lee Ingbar is professor of Family and Community Medicine, University of Massachusetts Medical School, and principal research associate, Department of Social Medicine and Health Policy, Harvard Medical School.

William F. Jessee is associate professor, Department of Health Administration, School of Public Health, and Department of Social and Administrative Medicine, School of Medicine, University of North Carolina, Chapel Hill.

Donald R. Korst is professor of medicine and chief, Section of General Internal Medicine, Evans Memorial Department of Clinical Research, Boston University Medical Center.

Jay Noren is director, Administrative Medicine, University of Wisconsin Medical School.

Frank T. Stritter is associate professor and director, Office of Research and Development for Education in the Health Professions, University of North Carolina, Chapel Hill.

John W. Williamson is visiting professor of international health, Department of Biostatistics, Harvard School of Public Health, and on leave from the School of Hygiene and Public Health, Johns Hopkins University.

## Senior Authors, Coordinating Editors, Project Staff

James I. Hudson, project director.

John W. Williamson, principal investigator.

Madeline M. Nevins, project coordinator (staff associate, Association of American Medical Colleges).

Renate Wilson, editorial coordinator (research associate, School of Hygiene and Public Health, Johns Hopkins University).

# Teaching Quality Assurance and Cost Containment in Health Care

*A Faculty Guide*

# Setting Goals
# and Objectives

*Frank T. Stritter*
*William F. Jessee*

১১১১১১১১১১১১১১১১১১১১১১১১১১

This chapter presents a comprehensive approach to planning a curriculum for teaching quality assurance and cost containment. Without appropriate and detailed curriculum planning, considerable faculty time may be invested in efforts that have little or no impact on student knowledge, skills, or attitudes. Conversely, attention to planning can often substantially reduce the trauma (for both faculty and students) associated with introduction of new material into the crowded medical school curriculum.

Definitions of *curriculum* are as numerous as those who write about it. For purposes of this chapter, *curriculum*, defined as *a structured series of intended learning outcomes,* can apply to a single course, a departmental program, or an institutionwide program. Curriculum here is distinct from *instruction,* which may be defined as *the means for achieving the learning outcomes specified in the curriculum plan.*

The process of planning the curriculum for a course or for broader programs involves arranging a series of goals and objectives in one of many possible patterns. It requires identifying, selecting, and organizing the concepts to be learned in accordance with the nature of these concepts, the needs of the learner, and the goals of the institution. The curriculum planning process results in a design that enables both the content and the process of instruction to be outlined.

No matter what its content, certain steps must be followed in developing a curriculum: The rationale of the curriculum must be articulated, curriculum goals must be developed, objectives based on the curriculum goals must be specified, and both goals and objectives must be clustered and/or sequenced. Each of these steps is discussed in detail and applied to the development of a quality assurance and cost containment curriculum. To illustrate their utility for planning, one aspect of a quality assurance and cost containment curriculum is examined.

### Articulating a Rationale: What It Must Include

Curriculum development begins with the statement of a well-articulated rationale defining the values on which the curriculum is based and justifying the learning to take place. A rationale thus defined serves as a basic building block for the entire curriculum and subsequent instruction. Without it, instructors might not understand why the curriculum should be planned and taught, nor students why they should learn.

Tyler (1975) has suggested that developing a rationale springs from an analysis of the specific problem that led to the decision to revise or build the curriculum. This problem might be a documented societal deficiency requiring correction, or it might be a recognition that certain societal values should be maintained. The problem may concern conflicting societal values or differing perceptions of societal responsibilities and constraints.

*Societal Problems.* In applying Tyler's theory to articulating a rationale for a quality assurance and cost containment curriculum in academic medical centers, one need only examine selected societal problems or values presently influencing health care. Consumers of health services have grown increasingly concerned with the quality of care. This concern is evident in the number of self-help groups that spurn the medical profession and turn to natural remedies for treating illness and disease. It is evident in the increase in malpractice suits and the frequent references to iatrogenic illnesses or diseases. Clearly, society is stating that it values good medical care and perceives current uncertainty about the quality of care as a problem.

Society is equally concerned about the costs of care. The media abound with reports on the effects of rising health services costs on federal spending, insurance premiums, and inflation. At the same time, highly sophisticated, expensive technology is in great demand. There is, then, a conflict of values: Consumers are seeking better quality of care and using more medical resources while also demanding that the costs of paying for this quality and these resources be held in check. Furthermore, physicians are being asked to examine their own role in increasing costs and dissatisfaction with the quality of care. Because one of the goals of medical education is to prepare students to assume the responsibilities that society imposes on them, one rationale for teaching quality assurance and cost containment might be expressed as follows:

> Societal demands for better quality of care, reduced costs, and greater satisfaction require that academic medical centers prepare students to participate in quality assurance and cost containment activities.

*Professional Needs of the Learner.* Another rationale derives from the learner's need to be prepared to meet the expectations of the medical profession. Members of the medical profession recognize the physician's need to be a self-assessing, self-correcting, lifelong learner—as witness the emphasis on continuing medical education of practicing physicians. One task of the academic medical center is to train students to view this continual self-assessment and lifelong learning as vital to their profession. A major function of quality assurance is to evaluate, through such mechanisms as peer review, the health professional's effectiveness in providing care. This evaluation of performance is a means of providing feedback to health professionals, allowing them to identify their own needs for additional knowledge and skills.

Furthermore, although many health care professionals have become involved in quality assurance and cost containment activities only in response to government regulation or other external pressures, most socially aware professionals recognize the benefit of peer review and accept their responsibility to contribute to the attempt to contain health care costs. Professional acceptance of Professional Standards Review Organizations (PSROs), participation in voluntary efforts to control hospital costs, and cooperation with the quality and cost reviews of the Joint Commission on Accreditation of Hospitals (JCAH) are some examples of the profession's acknowledgement of the importance of these issues. Perhaps the most important function of the quality assurance and cost containment curriculum in the academic medical center is to train students to view participation in these activities as an expected part of their professional behavior (Jessee and Goran, 1976).

A rationale based on the professional needs of the learner would consider such questions as: What will students need to achieve professional success? What will ensure that they are prepared for all their future professional responsibilities? In answering these questions, the following rationale might be formulated:

> Because students will be expected to become self-assessing and self-correcting professionals, to participate in activities designed to foster continuous self-evaluation and improvement, and to assume responsibility for maintaining standards of care and containing health care costs, the academic medical center must provide them with the knowledge and skills necessary to fulfill these professional obligations. Quality assurance and cost containment concepts and methodologies focus on the development of these attitudes and skills. Teaching quality assurance and cost containment, therefore, will develop this aspect of professionalism among students.

*Concerns of the Academic Medical Center.* A third rationale derives from the nature of the educational process at the academic medical center itself. Faculty members at such centers are viewed as role models and, as such, contribute to forming students' attitudes. In dealing with students at formative periods in their professional development, the medical faculty has a unique opportunity to foster positive attitudes toward professional responsibilities.

In addition, academic institutions are under increasing pressure to show that the disproportionate costs of health care in teaching hospitals are justified. Careful examination of both the cost of care and the quality of patient outcomes in the teaching hospital is central to the development of teaching programs in these areas. Self-examination by the academic medical center is essential in determining whether its costs can be reduced and the quality of its services improved. To respond to the continuing external criticism focused on the academic institution, it is incumbent on the faculty and staff to participate in its cost containment and quality assurance activities. Before medical schools can successfully train their students in quality assurance and cost containment, they must themselves be actively involved in ongoing internal quality assurance and cost control programs. Only when such programs become a normal part of the educational process will they be fully accepted by the physician-in-training and successful in ensuring high-quality but cost-effective care.

In applying this view to a rationale for teaching quality assurance and cost containment, one might say:

> To fulfill their responsibility as role models, medical faculty members must constantly reinforce those attitudes that will be required in students throughout their professional careers. By developing an ongoing curriculum for quality assurance and cost containment within both the medical school and the teaching hospital, the medical faculty will be contributing to the development of attitudes that are essential to the education of future physicians.

*Other Considerations.* Additional justification of a quality assurance and cost containment curriculum that could become part of the articulated rationale stems from the very nature of evaluation within any profession. For example, Brown and Uhl (1970) have proposed that performance evaluation is an ideal method for evaluating teaching programs. In the academic medical center, then, components of the curriculum in quality assurance and cost containment can serve as a mechanism for evaluating the efficacy of teaching programs in other areas. In addition, evaluation of students and house staff based on their performance in providing patient care can be a valuable addition to traditional methods of student evaluation, which have heretofore been based more on cognitive abilities than on patient care skills.

The problems, values, and needs that might be included in the rationale should, of course, be examined in the context of the entire institution. Possible resources for teaching the subject matter must be scrutinized to determine which of them would be useful and available. Factors within the institution that would act as constraints to solving the problems identified must also be considered. Individual faculty members or departments and segments in the institution's administration may be either resources to be utilized or constraints with which the curriculum planner must contend.

### Developing Curriculum Goals

Next in curriculum development is the identification of curriculum goals. Goals are the needs toward which the curricular efforts are directed; they are of long range and reflect the results that the entire experience is expected to achieve for the institution, the learner, and society. Goals are here defined as general statements of intended outcomes, in contrast to objectives, which are more specific statements of the recognizable changes in students that can be expected to result from instruction. Curriculum planning is concerned with goals, which are general and cover an extended time, whereas the planning of instruction is concerned with objectives, which are specific and apply to a discrete time period (for example, a day's work).

Saylor and Alexander (1974) indicate that curricular goals can be based on one or more of the following approaches to curriculum design:

*Specific Competencies of Graduates.* In this approach, often termed performance- or competency-based, the curriculum is built on skills required to perform a competent professional job. It requires a specific analysis of the responsibilities of the professional. Competency goals appropriate to a quality assurance and cost containment curriculum might be expressed as follows:

> Students will be able to participate effectively in medical and other quality assurance activities, such as peer review.

> Students will be able to participate in review and control of the use of services and cost of health care in their own medical practices.

*Disciplines/Subjects.* This approach uses the structure of knowledge as a basis for formulating goals and has been the dominant form of curriculum development over the years. The goals are based largely on the type and amount of organized knowledge available for curricular use. In applying this approach to a quality assurance and cost containment curriculum, one of the goals may be stated as:

> Students will be able to integrate and synthesize relevant knowledge and skills from such disciplines as epidemiology, biostatistics, sociology, and economics in participating in quality assurance and cost containment activities.

*Societal Activities and Problems.* An emphasis on society and its function and needs characterizes this approach. The goals might focus on life situations in our existence as social beings, on aspects or problems of community life, or on the improvement of society through direct application of the curriculum. Such a philosophical approach can both contribute directly to needs for societal improvement and be relevant to student needs and interests. A quality assurance and cost containment curriculum goal based on this approach might be:

> Students will be able to examine the issue of allocation of health care resources by applying quality/cost-benefit analyses to this societal problem.

*Process Skills.* The basic pattern for this approach is set by processes not unique to any particular professional field, such as observing, classifying, hypothesizing, and decision making. Parker and Rubin (1960) emphasize that "where the stress is upon process, the assimilation of knowledge is not derogated, but greater importance is attached to the methods of its acquisition and to its subsequent utilization." If this approach is used in planning the quality assurance and cost containment curriculum, one goal might be stated as follows:

> Students will acquire the necessary knowledge and
> skills to move sequentially through the stages of a quality
> assurance and cost containment study, from problem iden-
> tification through reassessment and verification of the ef-
> fects of the study.

*Individual Needs and Interests.* This approach, derived from
the philosophy of John Dewey, advocates a curriculum based on "a
coherent theory of experience" and "the experience learners already have" (Dewey, 1935). Goals based on this philosophy are
highly flexible, with built-in provisions for development and
modification to conform to individual learners' needs and interests
and with many options available to learners. In some instances, the
learner, with guidance, may develop his or her own curricular
goals. A goal appropriate to this approach might be expressed
as follows:

> Students will be able to select, from quality assur-
> ance and cost containment goals identified by the faculty,
> individual goals related to problems of cost and quality and
> will design their investigation on the basis of fundamental
> principles and methodologies in quality assurance and cost
> containment.

Although each of these approaches is quite different, curriculum goals are in fact often based on some combination of these
various schools of thought. Whatever the approach used, the curriculum planner should make sure that the goals are specific to the
articulated rationale and that they accurately reflect the intended
outcomes of the curriculum. Because the goals are essential to the
development of the specific objectives, which, in turn, guide the
development of instruction and form a basis for evaluating both
the students and the curriculum, this step in the curriculum planning process is extremely important.

## Instructional Objectives

The next step in curriculum planning is to refine goals derived from an articulated rationale into more specific statements,
termed instructional objectives. These are statements of what students should be able to know, do, or feel as a result of instruction.

Whereas goals pertain to the entire curriculum, instructional objectives pertain only to units within the curriculum and apply to days rather than years and to class sessions rather than semesters.

A well-stated objective specifies observable behavior that students will exhibit if they achieve the objective. Mager (1975) maintains that an objective is a statement that identifies the subject, or learner; the overall behavioral act, including action verb and observable result; any important conditions under which the behavior is to occur; and a criterion of acceptable performance. Other authorities offer different definitions of instructional objectives. However, Mager's suggestions will allow us to discuss curriculum planning just as well as any of the others would. Curriculum planners can then modify the components of their objectives using their own experience.

Precise statements of instructional objectives are useful for several reasons. First, they facilitate planning by the instructor in that they make possible informed curricular decisions about what should be included, how it should be taught, and how it should be evaluated. Second, they help students to learn more effectively and efficiently by informing them exactly what is expected and by enabling them to develop their own road maps to guide them through the planned curriculum. Third, they facilitate communication by enabling colleagues to ascertain the content of a particular portion of the curriculum and to coordinate their teaching of other aspects of the curriculum. Finally, objectives serve as a basis for evaluation of student performance and also of the curriculum. They give experienced evaluators and instructors explicit statements of what students should be able to do as a result of instruction, thus supplying the necessary ingredients for designing evaluation instruments and processes.

There are several approaches to developing objectives. The taxonomies proposed by Bloom (1956), Krathwohl, Bloom, and Masia (1964), and Harrow (1972) provide the best-known and most convenient scheme for organizing objectives, among which cognitive and affective objectives should be considered for the present purpose. Cognitive objectives are those having to do with thinking, knowing, and problem solving; affective objectives deal with attitudes, values, interests, and appreciation.

In a quality assurance and cost containment curriculum, cognitive and affective objectives might be distinguished and stated as follows:

### Cognitive

1.  Students will be able to state the stages to be followed in a comprehensive approach to quality assurance.
2.  Students will be able to describe in their own words why initial assessment is necessary in planning quality assurance and cost containment activities and indicate how it might be undertaken.
3.  Students will be able to understand the concepts of efficacy, efficiency, and effectiveness as they relate to particular health care interventions.
4.  Given a case study describing the management of a health care problem, students will be able to determine the appropriateness of each charge.
5.  Students will be able to design a quality assurance and cost containment study using a problem-oriented approach.

### Affective

1.  Students will be willing to consider the tenet that quality assurance and cost containment are essential to the practice of medicine.
2.  Students will acknowledge the value of peer review and self-evaluation in medical practice.
3.  Students will be willing to participate in quality assurance and cost containment programs in their academic medical centers.

## Clustering and Sequencing of Goals and Objectives

Before actual strategies for instruction can be determined, defined goals and objectives must be grouped into units around which instructional decisions can be made. Posner and Rudnitsky (1978) suggest five major points of emphasis around which the objectives may be clustered to form units for instruction: (1) the way the world is, (2) the way concepts are organized, (3) the way knowledge is generated, (4) the way students learn, and (5) the way learning can be used in one's profession.

*World-Related.* Objectives can be grouped in such a way that there is consistency between the grouping and empirical relations among events, people, and objects as they exist in the world. The relations may be temporal, spatial, or physical. For example, in an "Introduction to Clinical Medicine" course, quality assurance and cost containment objectives might be grouped to follow the history of quality assurance and cost containment legislation and its impact on medical practice over time.

*Concept-Related.* Objectives can be structured in a way that is consistent with some relations that exist among the concepts. The relations might be based on class (that is, concepts grouped according to common properties), on propositions (that is, combinations among the concepts that assert something such as theory/evidence or rule/example), on sophistication (concepts arranged according to complexity, abstractness, or level of refinement), or on logical prerequisite (the necessity to master the first concept in order to understand the second). For example, in a course on the economics of health care that incorporates cost containment teaching, students may need to understand basic economic principles and their application to the health care delivery system before studying how cost containment can be achieved in different practice settings.

*Inquiry-Related.* Here the objectives of curricular units might be based on the way knowledge is derived or, to put it more specifically, on the process of generating, discovering, or verifying knowledge. Units might be grouped according to the logic of inquiry (the science of valid agreement) or the empirics of inquiry (descriptions of how successful investigators actually proceed). For example, in teaching medical care evaluation, the instructor's first objective would be to have students learn how to identify problems. This would be followed by criteria development, then assessment strategies, and finally problem evaluation.

*Learning-Related.* This organizational focus is based on the psychology of learning that holds that the way people learn is more important than the nature of the subject matter. Relations among the objectives might be structured according to whether the learning of one skill is a prerequisite to the learning of another or according to familiarity (the frequency with which the learner has previously encountered an idea), difficulty (how difficult a concept is to learn), interest (the level of curiosity or challenge evoked by a particular concept), development (the stages of the psychological development and learning readiness of the learner), and internalization (the process by which a learner progresses from being open to examining a value to internalizing a value so that it becomes a characteristic of the learner). Organization around this focus is problematic, however, because the process of learning is highly individualized. Everyone learns differently. Although generalizations can often be made, it would be dangerous to assume that all learners conform to them. If this focus were the basis of organization for a course on quality assurance, the instruction would begin with an examination of the most recent case managed by the students and proceed to the introduction of quality assurance principles and systematic health care assessment and improvement procedures.

*Utilization-Related.* This focus organizes the objectives, and consequently the curricular units, in the manner in which learners will most likely use the concepts in the future. The arrangement of the objectives might reflect the stepwise progression in a particular procedure or the frequency with which the learner might be expected to use it. In teaching medical students how to conduct a quality assurance and cost containment study, for example, the instructor's first goals and objectives would be to develop the students' abilities to select topics and set priorities. The subsequent (and sequential) objectives would be to develop the knowledge and skills necessary for conducting an initial assessment, planning and implementing improvement actions, and reassessing the results of the study.

All of the foregoing are legitimate ways of clustering or sequencing curricular objectives. Before deciding on instruction strategies, however, the instructor should choose one as the main focus, although some overlapping is inevitable. To illustrate this portion of the curriculum planning process, Table 1.1 provides a number of possible objectives developed for teaching medical audit, utilization review, medical staff credentialing, and risk management, clustered according to the utilization-related focus described. In Table 1.2 some of the same objectives have been clustered according to a different set of principles, based on an instructional focus as described by Goodlad (1966), which groups objectives according to the types of instructional activities to be employed (such as projects, debates, field trips, papers, case studies, experiments, or literature review). In this approach the clustering is based on the teaching strategy or the available resources.

These two approaches to clustering/sequencing the goals and objectives of a quality assurance and cost containment curriculum have been selected as illustrations because they seem to have the characteristics needed for successful instruction. As organizing principles, they are *feasible;* they are *appropriate to the rationale and goals* already discussed; they are *appropriate to the learner's aptitudes;* and they offer the possibility of providing the learner with *a challenging and stimulating learning experience.* Curriculum planners who choose to use other organizational foci for clustering their objectives should ensure that the focus selected has these same characteristics.

## Conclusions

Much of the content of a medical curriculum in quality assurance and cost containment will be described in subsequent sections of this text. This chapter has laid out some basic principles of curriculum planning and provided examples that relate specifically to quality assurance and cost containment.

Using a systematic approach to curriculum planning for quality assurance and cost containment does not guarantee success. Clearly, implementing *any* new program of instruction in an academic medical center poses formidable political and practical problems that transcend the more easily addressed problems of educational philosophy and theory discussed in this chapter. Some of these political and practical problems will be discussed more fully in the next chapter. However, a systematic approach to planning, because of its rigor and logical progression from rationale to goals to specific objectives and to final instructional units, is more likely to result in institutional acceptance of the curriculum than is

**Table 1.1. Utilization-Related Clustering.**

---

*Partial list of objectives for curricular units in a quality assurance/cost containment curriculum clustered according to a utilization-related focus.*

I.    *Medical Audit*

   1.   Identify major problem areas in individual practice, institution, or community; in conjunction with other physicians and health care practitioners, set consensus priorities for study.
   2.   Develop explicit objectives for a medical audit that represent significant issues in quality or cost of care and are potentially soluble through the audit process.
   3.   Write and achieve consensus on screening criteria and definitions for use in the audit process.
   4.   Distinguish between screening criteria and clinical standards.
   5.   Analyze variations from screening criteria and explicitly describe a clinical or administrative rationale for determining whether each variation is justified or unjustified.
   6.   Analyze patterns and severity of variations and unjustified variations to determine the type of action to be taken.
   7.   State principles of individual and organizational behavior governing reactions to efforts to produce change.
   8.   Plan and conduct effective individual and organizational change programs to correct problems identified through audits.
   9.   Participate voluntarily in audit activities to evaluate care provided by the student and his or her colleagues.
  10.   Describe the relations between medical audit and other components of the quality assurance/cost containment system in individual practice, the hospital, and the community.

II.   *Medical Staff Credentialing*

   1.   Design a legally and professionally sound process for initial credentialing and annual review of hospital medical staff privileges.
   2.   Use information from medical audits, physician profiles, and other medical staff review activities in evaluation of individual physician performance and in decision making concerning privileges.
   3.   Describe the relations between medical staff privileges/credentialing and other components of the hospital quality assurance/cost containment system.

III.  *Utilization Review*

   1.   Define the levels of institutional care available within the community.

Table 1.1. Utilization-Related Clustering, Cont'd.

---

2.  Determine correctly 95% of the time the appropriate level of care for a given patient, based on review of information in the medical record.
3.  Analyze profiles of health care utilization (by practitioner, institution, and patient) to identify problem areas in which review should be intensified and areas of appropriate utilization where review can be reduced.
4.  Monitor personal practice patterns to reduce or eliminate inappropriate utilization of facilities and services.
5.  Correlate utilization of facilities and services with costs of health care.
6.  Develop and implement effective corrective actions to improve individual and institutional utilization patterns.
7.  Know the relations between utilization review and other components of the quality assurance/cost containment system in individual practice, the hospital, and the community.

IV.  *Risk Management*

1.  Know the relations among quality of care, utilization of services, patient and physician attitudes, and malpractice liability.
2.  Design and implement a system for identifying and reducing risks of patient injury and risks of physician/institution liability in hospitals.
3.  Discuss the relations between accuracy and completeness of medical records and liability experience.
4.  Describe the influence of malpractice actions and judgments on costs of hospital and nonhospital care.
5.  Show the relations between risk management and other components of the quality assurance/cost containment system in individual practice, the hospital, and the community.

---

a less clearly articulated approach. In addition, having followed this developmental pattern, the planner can move easily into the role of the instructor, with a curriculum in which student evaluation is facilitated and in which the desired student behaviors have an optimal chance of being taught. Less rigorous approaches, though occasionally very successful, are much more dependent on the whims of fortune and subject to the changing moods of the academic environment.

**Table 1.2 Instruction-Related Clustering.**

*Partial list of objectives for a quality assurance/cost containment curriculum clustered around an instructional focus and compared with utilization-related clustering from Table 1.1. (Note that some objectives overlap multiple instructional modes.)*

| *Instructional-Related Clustering* | *Utilization-Related Clustering[a]* | |
|---|---|---|
| I. *Journal articles and government publications* | | |
|    1. State principles of individual and organizational behavior governing reactions to efforts to produce change. | M.A. | 7 |
|    2. Describe the relations between medical audit and other components of quality assurance/cost containment system in individual practice, the hospital, and the community. | M.A. | 10 |
|    3. Define the levels of institutional care available within the community. | U.R. | 1 |
|    4. Correlate utilization of facilities and services with costs of health care. | U.R. | 5 |
|    5. Know the relations between utilization review and other components of the quality assurance/cost containment system in the individual practice, the hospital, and the community. | U.R. | 7 |
|    6. Describe the relations between medical staff privileges/credentialing and other components of the hospital quality assurance/cost containment system. | M.S.C. | 3 |
|    7. Know the relations among quality of care, utilization of services, patient and physician attitudes, and malpractice liability. | R.M. | 1 |
| II. *Role-playing exercises* | | |
|    1. Plan and conduct effective individual and organizational change programs to correct problems identified through audits. | M.A. | 8 |

[a]Numbers refer to placement in the list of objectives in Table 1.1.
M.A. = Medical Audit, U.R. = Utilization Review, M.S.C. = Medical Staff Credentialing, R.M. = Risk Management.

**Table 1.2. Instruction-Related Clustering, Cont'd.**

|  |  |  |  |
|---|---|---|---|
| | 2. Develop and implement effective corrective actions to improve individual and institutional utilization patterns. | U.R. | 6 |
| III. | *Case studies* | | |
| | 1. Identify major problem areas in individual practice, institution, or community; in conjunction with other physicians and health care practitioners, set consensus priorities for study. | M.A. | 1 |
| | 2. Analyze patterns and severity of variations and unjustified variations in order to determine the type of action to be taken. | M.A. | 6 |
| | 3. Determine correctly 95% of the time the appropriate level of care for a given patient, based on review of information in the medical record. | U.R. | 2 |
| | 4. Analyze profiles of health care utilization (by practitioner, institution, and patient) to identify problem areas in which review should be intensified and areas of appropriate utilization where review can be reduced. | U.R. | 3 |
| IV. | *Projects* | | |
| | 1. Design and implement a system for identifying and reducing risks of patient injury and risks of physician / institution liability in hospitals. | R.M. | 2 |
| V. | *Committee participation* | | |
| | 1. Develop explicit objectives for a medical audit that represent significant issues in quality or cost of care and are potentially soluble through the audit process. | M.A. | 2 |
| | 2. Write and achieve consensus on screening criteria and definitions for use in the audit process. | M.A. | 3 |

## Table 1.2. Instruction-Related Clustering, Cont'd.

| | | | |
|---|---|---|---|
| 3. | Analyze variations from screening criteria and explicitly describe a clinical or administrative rationale for determining whether each variation is either justified or unjustified. | M.A. | 5 |
| 4. | Plan and conduct effective individual and organizational change programs to correct problems identified through audits. | M.A. | 8 |
| 5. | Participate voluntarily in audit activities to evaluate care provided by the student and his or her colleagues. | M.A. | 9 |
| 6. | Analyze profiles of health care utilization (by practitioner, institution, and patient) to identify problem areas in which review should be intensified and areas of appropriate utilization where review can be reduced. | U.R. | 3 |
| 7. | Monitor personal practice patterns to reduce or eliminate inappropriate utilization of facilities and services. | U.R. | 4 |
| 8. | Use information from medical audits, physician profiles, and other medical staff review activities in evaluation of individual physician performance and in decision making concerning privileges. | M.S.C. | 2 |

# Implementing the Changes

## Donald R. Korst

ΚΩΚΩΚΩΚΩΚΩΚΩΚΩΚΩΚΩΚΩΚΩΚΩΚΩΚΩΚΩΚΩ

Several years ago members of the Workshop on Medical School Curricula made a series of recommendations that resulted from their study of the process of physician education in medical school. They concluded their recommendations by stating: "The costs of medical care must be controlled if the present system is to retain its credibility. Research must be undertaken by medical schools to develop alternatives to hospitalization. The cost-benefit relation of the physician's decision must become a part of the evaluation of the appropriateness of those decisions in the educational programs of our medical schools. The problem of maintaining quality and effectiveness of health services while developing more efficient organization, more general availability, and more reasonable costs is one that will not be solved without the participation of the medical schools" (Hubbard, Gronvall, and DeMuth, 1970, p. 9).

During the past decade, other and stronger statements on the need to include quality assurance and cost containment throughout the medical school curriculum and residency programs have been made by such organizations as the Association of American Medical Colleges and the American Medical Association. Many of the societal, professional, and personal needs outlined in the preceding chapter as a basis for developing the curriculum rationale are equally pertinent to an institutional rationale for planning such a curriculum. Regardless of the persuasiveness of these rationales, there are numerous obstacles to implementing the proposed curriculum, however—ranging from such practical matters as the lack of money, resources, and time to devote to new curriculum needs to less tangible and tractable problems, such as resistance to any changes in existing curricula by faculty members with different orientations. Those involved in planning a quality assurance and cost containment curriculum must, therefore, develop implementation strategies that will address these obstacles.

This chapter concentrates on ways and means of obtaining administrative and interdepartmental support and approval required for successful implementation. In addition, it reviews approaches to translating the goals and objectives of the quality assurance and cost containment curriculum into specific instructional units to be integrated into the existing medical curriculum. Because each academic medical center differs in its approach to curriculum planning and implementation, no specific courses or programs are proposed. Rather, this chapter considers the extent to which the relevant quality assurance and cost containment objectives are compatible with the objectives of other portions of the medical school curriculum or residency programs, so as to show where integration is feasible. It also suggests a decision-making process to help determine whether to integrate quality assurance and cost containment into the existing curriculum or to add new instructional units.

## Ensuring Institutional Support

*Forming the Committee.* Broad institutional support will be required to integrate instruction in quality assurance and cost containment into the continuum of education from the first year of undergraduate medical school through the residency years. One approach would be an interdisciplinary and interdepartmental planning committee composed of interested faculty members. To be effective, this committee should be given official recognition— for example, by having the members appointed by the dean and the chair of the curriculum committee. Once officially recognized, the committee would have two major responsibilities: (1) to elicit the approval and consolidate the support of other members of the academic medical center who would be affected by the decision to teach quality assurance and cost containment and (2) to plan the curriculum.

*Obtaining Approval and Support.* It is advisable to identify those whose approval and support are critical if the curriculum is to be implemented efficiently and to keep them informed of the curriculum planning process. Within the medical school, this group includes faculty members who are responsible for overseeing curriculum development: the dean, department heads, section chiefs, members of the curriculum committee, instructors, and those in charge of disseminating data. In the teaching hospital, similar approval is required from hospital administrators, department heads, section chiefs, directors of nursing, medical directors, and course instructors, since quality assurance and cost containment instruction will inevitably, and in some instances dramatically, affect their areas of responsibility. Cooperation and support from a number of other sources will also be required. For example, because of the type and range of information needed for teaching quality assurance and cost containment, it would be impossible, or at least very difficult, to obtain necessary information for reviewing patient charts or hospital charges without the full support of the medical records director. Active support by the hospital PSRO committee, the patient advisory committee, the hospital chiefs of staff, and the house staff is needed to ensure access to important information and to provide guidance in carrying out quality assurance and cost containment activities required by the curriculum. Informing the chief pharmacist, the continuing medical education (CME) committee, the hospital attorney, and members of the board of trustees will smooth the way for program implementation and may well produce important feedback.

Means of obtaining support and establishing a mechanism for disseminating information about quality assurance and cost containment teaching might include the following:

- Enlisting cooperation of the quality evaluation committee at affiliated hospitals.
- Inviting house staff and students to attend committee planning meetings.
- Offering the services of members of the planning committee to faculty members who are developing specific instructional units.
- Reporting regularly on the successes and shortcomings of the new programs to key members of various departments and administrative offices.

While the instructional planning is in process, it is important to keep the issue of quality assurance and cost containment teaching in the forefront both at the administrative level and within other departments. Periodic reports to the faculty and dean on the process of the planning and on the design and results of any pilot projects would be one way of obtaining additional support. Providing special educational programs or seminars for the faculty on quality assurance cost containment issues may also be helpful. Both approaches might reduce opposition that springs from fear of overloading the curriculum or unawareness of the need to teach quality assurance and cost containment activities.

### Organizing Curriculum Implementation

While establishing lines of communication is important, the planning committee must at the same time proceed with actual curriculum planning. As a first step, it is advisable to identify resources within the academic medical center to be utilized. Next, the curriculum plan would be developed, using a combination of the educational principles outlined in Chapter One: articulating the rationale, developing curriculum goals and objectives, and clustering or sequencing the objectives. With this plan in hand, specific instructional units can be developed. Although ideally the undergraduate curriculum and residency programs should be implemented institutionwide, it is more practical to assume that the instructional units in quality assurance and cost containment will first be introduced in several departments as pilot projects, electives, or demonstration models, later to be integrated into the overall medical school curriculum and residency programs.

## Integration into the Medical Curriculum and Residency Programs

The instructional units may be incorporated into any of a number of department programs. It is important, therefore, to identify possible points of integration and implementation throughout the educational continuum.

*The Preclinical Years (I, II).* Generally, the emphasis for first- and second-year students is on the content of the basic sciences and the pathophysiology of organ systems. Information on physical diagnosis and epidemiology is also frequently included in instruction at this level through such course offerings as "Introduction to Clinical Medicine" and "Preventive Medicine." Through these learning experiences the student develops skills in interviewing techniques, physical diagnosis, data gathering, physician/patient communication, and case presentation.

Aspects of quality assurance and cost containment that are compatible with this level of the medical curriculum include knowledge of the physician's role in assuring quality of care and containing health care costs and of the history of quality assurance and cost containment legislation (see Appendix A). Instructional units on these quality and cost issues can be designed for inclusion in preclinical courses such as "Introduction to Clinical Medicine," 'Introduction to Health Care," "Humanities in Medicine," and "Social Aspects of Medicine." Such courses are particularly useful for forming basic attitudes and values and creating consciousness of social issues among physicians-in-training. Accordingly, the instructional objectives may be both cognitive and affective (see Chapter One) and might be expressed as follows:

- Students will be able to trace the development of quality assurance and cost containment legislation.

- Students will be able to demonstrate methods for acquiring information about the extent and costs of health care problems.
- Students will accept that quality assurance and cost containment are essential components of contemporary medical practice.
- Students will accept that the principles of deductive problem solving that relate to clinical diagnosis also apply to quality assessment methods.
- Students will accept that, for quality assurance practitioners, the "patient" is a population consisting of both providers and consumers of health care interacting in a defined geographic and organizational environment.

Information on the frequency of health problems and the costs related to individual disease categories can be integrated into such courses as "Public Health," "Community Health," "Epidemiology," and "Biostatistics." These courses offer an ideal opportunity for teaching quality assurance and cost containment objectives, establishing the validity and reliability of data, or identifying information sources on the extent and costs of health care problems. Even courses such as pathology and pharmacology can address quality and cost issues by introducing information on how to identify problems in the delivery of care relevant to diagnostic performance and the safety and efficacy of drugs and on the costs of laboratory tests and prescribing.

In reviewing the overall preclinical curriculum, those planning the instructional units can determine whether specified quality assurance and cost containment objectives can be met in existing courses or whether it will be necessary to create a new course (or courses) to meet these objectives.

Figure 2.1 illustrates a decision process that will lead to identification of points of implementation and integration at the preclinical level. It is also useful to consider learning activities appropriate to attainment of the instructional objectives. For example, if it is determined that the objective of tracing the development of quality assurance and cost containment legislation can be met in a course such as "Introduction to Clinical Medicine" or "Health Care," the committee can suggest that readings on this

Content of the Basic Curriculum

Basic Sciences, Pathophysiology of Organ Systems, Courses in Introduction to Clinical Medicine and Preventive Medicine

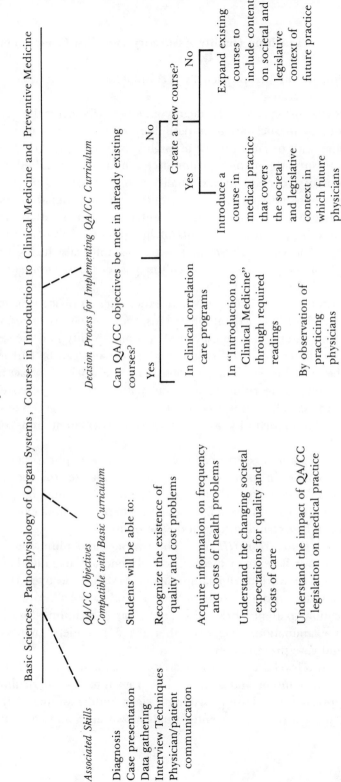

*Associated Skills*

Diagnosis
Case presentation
Data gathering
Interview Techniques
Physician/patient communication

*QA/CC Objectives*
*Compatible with Basic Curriculum*

Students will be able to:

Recognize the existence of quality and cost problems

Acquire information on frequency and costs of health problems

Understand the changing societal expectations for quality and costs of care

Understand the impact of QA/CC legislation on medical practice

*Decision Process for Implementing QA/CC Curriculum*

Can QA/CC objectives be met in already existing courses?

Yes

In clinical correlation care programs

In "Introduction to Clinical Medicine" through required readings

By observation of practicing physicians

No

Create a new course?

Yes

Introduce a course in medical practice that covers the societal and legislative context in which future physicians will practice

No

Expand existing courses to include content on societal and legislative context of future practice

**Figure 2.1. Implementing the Quality Assurance/Cost Containment Curriculum: The Preclinical Years.**

legislation or on the physician's accountability to society be included in the course.

Recognizing that many faculty members who offer the standard courses in such areas as pathology or biostatistics may be unfamiliar with or lack interest in quality assurance and cost containment issues, the planning committee can identify qualified faculty members to assist in the quality and cost aspects in these courses. These persons can be designated an interdepartmental quality assurance and cost containment team that assists course instructors in planning the points of integration, is available for conducting individual classes at appropriate intervals during the course itself, or prepares a curriculum packet for dissemination among clinical teaching faculty.

Where students are provided experience in office practice settings to observe practicing physicians, they can be instructed to give specific attention to questions of cost and quality in these settings. Overall awareness of quality and cost issues can be further strengthened while students are observing the work-up of actual patients and are learning to examine patient charts. Moreover, many of the so-called clinical correlation courses taught at this level offer ample opportunity to stress quality assessment and cost awareness.

Should a new course be necessary, it may be appropriate to suggest a course in medical practice that emphasizes the societal and legislative context for which future physicians must be prepared. Or the committee might suggest where and how existing courses can be expanded to include these topics.

*The Clinical Years (III, IV).* The overall curriculum for the third and fourth years of medical school generally includes basic clerkships in the various clinical specialties, as well as electives. During these years, students are expected to develop skills in problem identification; patient work-up; chart keeping, including history, physical examination, diagnosis, therapy, and patient management; and case presentation.

At this level the most appropriate quality assurance and cost containment content and skills to integrate into the curriculum would appear to be those providing a clear understanding of the basic steps of a problem-oriented quality assurance and cost containment study. Appropriate instructional objectives might include the following:

- Students will apply quality assurance and cost containment principles, such as priority setting, problem identification and assessment, improvement planning and implementation, and reassessment, to various methods for assessing the quality and costs of care.
- Students will assess the costs of individual procedures as part of their patient management.
- Students will be able to develop and write structure, process, and outcome criteria.
- Students will develop positive attitudes toward self-assessment and peer review.
- Students will understand the relationship between quality assurance and cost containment activities and the practice of medicine in office practice, hospitals, and the community, especially in terms of Professional Standards Review Organizations (PSROs) and Joint Commission on Accreditation of Hospitals (JCAH) requirements.

The committee planning quality assurance and cost containment instruction can determine where the objectives can be met in the existing curriculum and where new learning experiences need to be added.

Clerkships seem particularly feasible as a means of integrating cost and quality issues, since the patient's work-up is prepared and entered into the chart by the student and reviewed by the ward staff with the student. This review covers the history, physical examination, diagnosis, and management plan, with the last two aspects discussed in depth during the ward conference.

To promote cost consciousness at this level, computer printouts of hospital charges to patient bills may be distributed to students to acquaint them with diagnostic charges (laboratory procedures, x rays, EKGs, and so on) and other costs of care. As most students are primarily concerned with learning experiences in patient management, case simulations that promote discussion of quality and cost can be used. Simulations can be developed from actual charts and students directed to determine and solve the problem. Each student receives feedback on this problem-solving process. Although this type of instruction is intended to improve clinical problem-solving skills, it also holds promise for illustrating quality of care and cost containment decision processes. However, it cannot substitute for educational exercises that address cost containment in aggregated patient populations, nor can it replace instruction on how to develop quality assurance programs for aggregate populations in a group practice, a clinic, or an inpatient institution. Topic-oriented conferences and field exercises using aggregated patient data also need to be included during this phase of the curriculum.

Finally, students in the third and fourth years might observe PSRO committee activities at the academic medical center or at local community hospitals. If this is not possible because of time constraints or scheduling difficulties, PSRO committee members can participate in the clerkship conferences, describing how quality assurance is conducted locally.

It may yet be necessary to add further learning experiences to the curriculum at this level. Case studies may be developed that are specifically designed for discussion of quality assurance and cost containment issues. Regular sessions may be introduced in which peer review of charts and work-ups is conducted; and students may be trained to develop process and outcome criteria for particular problems. In addition, primary care experience may be required for all students so that they can observe various quality assurance and cost containment activities in a practice setting that is particularly effective for role modeling. Funds can also be made available to allow students to do research or independent reading in methods of measuring quality and examining costs of health care or to develop protocols for tracking and evaluating care for individual health problems. Hip fractures, asthma, coronary artery occlusion, urinary tract infection, infections treated with antibiotics, and alcoholism would make excellent topics for research because much remains to be studied on the effectiveness of present therapeutic methods for these conditions.

Figure 2.2 compares the content and skills required in the overall curriculum and those of the quality assurance and cost con-

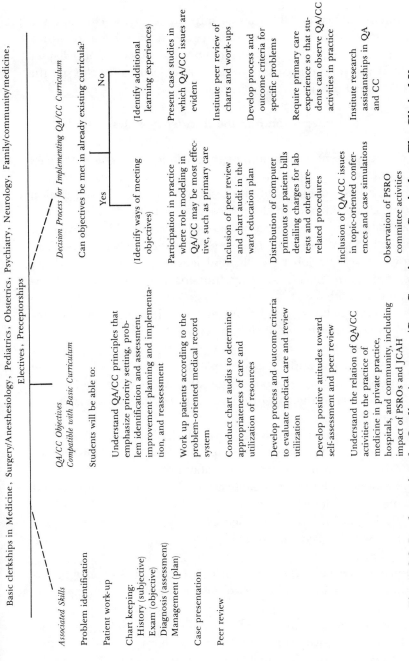

**Figure 2.2. Implementing the Quality Assurance/Cost Containment Curriculum: The Clinical Years.**

tainment curriculum that can be introduced at the clinical level. Again, note that once points of integration have been identified and goals have been clustered/sequenced as described in Chapter One, it will still be necessary to develop objectives for the specific instructional units.

## Integration into the Residency Years

At present a minimum of three clinical postgraduate years is required for certification in all medical specialties. Residents participate in rotations within the hospital and in certain clinical settings, concentrate on their chosen specialties, and master the material required for specialty board certification. These years are devoted to perfecting the skills taught in the medical school, improving problem-solving skills, and learning to interact with all members of the health care team (nursing staff, pharmacists, technicians, and others).

The quality assurance and cost containment goals most appropriate to the residency years are these:

- Residents will apply the principles and processes of deductive problem solving to a population of health care providers and consumers in their own practice setting, such as a hospital or clinic.
- Residents will accept that, as role models for medical students and interns, they have a responsibility to stress the importance of quality assurance and cost containment.
- Residents will provide quality assurance training to interns and medical students in their charge.
- Residents will accept that self-evaluation and peer review are necessary ingredients in their professional practice.

To give credence to the importance of these issues, it may be appropriate to hold residents accountable for demonstrating their knowledge and skills in quality assurance and cost containment as part of the requirement for board certification. Residents may also be required to give evidence of their familiarity with the various techniques for assessing quality and reducing costs where appropriate, particularly with respect to measuring and improving patient outcomes.

There are several ways to address quality assurance and cost containment in already existing residency programs: Residents may be encouraged to participate on hospital chart audit or quality assurance and cost containment committees or be asked to address quality assurance and cost containment issues in the daily report of cases (a form of peer review). It may also be necessary to introduce additional learning experiences in the residency programs—that is, to expand the training programs to include community settings where there are established quality assurance and cost containment systems. Consideration should also be given to providing elective time for residents to take additional courses in quality assurance and cost containment at schools of public health or in departments of preventive medicine.

At the residency level, the availability of research fellowships (similar to those suggested for the clinical clerkships) will expand the educational program in quality assurance and cost containment, particularly if these assistantships are designated for those specializing in primary care. This does not mean that quality assurance and cost containment should be limited to primary care. Rather, since there is no area of academic research that is particular to primary care specialties at present, it suggests that the academic research might best be carried out by primary care specialists whose investigations would benefit the other specialties.

Figure 2.3 illustrates a suggested approach for deciding how to integrate quality assurance and cost containment in residency programs. Attention is also given to possible new approaches that might be feasible at this level.

## Conclusions

The approach to implementing a quality assurance and cost containment curriculum described in this chapter emphasizes integration of specific instructional units at all levels of medical education—from the first year of medical school through the last year of residency. During the preclinical years, the goals and objectives would focus on learning basic concepts and terminology and

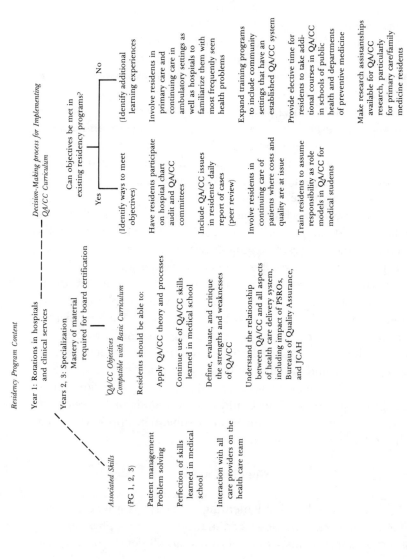

Residency Program Content

Year 1: Rotations in hospitals and clinical services

Years 2, 3: Specialization
Mastery of material required for board certification

*Decision-Making process for Implementing QA/CC Curriculum*

Can objectives be met in existing residency programs?

Yes

No

*Associated Skills*
(PG 1, 2, 3)

Patient management
Problem solving

Perfection of skills learned in medical school

Interaction with all care providers on the health care team

*QA/CC Objectives*
*Compatible with Basic Curriculum*

Residents should be able to:

Apply QA/CC theory and processes

Continue use of QA/CC skills learned in medical school

Define, evaluate, and critique the strengths and weaknesses of QA/CC

Understand the relationship between QA/CC and all aspects of health care delivery system, including impact of PSROs, Bureaus of Quality Assurance, and JCAH

(Identify ways to meet objectives)

Have residents participate on hospital chart audit and QA/CC committees

Include QA/CC issues in residents' daily report of cases (peer review)

Involve residents in continuing care of patients where costs and quality are at issue

Train residents to assume responsibility as role models in QA/CC for medical students

(Identify additional learning experiences)

Involve residents in primary care and continuing care in ambulatory settings as well as hospitals to familiarize them with most frequently seen health problems

Expand training programs to include community settings that have an established QA/CC system

Provide elective time for residents to take additional courses in QA/CC in schools of public health and departments of preventive medicine

Make research assistantships available for QA/CC research, particularly for primary care/family medicine residents

**Figure 2.3. Implementing the Quality Assurance/Cost Containment Curriculum: The Residency Years.**

becoming familiar with quality assurance and cost containment legislation. Quality assurance and cost containment methodologies would be taught during the clinical years. At the residency level, the emphasis would be on applying quality assurance and cost containment principles and methods to actual assessment and improvement of care.

Strategies suggested for successful implementation include establishing an interdepartmental planning committee that has official status in the academic medical center, developing a strong universitywide support base, and identifying useful resources. Among the most promising faculty resources are those who are familiar with quality assurance and cost containment legislation, those who specialize in primary care and community health programs, and those who teach methods for evaluating and improving performance. Ideally, designated faculty members from departments of health services research, the behavioral sciences, and medical humanities would join with selected clinicians from departments of preventive medicine and the primary care specialties as well as faculty members from schools of public health to form a team that could be called on to teach course segments throughout the curriculum. This approach may not be practical in every institution, but at least these faculty members should be consulted regularly, as they can help the planning committee develop programs and methods for quality assurance and cost containment instruction.

Throughout the implementation process, special attention should be given to relating quality assurance and cost containment education to the immediate needs and concerns of the learners and the goals and objectives of their clinical education.

〿〿〿〿〿〿〿〿〿〿〿〿〿〿〿〿〿〿〿〿〿 3

# Evaluating
the Effects

*Daniel M. Barr*

〿〿〿〿〿〿〿〿〿〿〿〿〿〿〿〿〿〿〿〿〿〿

No curriculum plan is complete without a component that provides methods to evaluate the curriculum. Like the other steps in curriculum development—identifying a problem that the educational process should address, articulating a rationale, developing goals and objectives, and clustering instructional objectives—evaluation should be planned even before instruction begins.

Early evaluation planning will enable those who develop the curriculum to identify what each component of instruction addresses and what has been purposely omitted. It will also help to determine the kinds of data needed by evaluators to conduct before-and-after studies of student attitudes, knowledge, and skills; selection criteria to be used for comparison studies; and factors affecting the external and internal validity of evaluation instruments. Furthermore, the evaluation plan will serve as a road map showing the most appropriate points in the curriculum for evaluating progress.

Curriculum evaluation is conducted to assess the effectiveness of the curriculum in producing the desired outcomes in the learner (knowledge, attitudes, and skills), the quality of the instruction, or both (Fink and Kosecoff, 1978). In evaluating the effectiveness of a quality assurance and cost containment curriculum, for example, it is important to ascertain whether the students developed positive attitudes toward self-evaluation, peer review, and quality assurance and cost containment activities and whether they acquired the knowledge and skills necessary to participate in studies of quality and costs. In conducting an evaluation to identify ways of improving the curriculum, the emphasis is on quality of the learning experiences, efficiency with which the programs were run, degree to which the immediate needs of the learners were met, and progress made toward meeting the stated instructional objectives. Results of this assessment will indicate how the curriculum and the associated learning experiences can be upgraded, modified, refined, reduced, or expanded.

Whether the intent is to evaluate the effectiveness of the curriculum or to determine how to improve it, similar information may be collected at the same stages of the evaluation process (Fink and Kosecoff, 1978). This chapter addresses some approaches and methods that can be used in evaluating a quality assurance and cost containment curriculum and provides illustrations of evaluation instruments currently used in existing programs.

## Approaches to Evaluating Curriculum Effectiveness

*Evaluating Long-Term Effectiveness.* The goals of a quality assurance and cost containment curriculum include inculcating cost consciousness, awareness of quality, and concern for professional self-regulation that will remain with and influence the behavior of students and residents throughout their professional lives. Such goals clearly embody the long-term needs of students and residents and respond to professional and societal problems, external to medical education and to any particular medical school, that gave rise to one of the rationales underlying the curriculum.

Evaluation of curricular effectiveness will involve determining the extent to which the curriculum affects the societal or professional problems to which it is a response:

- Do medical students and residents remain cost conscious and aware of quality?

- For how long?
- Under what circumstances?

Evaluations responsive to such questions are perhaps of limited immediate value to a given institution, but they are of great value to the medical profession generally. Conducting such evaluations is difficult, however, since they require measuring long-term effectiveness. Quality assurance and cost containment curricula are of too recent origin to make it possible to conduct such studies as yet. Garg estimates that "between 5 and 10 percent of the graduates . . . will remain outspoken on the subject and dedicated to its concepts" (Friedman, 1979). Obviously, it will be necessary to wait until currently enrolled students and residents have become practicing physicians to conduct a true effectiveness evaluation to confirm this projection. As will be discussed later, there are problems associated with large studies, due mainly to the high probability of intervening variables.

*Evaluating Short-Term Effectiveness.* It is possible, however, to evaluate curriculum effectiveness within the academic medical center in the short term. The degree to which students and residents recognize problems of cost and quality during rounds, case presentations, or discussions of simulated patient cases can be observed and evaluated, as can their willingness to participate in peer review and quality assurance/cost containment activities. In fact, there have been a few published reports of the effectiveness of such activities in developing positive attitudes toward quality assurance and cost containment curricula (Barr, Wollstadt, and Kinast-Porter, 1979; Zeleznik and Gonnella, 1979).

It is also possible to evaluate curriculum effectiveness in developing required knowledge and skills. These evaluations may be in the form of before-and-after tests of mastery of the principles and processes of quality assurance and cost containment, or they may document improvement in quality of care or reduction of costs when students or residents are closely involved with and share responsibility for patient care. An evaluation of a quality assurance program in ambulatory care, for example, documented increases in the use of streptococcal screening cultures and in immunization levels (Barr and others, 1976). A similar effectiveness evaluation of a hospital-centered program documented increased adherence to pneumonia criteria (Mulligan, 1979). Both evaluations were conducted to assess whether the stated program goals and objectives had been attained.

*Evaluation Design.* It is difficult to design evaluations that show clearly that desired learning outcomes can be attributed specifically to the impact of a curriculum. If costs are the buzzword at a given moment in medical history, cost consciousness may be as much the result of exposure to environmental influences, such as the media or discussions with faculty members, relatives, and peers, as an outcome of the curriculum. It is also possible that concern with quality and costs is due to the increased knowledge and skill that naturally accompany progression from early to more advanced levels of medical education. During the preclinical and clinical years, students are still concerned primarily with learning how to be physicians and are struggling to grasp details about the process of care; as residents, they are actually providing care rather competently and are psychologically more prepared to examine issues of cost and quality.

To counteract this difficulty in attributing outcomes to the curriculum, particularly for new curricula such as those in quality assurance and cost containment, evaluations of curriculum effectiveness should probably include some type of comparison study. Comparison studies may include historical, observational, or allocated control groups. Each of these methods has advantages and disadvantages.

The typical before-and-after study involving historical control groups (Barr and others, 1976) can be used for any curricular activity and does not require an experimental design. In evaluations that are observational, a group with a particular characteristic—such as enrollment in the quality assurance curriculum—can be identified, and a comparison group can be composed of those who do not possess that characteristic. The two groups can then be compared before, during, and after participation in the curriculum activities (Barr, Wollstadt, and Kinast-Porter, 1979). A similar evaluation can be conducted by comparing those enrolled in an elective program with those not enrolled (Zeleznik and Gonnella, 1979). The use of observational controls has the principal advantage of requiring no extra effort to allocate students. All that is needed for such evaluations is data from the groups without the specified characteristic or from those not enrolled in the elective program. There are disadvantages, however, that may threaten the validity or reliability of the evaluation. For example, the comparison groups may differ in respects other than not possessing the characteristic of being enrolled in the elective program, although the effects of these additional differences may be countered in part by pretest comparisons or matching controls. Despite the economy of effort and the initial usefulness of these types of comparison-group evaluations, however, they fail to supply the amount of data needed to establish definitively the relation between the curriculum and the outcome and hence do not prove the value of a given curricular activity.

Random allocation of students to participate in the curricular activities should produce the most reliable evaluation results. However, there are pitfalls even in this approach, as Haggerty (1962) points out. Random allocation to medical school courses produces resentment among the students, and discussions between those in the control groups and those in the experimental groups often bias the results. Medical schools fortunate enough to allocate clerkships on a truly random basis as standard operating procedure have a considerable advantage in evaluating the effectiveness of a new curriculum (Zeleznik and Gonnella, 1979). Student resentment is then directed only to school policy and is not attributed to the curriculum, even though the problems created by interaction of the students from the control and experimental groups and other problems described by Haggerty are not obviated. The principal advantage of random allocation remains, however: The observed differences between the groups can be reasonably attributed to the impact of the curriculum and not to any bias of selection.

## Approaches to Curriculum Improvement Evaluation

Other purposes of conducting an evaluation are to assess how well the curriculum meets the learner's perceived needs and how efficiently it is being run.

*Needs of the Learner.* Medical faculty members, with considerable expertise in their own specialties, have little or no trouble in recognizing the future needs of students in these specialties. The faculty may also be adept at seeing how quality assurance and cost containment correspond to students' long-term professional needs. In fact, Chapter One recommends that curriculum goals and objectives reflect these long-term needs, and I have mentioned the importance of including them in the evaluation of curriculum effectiveness. It may be more difficult for faculty members to identify what the students perceive to be their own immediate needs and consequently more difficult not only to develop goals and objectives that reflect these immediate needs but also to evaluate how well they have been met in the curriculum. Yet programs or courses within a curriculum or even the curriculum itself frequently fail or are less successful than they might be because the objectives do not correspond to the learners' immediate needs.

For example, second-year students feel a need to know "the questions to ask" of patients on whom they practice physical diagnosis and frequently ask these questions in a stereotyped, listlike fashion. If the faculty member attempts to emphasize the patient's psychosocial needs at the expense of data collection at this point in learning, some students become hostile, even though these same students, when confronted with the necessity to attend to psychosocial needs later in their education, respond with great interest. A similar lack of compatibility between student needs and curricular goals and objectives may limit the effectiveness of the quality assurance and cost containment curriculum. Emphasizing patient outcomes at a point in the educational process when the learner is struggling to grasp details of the process of care could adversely affect the student's evaluation of the curriculum, as could negative feedback about excessive charges with no recognition of or reward for appropriate behavior in diagnostic test ordering at admission. The approach to implementation suggested in Chapter Two, where quality assurance and cost containment objectives were examined in light of the objectives of the total curriculum, should increase the likelihood of developing a curriculum that responds to the learner's immediate needs. Certainly one purpose of evaluating the curriculum to determine where improvement could be made is to see whether both the perceived and unrecognized needs of the program's constituents have been met. If the evaluation shows that the curriculum fails in this respect, the evaluators have some indication of what needs to be done to improve it.

*Curriculum Efficiency.* Evaluation for improvement should also assess the feasibility of the curriculum in terms of costs and scheduling. It is important to ascertain whether the new activities sufficiently reduce charges generated by students and residents to compensate for the additional expense incurred. It may also be important to determine whether these projects can be carried out without overburdening the student or placing a strain on institutional resources. In evaluating costs and the strain on resources, however, one should be mindful that quality assurance and cost containment programs contribute a great deal to learning about health care—a benefit that may offset some of their costs.

In addition to collecting data for evaluating curriculum effectiveness and efficiency and for determining ways of improving the curriculum, the evaluator may gain important insights into the value that the learners place on the curriculum. Examining attendance records, observing the curriculum activities themselves, and eliciting learners' reactions and opinions by means of discussions with student groups, opinion polls, and questionnaires are useful means for gathering information to guide decisions about how programs or the curriculum could be modified.

## Evaluation Instruments

Unfortunately, no generally applicable instruments have been developed and assessed for reliability and validity that could assist quality assurance and cost containment curriculum evaluators. The instruments and illustrations provided here have been developed for use in particular programs and are offered by way of example of what can be used for evaluating specific facets of a curriculum.

*Knowledge.* Several programs have assessed student knowledge of the contents of a quality assurance and cost containment curriculum. Tables 3.1 and 3.2 provide examples of evaluation instruments developed by individual faculty members for specific programs. Table 3.3 is a questionnaire developed to assess student

### Table 3.1. Evaluating Knowledge of the Content of a Quality Assurance Program.

1. Describe as briefly as possible what is meant by *explicit* criteria:

2. Describe as briefly as possible what is meant by a *process* audit:

3. The percentage of mortality as a result of appendectomy would be a "process" result:

    _____ True       _____ False       __|__ ?

4. A study was designed to see the proportion of patients who, after having an abnormal hospital admission urinalysis, received appropriate work-up of this problem. Hospital house staff developed criteria on what an "abnormal" urinalysis was and what could be considered a "work-up" of this problem. This study would be considered a "diagnostic process" audit:

    _____ True       _____ False       _____ ?

5. In a nursing home in Florida the staff underwent an audit. Topic: Initial assessment of patients. Objective: To ensure that all disciplines document an initial assessment before the initial patient care conference.

    *Part of the Criteria List*

    | Criterion | Where to Find in Record |
    |---|---|
    | a) Vitals taken and recorded every 4 hours for first 24 hours | Nurse's record and progress notes |
    | b) Weight taken and recorded on admission | Patient admission data |
    | c) Bowel and bladder function | Nursing assessment, labeled "bowels" and another "bladder" and both documented |

    This is an audit using explicit criteria:

    _____ True       _____ False       _____ ?

    This a process audit:

    _____ True       _____ False       _____ ?

6. There is more variance between peers in the judgment of what is good, fair, or poor care in an explicit audit than in other audits:

    _____ True       _____ False       _____ ?

Table 3.1. Evaluating Knowledge of the Content of a
Quality Assurance Program, Cont'd.

---

7.  One of the objectives of self-review is to permit the student/physician
    to see his own progress over time by reviewing the care he has
    provided:

    _____ True          _____ False          _____ ?

8.  One of the objectives of self-review is to bring the student/physician
    up to date on information received since the student/physician last
    saw the patient and to permit him to follow up on any loose ends
    discovered in the care:

    _____ True          _____ False          _____ ?

9.  Audit programs are done to (Rank 1–5 with 1 highest priority and 5
    lowest priority):

    _____ Improve care

    _____ Provide continuing education

    _____ Recertify physicians

    _____ Determine deficiencies in care

    _____ Reduce the cost of care

10. It is a right of the patient to ask if his physician engages in peer
    review in order to assure the patient that specified standards of care
    are being met:

    _____ Yes          _____ No

    Why?

---

Source: Silva (1979). Rockford School of Medicine, University of Illinois
College of Medicine, Rockford, Illinois, 1978.

knowledge about selected charges for interventions that might be
used for a patient with congestive heart failure (answers provided).
Table 3.4 is taken from a recently published report of an assessment of costs of care (Dresnick and others, 1979).

*Skills.* Instruments for evaluating quality assurance and cost
containment skills of students and residents as applied in case
studies or in actual clinical practice have not been published. One
faculty questionnaire is available from Zeleznik and Gonnella at
Jefferson Medical College (Zeleznik and Gonnella, 1979). This area
of education evaluation needs attention.

**Table 3.2. Evaluating Knowledge of the Content of a Cost Containment Program: An Instrument Used at Thomas Jefferson Hospital.**

1.  What is the charge for one day in a semi-private room in Thomas Jefferson University Hospital? _____

2.  What is the charge for one day in the coronary intensive care unit in Thomas Jefferson University Hospital? _____

3.  What is the charge for one day in the intensive care nursery unit? _____

4.  What is the average hospital charge (that is, exclusive of physician fees) for a patient who has been treated for stage I appendicitis (that is, uncomplicated appendicitis)? _____

5.  What is the average hospital charge for such a patient treated for stage II appendicitis (that is, perforated or gangrenous appendix)? _____

6.  What is the average hospital charge (mother and child, exclusive of physician's fees) for a normal delivery (first-born)? _____

7.  What is the average hospital charge (mother and child, exclusive of physician's fees) for a Caesarean delivery (first-born)? _____

8.  What is the charge for a chest x ray? _____

9.  What is the charge for an SMA-12? _____

10. What is the charge for a culture and sensitivity of the sputum? _____

11. What is the charge for a liver scan? _____

12. What is the mean length of stay in the hospital of all patients? _____

13. What is the mean length of stay in the hospital of patients treated with a discharge diagnosis of cholecystitis, acute? _____

14. What is the charge for an EKG? _____

15. What is the charge for an upper GI study? _____
                                    lower GI study? _____
                                    gall bladder study? _____

*True or False*

1.  The government has no right to interfere in any way with how a physician wishes to provide care for patients he treats.

2.  The main reason for increased health care costs is increased labor costs by hospital nonprofessional workers.

**Table 3.2. Evaluating Knowledge of the Content of a Cost Containment Program: An Instrument Used at Thomas Jefferson Hospital, Cont'd.**

3. Good medical care is necessarily more expensive than poor medical care.

4. The major effects of technological advances in medicine have been to reduce medical costs.

5. Relatively few hospitals have active physician committees concerned with monitoring the costs of care provided within the hospitals.

6. The main reason that length of stay in university hospitals is greater than in community hospitals is that the costs of providing education add so much to the university hospitals' costs.

7. There is no way to establish objective criteria to guide utilization review committees in reviewing the care given to hospitalized patients.

8. Utilization review regulations do not apply to emergency room or outpatient visits.

9. There are no significant differences in length of stay for a given disease in different parts of the country.

10. Utilization review is really the same thing as quality review.

11. It is very difficult to determine what the actual costs of a laboratory test are in most hospitals (that is, as opposed to costs charged to patients and third parties).

12. It is often to a hospital administrator's advantage for laboratory facilities in a hospital to be fully utilized.

13. Much of the conflict concerning increases in medical costs arises from the fact that different people have different perspectives and different interests.

14. A significant portion of the costs of providing health care to individuals with negative health habits has to be paid by individuals who have positive health habits.

15. Currently, about 10 percent of the gross national product of the United States is devoted to providing people with health care.

(A total of 48 items were listed in the original questionnaire.)

*Source:* Zeleznik (1979). Jefferson Medical College, Thomas Jefferson University, Philadelphia, 1978.

Table 3.3. Evaluating Knowledge of Selected Charges for Interventions
Employed for Congestive Heart Failure: Answer Sheet.

I.  Estimate to nearest dollar the hospital charge for each item:

| Blood gases | $30.00 | SMA-6 | $13.00 |
|---|---|---|---|
| Creatinine | 5.00 | Urinalysis | 6.00 |
| Electrolytes | 10.00 | Chest x ray (single view) | 11.00 |
| Potassium only | 5.00 | EKG | 22.00 |
| T-4 | 10.00 | Ave. cost of bed per day | 83.00 |
| SGOT | 5.00 | Protime | 5.00 |
| CBC | 8.00 | CPK | 6.00 |
| SMA-12 | 15.00 | HBD | 12.00 |

II.  Estimate to nearest dollar the charge to the patient for each
     medication:

| (Aldactone) spironolactone<br>25-mg tablet: 4 tablets daily for 30 days | $3.00 |
|---|---|
| (Lasix) furosemide<br>40-mg tablet: 1 tablet daily for 30 days | 5.00 |
| (Hydro-Diuril) hydrochlorothiazide<br>50-mg tablet: 1 tablet daily 30 days | 4.00 |
| (Choledyl) oxtriphylline<br>200-mg tablet: 2 tablets 4 times daily for 30 days | 14.00 |
| (Lanoxin) digoxin<br>0.25-mg tablet: 1 tablet daily for 30 days | 2.00 |
| nitroglycerin<br>0.4-mg tablet: 10 tablets/month | 4.00 |
| quinidine sulfate<br>200-mg tablet: 2 tablets 4 times daily for 30 days | 4.00 |

*Source:* Mulligan (1979). University of Missouri School of Medicine, Kansas
City, Missouri, December 1976.

**Table 3.4. Response Error Rate In Estimating Actual Hospital Charges Before Education Interventions[a].**

| | Actual Hospital Charge ($)[b] | Range ($) | Percentage Within 10% of Correct Charge | | | Percentage Within 25% of Correct Charge | | |
|---|---|---|---|---|---|---|---|---|
| | | | Medical Students | House Staff | Faculty | Medical Students | House Staff | Faculty |
| CBC | 15 | 13–17 | 36 | 26 | 29 | 44 | 37 | 57 |
| Hemoglobin and hematocrit levels | 10 | 9–11 | 19 | 21 | 15 | 46 | 35 | 32 |
| Urinalysis | 15 | 13–17 | 17 | 17 | 8 | 30 | 23 | 20 |
| Urine culture | 24 | 22–28 | 19 | 18 | 30 | 43 | 45 | 58 |
| EKG | 25 | 22–28 | 26 | 37 | 34 | 59 | 57 | 78 |
| Piped oxygen per 24 hr | 48 | 43–53 | 17 | 26 | 12 | 29 | 46 | 25 |
| Semiprivate room | 111 | 100–122 | 34 | 45 | 46 | 47 | 60 | 68 |
| Intermittent positive pressure breathing | 15 | 13–17 | 3 | 8 | 10 | 3 | 11 | 17 |
| Operating room | 200 | 180–220 | 20 | 23 | 24 | 30 | 45 | 51 |
| Blood per unit type, cross, and processing | 61 | 55–67 | 6 | 6 | 10 | 44 | 50 | 54 |
| Intravenous solution per liter | 15 | 13–17 | 29 | 14 | 22 | 34 | 20 | 32 |
| Upper GI series | 64 | 58–71 | 13 | 8 | 27 | 46 | 47 | 68 |
| Intravenous pyelogram | 59 | 53–65 | 7 | 11 | 17 | 16 | 32 | 49 |
| Chest (posterior-anterior and lateral) | 27 | 25–31 | 43 | 43 | 46 | 49 | 53 | 61 |
| Laboratory profile 6 | 28 | 25–31 | 27 | 24 | 26 | 39 | 29 | 41 |
| Potassium only | 11 | 10–12 | 27 | 22 | 20 | 40 | 29 | 29 |
| Clinic visit | 24 | 21–27 | 27 | 32 | 32 | 54 | 57 | 60 |

[a]Medical students, N = 70; house staff, N = 319; faculty, N = 41.

[b]All prices are billing prices. Radiology procedures do not include radiologist fees.

Source: Dresnick and others (1979). Jackson Memorial Hospital and the University of Miami School of Medicine, 1979.

*Attitudes.* Kane (1973a) developed a sixteen-item set to assess learner attitudes toward quality assurance. Although not tested for reliability and validity, this evaluation instrument has been widely used. A modified version was administered to students at the Rockford School of Medicine; the results are shown in Table 3.5.

*Clinical Behavior.* The basic approach to quality assurance and cost containment involves an assessment of quality and costs, the development and implementation of certain actions to alter what has been observed (if alteration is required), and a reassessment of quality and costs to determine whether any improvement has occurred. Several reports have been published that document the results of such assessments of clinical behavior (Williamson, 1977). One tool frequently used to influence clinical behavior prospectively is a criteria list that has been honed by repeated assessments and interventions. Table 3.6 shows a criteria list that addresses both quality assurance and cost containment. Though not an evaluation instrument specifically developed to measure the effectiveness of a curriculum, it does illustrate a tool that could be used to assess the clinical behavior of learners. In addition, an internal medicine group practice has reported interesting cost and anecdotal quality results derived from a problem-oriented approach (Tufo and others, 1977).

*Other Attributes.* Course evaluation forms, individual and group critiques, attendance records, and estimated program costs have been developed for various programs (Dennis and others, 1977; Lawler and others, 1978). Again, no generally useful instruments are available. The absence of an instrument to assess the costs of curricular activities in quality assurance and cost containment that could be used to compare costs between institutions poses a particular problem.

## Conclusions

Faced with a diversity of approaches and methods for evaluating a quality assurance and cost containment curriculum and with a lack of evaluation instruments that have been tested for reliability and validity, evaluators may feel at a loss about where to begin to assess the effectiveness of the curriculum or to determine

**Table 3.5. Quality Assurance Attitude Index Administered to
Rockford Medical Classes, 1975–1977.**

---

Attitudes of students toward quality assurance were measured before and after participation in a quality assurance program. Column A reflects the percentage of students in agreement with the items in the quality assurance index; Column B, the percentage of students who believed that participation in the quality assurance program was worthwhile and who were in agreement with the items; Column C, the percentage of those who felt participation was not worthwhile but who were in agreement with the items.

| *Item* | *A*<br>*All Students*<br>*(N = 60)* | | *B*<br>*Worthwhile*<br>*(N = 30)* | | *C*<br>*Not Worthwhile*<br>*(N = 29)[a]* | |
|---|---|---|---|---|---|---|
| | *Before* | *After* | *Before* | *After* | *Before* | *After* |
| Auditing is a basic medical skill | 65.0 | 58.5 | 66.7 | 80.0 | 65.5 | 37.9 |
| Auditing is a basic medical skill which each physician should learn | 68.3 | 63.3 | 73.4 | 86.5 | 65.5 | 41.4 |
| Physicians should be required to be involved in audits | 65.0 | 46.7 | 70.0 | 60.0 | 58.6 | 34.5 |
| Medical audits do more than just confirm what is already known | 70.0 | 70.0 | 70.0 | 76.7 | 72.4 | 65.5 |
| Medical audit is the best way to determine a physician's need for continuing education | 55.0 | 25.0 | 56.7 | 30.0 | 55.1 | 20.6 |
| Physicians should be required to recertify on the basis of medical audits | 64.4 | 42.4 | 63.3 | 60.0 | 64.3 | 25.0 |
| Medical audits can pay for themselves in eventual cost savings | 55.0 | 38.3 | 56.6 | 53.4 | 55.1 | 24.1 |

**Table 3.5. Quality Assurance Attitude Index Administered to
Rockford Medical Classes, 1975-1977, Cont'd.**

| | | | | | | |
|---|---|---|---|---|---|---|
| Not auditing one's practice regularly means not practicing good medicine | 45.0 | 26.7 | 53.3 | 36.7 | 37.9 | 17.3 |
| Mean (index score) | 61.0 | 43.3 | 62.1 | 60.9 | 59.3 | 33.3 |
| S.D. | 8.5 | 16.5 | 10.2 | 19.6 | 20.5 | 15.6 |

[a]One student did not respond to the item rating problem worth.

*Source:* Kinast-Porter, Barr, and Wollstadt (1978). Rockford School of Medicine, University of Illinois College of Medicine, Rockford, Illinois.

**Table 3.6. Acute CVA/Stroke Audit Criteria: Used for a Department of
Medicine Audit on Records.**

The following criteria were used for a Department of Medicine audit on records from June to October, 1977. The Department of Medicine has recommended that copies of the criteria be posted in all inpatient and outpatient medicine units with copies available to be placed in appropriate records.

The criteria have been professionally developed to identify those considerations that generally should be addressed in the care of this particular condition. The criteria should not be considered as standards that must be implemented in the care of all patients with the specific problem or disease. The unique condition of the patient, coupled with the medical judgment of physicians and other health professionals, may indicate that certain deviations are appropriate and within the exercise of proper patient care.

If your care is an exception to a criterion, please explain in progress note the reason it is not applicable to your patient. If you have any recommendations for revisions, please inform the Accredited Record Technician or Dena Strum Klein, Quality Assurance Program Administrator for the Department of Medicine and Division I (UMKC School of Medicine, Room M5-425, Ext. 526). All recommendations will be directed to Dr. Jack Mulligan, Vice-Chairman, for Dr. William Sirridge, Chairman, Department of Medicine.

**Table 3.6. Acute CVA/Stroke Audit Criteria: Used for a Department of Medicine Audit on Records, Cont'd.**

| Criteria | Total Charges to the Patient* |
|---|---|
| *JUSTIFICATION FOR ADMISSION* | |
| 1.   Recent or sudden onset of neurological deficits | |
|      *Exception:* Hospital-occurring CVA | |
| *JUSTIFICATION FOR DIAGNOSIS* | |
| 2.   Findings consistent with compromised cerebral circulation | |
| *INDICATIONS FOR SURGERY AND OTHER SPECIAL PROCEDURES* | |
| 3.   LP | $82.00 |
| 4.   Skull x ray | 56.50 |
| 5.   EKG | 34.00 (routine 12-1e) |
|      *Exception 3–5:* Decision statement re reason not done | |
| *DISCHARGE STATUS* | |
| 6.   Stable for 3–4 days after progression of deficits has ceased | |
|      *Exception:* Concurrent disease(s) and/or complication(s) | |
| 7.   Rehab. eval. within 24 hrs. after pt. is stable (PT or OT & Speech Therapy if pt. has speech problem) and documentation that follow-up has begun on recommended actions if indicated (by Rehab. evaluation) | 13.00 (PT evaluation) 13.00 (OT evaluation) 40.00 (Speech evaluation) |
|      *Exception:* Justifying statement why evaluation and/or follow-up was not ordered | |
| 8.   Patient and/or family instruction re diet (if special or modified diet given), meds, therapy, physical limitations and follow-up treatment | |
|      *Exception:* Instructions given to nursing home, Visiting Nurse Association, or other responsible party | |
|      *Exception 6–8:* Patient left a.m.a. or was transferred | |

*Total charges to the patient include both hospital and physician services if applicable.

**Table 3.6. Acute CVA/Stroke Audit Criteria: Used for a Department of
Medicine Audit on Records, Cont'd.**

*LENGTH OF STAY*

9.   Maximum 14 days                        102.00 (regular room
     *Exception:* a. Placement problem,      charge per day)
     b. Concurrent disease(s) and/or
     complication(s)

*MORTALITY*

10.   Review all deaths

### COMPLICATIONS AND THEIR MANAGEMENT

11.   Ventilatory problems
      **a.   Head of bed elevated unless patient ambulatory or able to
             turn self
      **b.   Suction unless patient is able to mobilize own secretions
      **c.   Turn, cough and deep-breathe bedridden patients unless
             patient is unable to cooperate
        d.   Chest x ray
        e.   Appropriate antibiotics
12.   Contractures
      **a.   Turn q 4 hours if patient bedridden or q 2 hours if patient
             comatose or on respirator
      **b.   ROM exercises × 2 daily if patient bedridden

13.   Decubiti
      **a.   Turn q 2 hours if patient bedridden
      **b.   Air mattress if patient bedridden
      **c.   Sheepskin and/or heel pads and/or elbow pads if patient
             bedridden

14.   Shoulder subluxation
      **a.   Hemi-sling if patient in danger of subluxation (that is,
             weakened or flaccid extremity in patient who is able to sit or
             ambulate)

15.   Infection due to indwelling catheter
        a.   C & S
        b.   Appropriate anti-infectives

**Preventive measures.

### REFERENCES

1.   Van Horn, Gage, *Disease of the Month: Cerebrovascular Disease*, 1–46,
     June 1973.

2.   Mohr, Jay P., Fisher, D. Miller, Adams, Raymond D. Cerebrovascular
     Diseases. Chapter 334, *Principles of Internal Medicine*, Thorn, George
     W., et al. (Eds.). McGraw-Hill, 1977, 1832–1868.

**Table 3.6. Acute CVA/Stroke Audit Criteria: Used for a Department of Medicine Audit on Records, Cont'd.**

3. Hoff, Julian T., M.D., Intracerebral Hemorrhage. *Current Therapy,* Conn, Howard F., M.D. (Ed.) Saunders, 1978, 675–677.

4. Hass, William K., M.D., Acute Ischemic Cerebrovascular Disease. *Current Therapy,* Conn, Howard F., M.D. (Ed.). Saunders, 1978, 677–679.

5. Brennan, Robert W., M.D., Rehabilitation of the Patient with Hemiplegia. *Current Therapy,* Conn, Howard F., M.D. (Ed.). Saunders, 1978, 679–681.

*Source:* Mulligan (1979). University of Missouri School of Medicine, Kansas City, Missouri, December 1978.

how to improve it. In this situation, it would perhaps be best to apply the general principles involved in institutional evaluation. Following this approach, one would develop evaluation design alternatives as part of the curriculum process, thus ensuring that the evaluation took into account the curriculum objectives and the feasibility of implementing them in specific instructional units. The evaluation, then, would cover the following assessments, ranked in order of increasing difficulty:

1. Assessment of the participants' reactions to the curriculum and the learning experiences.
2. Assessment of the actual operation of the curriculum (scheduling, events, attendance) and its utility.
3. Assessment of the effect of the curriculum on quality and costs of care within the academic institution itself.
4. Assessment of the degree to which the goals were attained.
5. Assessment of the modifications needed to improve the curriculum.
6. Assessment of the long-range effects on participants' knowledge, attitudes, and skills.

There would be additional advantages if comparisons could be made between institutions with and without programs to evaluate the effects of a QA/CC curriculum. Such comparisons would allow evaluators to compare participating students and those who had not participated, without becoming entangled in the difficulties associated with random allocation within a single institution. To date, this type of cross-institutional evaluation has not been conducted for quality assurance and cost containment curricula. A regional or national study of this kind could serve as a prototype for cooperation among institutions and would be potentially beneficial to all involved.

Unlike biochemistry, pathology, internal medicine, and surgery, quality assurance and cost containment are far from being curricular mainstays at academic medical centers. To conduct these currently "marginal" activities without evaluation is dangerous to their future growth and development. Health care evaluation has become to medicine what pathology was a few decades ago: the source of the final answers, if there are any. Those of us who teach evaluation or who want to learn to must continually retune our ears to the needs of the audience, as well as learn to listen to the cries of dismay when medical students and physicians don't like "our results" or "our curricula."

Although health care evaluation needs a better microscope—or, better still, an "autoanalyzer"—we must use what we have. Yet while we employ our meager tools, we must assure ourselves and others that, crude as they are, we are using them well.

# 4

# Using Health Problems as the Organizing Framework

*John W. Williamson*

Many components of health care delivery could provide the focus of quality assurance: health care providers, health care facilities and their administration, clinical interventions, and costs. However, the most fundamental aspects of all these components are the specific health care problems that people bring to the health profession. Patients seek care because of manifestations or symptoms of a health problem, or a desire to avoid them; providers decide on a particular diagnostic strategy on the basis of the type of suspected problem; the nature of the health problem determines the preventive or therapeutic intervention to be used; and the type or severity of a health problem influences the costs involved in managing it.

This chapter discusses the use of health problems as the organizing framework for establishing quality assurance priorities and shows how understanding the broad range of problems encountered by physicians in various medical settings is a necessary and practical first step in understanding the total quality assurance process. For this purpose, it reviews health problem nomenclature and coding classifications and indicates the most important classification sources presently available. It also compares current national data classifications of health problems with those used in local hospitals to indicate areas of compatibility.

## Implications of a Health Problem Framework for Quality Assurance

There are many ways of classifying health problems. The anatomist develops his nosology according to body location of organs and tissues, the physiologist by functional body systems, and the practitioner according to whether care is mainly medical or surgical. In the public health arena, the emphasis is on classifying diseases that occur in epidemics or those of a more common sporadic nature, injuries resulting from external causes, and health problems related to environmental causes. Although ideally it would be desirable to have a classification scheme based on a single dimension, such as etiology, most nosologies must involve compromises if they are to be practical. Current diagnostic categories are a mixture of classifications based on etiology, anatomic site, patient age, and circumstances of onset. Consequently, researchers, practitioners, and quality assurance personnel must adapt to their own needs the heterogeneous systems by which current health problem data are compiled and classified.

For quality assurance purposes, two health problem categorizations are important: (1) patient reasons for contacting the medical profession, or "patient reasons for visit," and (2) the diagnostic categories used by medical providers. Each of these has a separate and specific use in the assessment of care.

Patient reasons for contacting providers are the starting point for assessing the effectiveness and efficiency of *diagnostic performance*. The inductive reasoning process used to identify specific medical entities that explain presenting complaints requires that multiple hypotheses be tested in terms of their relative probabilities. Thus, the process of forming a diagnostic judgment starts with initial patient complaints, signs, symptoms, or "self-diagnosis" (for example, "my asthma," which may in fact be congestive heart failure).

Once a diagnosis has been formulated, at least tentatively, it is necessary to deduce the essential actions to be implemented in treating the health problem, a process that involves planning and implementing the timing, quantity, modality, and type of treatment. Assessment of the effectiveness and efficiency of therapeutic or preventive performance must, therefore, use diagnostic categories for the assessment of *therapeutic performance*.

Quality assurance personnel must, therefore, understand and be able to apply and distinguish between these two types of health problem classifications. For example, since current health problem coding is generally restricted to final diagnoses, and a review of medical records will therefore yield information mainly on therapeutic care, the assessment emphasis has been on therapeutic management. However, patients do not present with health problems in terms of diagnostic categories, such as "acute myocardial infarction." Rather, they present with acute chest pain and shortness of breath, symptoms for which acute myocardial infarction is one of many possible diagnoses. Thus, approaches such as medical audits based entirely on patient charts containing provider diagnostic labels are inadequate for assessing diagnostic performance. This approach may discover false positive diagnoses in a group of patients (for example, those not having a myocardial infarction who were erroneously diagnosed as such), but it cannot assess skills in avoiding false negative diagnoses (for example, myocardial infarctions diagnosed as a more innocuous health problem). Thus, patient complaint coding is required to identify a patient sample that can provide the data for assessing deficient diagnostic performance.

Both systems of classifying health problems (that is, from the points of view of both patient and provider) are needed for quality assessment; therefore, quality assurance personnel must become aware of the scope and depth of existing classification schemes derived from diagnostic categories and from the patient's reason for contacting a provider of care. The following section describes coding schemes in general use today that reflect these health problem classifications.

### Health Problem Classification Systems

An important reason for understanding classification systems for health problems is that extensive data exist indicating the frequency of various health problems (see also Chapter Five). These data provide an invaluable resource for identifying problems relevant to quality assurance study and establishing priorities among such problems. If quality assurance personnel are to locate and understand these data, the structure of existing nosologies must be accurately understood and applied.

*Provider Diagnostic Categories.* Modern health problem classification by diagnostic categories is generally attributed to François Bossier de Lacroix (1706–1777). Earlier nosologies were developed primarily as a means of classifying causes of death—John Graunt's "Natural and Political Observations upon the Bills of Mortality in London" (1662) being the most famous instance. Work begun by the First International Statistical Congress in 1853 was carried on by the International Statistical Institute under the direction of Jacques Bertillon (1851–1891). By 1900 most nations had accepted the "Bertillon Classification of Causes of Death." The American Public Health Association recommended decennial revisions of this classification scheme, and in 1948, at the Sixth Decennial Revision Conference, the combined morbidity/mortality classification developed by the U.S. Committee on Joint Causes of Death was adopted internationally. This classification provided the general structure that now is part of the standard nomenclature and coding system for classifying health problems, the *International Classification of Diseases,* or ICD, which is revised every decade; the most recent revision is the ninth (World Health Organization, 1977). The U.S. National Commission on Vital and Health Statistics, in collaboration with the American Hospital Association, subsequently developed a slightly modified version of this classification for use specifically in the United States. This version, the *International Clas-*

*sification of Diseases, Adapted* (ICDA), is the official classification code for the U.S. National Center for Health Statistics (NCHS). It is also updated regularly, the present revision being the eighth (National Center for Health Statistics, 1977). Unfortunately, the Commission on Professional and Hospital Activities (CPHA) has decided to continue developing its own version, the *Hospital Adaptation of the International Classification of Diseases, Adapted for Use in the United States,* or H-ICDA (Commission on Professional and Hospital Activities, 1973). Consequently, statistics generated by the Professional Activities Study (PAS) and Medical Audit Program (MAP), the quality assurance programs of the CPHA, are based on a somewhat different coding scheme from that used by NCHS. However, the first three digits of the ICD and ICDA are the same, and the fourth digit differs only in certain codes. The H-ICDA generally differs from both other versions in the third and fourth digits.

The content of the seventeen major categories of the ICDA is reflected in Table 4.1 by a listing of the types of diseases included in each category. A final category (Supplementary Classifications) is not officially labeled as such by the ICDA but is frequently used to refer to nondisease states—that is, for persons who were not sick, live-born infants by type of birth, and fetal deaths (as in an abortion).

It has been recognized that this classification is mainly topographical and oriented to body systems and that functional aspects and levels of severity are not sufficiently reflected in present ICDA categories. An example of a classification scheme that places greater emphasis on a multiaxial approach and relates more specifically to prognosis and treatment needs is the classification developed by the American Psychiatric Association's Task Force on Nomenclature and Statistics in its *Diagnostic and Statistical Manual of Mental Disorders* (DSM III; American Psychiatric Association, 1980). Whereas the ICDA category on mental disorders (Category V) is limited to major subcategories (organic psychotic conditions; other psychoses; neuroses, including personality disorders and other nonpsychotic mental disorders such as sexual problems and drug addictions; and mental retardation), DSM III requires categorization of each patient on five independent axes: (1) clinical syndromes, (2) personality disorders and specific developmental disorders, (3) physical disorders and conditions, (4) severity of psychosocial stressors, and (5) highest level of adaptive functioning in past year. Clearly, such a classification is much more suitable for quality assurance purposes, because it can provide a greater range of data on the type and quality of care provided.

*Patient Reasons for Contacting Provider: A Classification Scheme for Ambulatory Care.* The ICDA provided a widely used diagnostic coding scheme for both hospital and ambulatory use. What this scheme does not reflect (apart from Category XVI, "Symptoms and Ill-Defined Conditions") is specific patient complaints underlying the eventual diagnosis. Such a scheme emerged only recently in an effort to provide national baseline data on the use of ambulatory medical services. In 1974, the National Center for Health Statistics (NCHS) published its *Symptom Classification* for use in coding patient complaints in the National Ambulatory Medical Care Survey (NAMCS), which was developed by Meads and McLemore, building on earlier symptom classification schemes such as those of Bain and Spaulding (1967) and Renner and Piernot (1972). This symptom classification (National Center for Health Statistics, 1974) was used for NAMCS from 1973 to 1976.

At the same time, a refined and more comprehensive system of classifying and coding patient reasons for seeking care was being developed and tested. Designed to meet not only the needs of the NAMCS but those of a variety of other users, this scheme, the *Reason for Visit Classification* (RVC), by Schneider, Appleton, and McLemore (National Center for Health Statistics, 1979a) has been in use since 1977 and employs a modular structure that accommodates the patient's reason for seeking care as well as the provider's response to that reason (Table 4.2). The strength of this classification lies in its flexibility (each module can be expanded to provide greater specificity) and its compatibility with other systems, such as sections of the ICDA or the *International Classification of Health Problems in Primary Care* (American Hospital Association, 1975). In addition, the fact that the RVC has been designed for a range of ambulatory care settings and offers many specific applications (for example, to facilitate assignment of patients to individual members of the health care team and, consequently, more efficient resource allocation and patient scheduling) makes it particularly useful for quality assurance application (see also Schneider and Appleton, 1977).

**Table 4.1. Classification of Health Problems into Major Disease Categories, from ICDA 8.**

| | Category | Sample of Health Problems Included |
|---|---|---|
| I. | Infective and parasitic diseases | Restricted to communicable diseases considered transmittable; localized infections (for example, abscesses) classified with organ systems in which they occur |
| II. | Neoplasms | Classified by anatomic site in two major divisions: malignant and benign |
| III. | Endocrine, nutritional, and metabolic disease | Endocrine disease classified by anatomical tissue of glands; nutritional disorders by specific vitamin and protein deficiency; other metabolic diseases by metabolic substances, predominantly those missing in certain congenital disorders |
| IV. | Diseases of the blood and blood-forming organs | Anemia, coagulation defects, and other conditions (for example, polychthemia), exclusive of anemia associated with pregnancy and puerperium |
| V. | Mental disorders | Organic psychotic conditions, other psychoses, neuroses as well as personality disorders and other nonpsychotic mental disorders (for example, sexual problems and drug addiction); mental retardation, even if associated with or secondary to physical conditions |
| VI | Diseases of the nervous system and sense organs | Inflammatory and other diseases of central nervous system; diseases of nerves and peripheral ganglia; inflammatory and other eye diseases; diseases of ear |
| VII. | Diseases of the circulatory system | Active rheumatic fever, chronic rheumatic heart disease, hypertension; ischemic and other forms of heart disease; diseases of arteries, arterioles, capillaries, veins, and lymphatics; other diseases of the circulatory system, including gangrene |
| VIII. | Diseases of the respiratory system | Acute upper respiratory infection; influenza; pneumonia, bronchitis, emphysema, and asthma; other diseases of upper respiratory tract and respiratory system |

| | | |
|---|---|---|
| IX. | Diseases of the digestive system | Oral cavity, salivary gland and jaw diseases; those of the esophagus, stomach and duodenum; appendicitis; hernia of abdominal cavity; other diseases of intestine and peritoneum as well as diseases of liver, gall bladder, and pancreas |
| X. | Diseases of the genitourinary system | Nephritis, nephrosis, and other diseases of urinary system, including urinary tract infections; diseases of male and female genital organs; breast diseases |
| XI. | Complications of pregnancy, childbirth, and the puerperium | Complications of pregnancy; urinary infections and toxemia of pregnancy and the puerperium; abortion; delivery; puerperium complications |
| XII. | Diseases of the skin and subcutaneous tissue | Infections and inflammations as well as other diseases of skin and subcutaneous tissue, excluding viral warts and other local infections classified under Category I |
| XIII. | Diseases of the musculoskeletal system and connective tissue | Arthritis and rheumatism except rheumatic fever; osteomyelitis and other diseases of bone, joint, musculoskeletal system, and connective tissue |
| XIV. | Congenital anomalies | Classified by anatomic location of anomaly |
| XV. | Certain causes of perinatal morbidity and mortality | Classified by combination of anatomic location and etiology |
| XVI. | Symptoms and ill-defined conditions | Classified by systems or organs and including senility |
| XVII. | Accidents, poisonings, and violence | Incorporate dual classification according to nature of injury and external cause |

*Source:* National Center for Health Statistics (1977).

**Table 4.2. NCHS Reason for Visit Classification.**

*Symptom Module*

General symptoms

Symptoms referable to psychological and mental disorders

Symptoms referable to the nervous system (excluding sense organs)

Symptoms referable to the cardiovascular and lymphatic systems

Symptoms referable to the eyes and ears

Symptoms referable to the respiratory system

Symptoms referable to the digestive system

Symptoms referable to the genitourinary system

Symptoms referable to the skin, hair, and nails

Symptoms referable to the musculoskeletal system

*Disease Module*

Infective and parasitic diseases

Neoplasms

Endocrine, nutritional, and metabolic diseases

Diseases of the blood and blood-forming organs

Mental disorders

Diseases of the nervous system

Diseases of the eye

Diseases of the ear

*Disease Module* (Continued)

Diseases of the circulatory system

Diseases of the respiratory system

Diseases of the digestive system

Diseases of the genitourinary system

Diseases of the skin and subcutaneous tissue

Diseases of the musculoskeletal system and connective tissue

Congenital anomalies

Perinatal morbidity and mortality conditions

*Diagnostic, Screening, and Preventive Module*

General examinations

Special examinations

Diagnostic tests

Other screening and preventive procedures

Family planning

*Treatment Module*

Medications

Preoperative and postoperative care

Specific types of therapy

Specific therapeutic procedures

Medical counseling

Social problem counseling

Table 4.2. NCHS Reason for Visit Classification, Cont'd.

| | |
|---|---|
| Program visit, N.E.C. | Poisoning and adverse effects |
| *Injuries and Adverse Effects Module* | |
| Injury by type and/or location | *Test Results Module* |
| | *Administrative Module* |
| Injury, not otherwise specified | *Uncodable entries* |

*Source:* National Center for Health Statistics (1979b).

## Health Problem Coding Systems in Quality Assurance Studies

*Local Use of National Data.* While both ICDA and RVC provide coding schemes for national statistics that can be adapted to local quality assurance needs, present developments have centered mainly on short-stay hospital use and, therefore, on ICDA categories. The ICDA is currently being used in federally mandated and professional hospital quality assurance programs, resulting in the availability of local data arranged according to the ICDA categories and in a growing body of quality assessment criteria related to them.

For example, partly as a consequence of Medicare and Medicaid reimbursement programs, short-stay hospitals throughout the country have been required to provide statistical information on hospital discharges. In addition, hospitals participating in the Commission on Professional and Hospital Activities (CPHA) have generated health problem data as part of the CPHA hospital discharge abstracting services. Compilations of major diagnoses managed in short-stay hospitals and coded to the ICDA are almost universally available at the local level. Most hospitals have copies of the ICDA codebook and provide periodic statistics in the formats prescribed by federal quality assurance requirements as well as those of CPHA.

Data on length of stay in short-stay hospitals are also available as a result of CPHA's massive accumulation of length-of-stay statistics. These statistics, though not representative of the United States as a whole, were used as a national standard for quality assurance purposes. For each health problem category (in specified ICDA code inclusions and exclusions), CPHA has statistics on average length of stay in percentiles by patient age and sex, further categorized by whether surgery was performed. Professional Standards Review Organizations (PSROs), the federally established quality review program for Medicare and Medicaid patients, require that each hospital provide direct data on hospital utilization classified by discharge diagnoses. The Joint Commission on Accreditation of Hospitals (JCAH), which has a similar utilization review requirement, also requires basic statistical compilations in hospitals participating in its voluntary certification program. The American Medical Assocation (AMA), through a contract with the national PSRO program, has developed authoritative, diagnostic-specific screening criteria for establishing appropriateness of hospital admissions. Thousands of medical audits have been conducted on basic diagnostic categories of diseases seen in short-stay hospitals.

   *Methods for Developing Local Data: The Case-Mix Approach.* In addition, a number of methods are being developed to provide regional or local data on differences in costs of care and services provided to patients with the same discharge diagnosis. A recent development in health problem coding, the case-mix approach, owes its origin to current concern with cost containment. It considers health problem categories in conjunction with case characteristics (for example, age, patient complications, secondary diagnoses) for assessing the cost of care. Promoted by state hospital rate-setting review boards and more recently by the Health Care Financing Administration (HCFA) in efforts to develop equitable reimbursement policies for hospitals participating in Medicare/Medicaid programs, a number of measures have been designed that allow such case-mix comparisons to be made among different hospitals. The purpose of these comparisons is to examine the feasibility of reimbursing hospitals on the basis of the complexity or severity of cases (case mix) rather than on the number of hospital beds, ratio of residents to beds, or average days of hospitalization.

An extensive review has recently been completed of a number of case-mix measurement approaches presently being proposed or developed (Bentley and Butler, 1980). One is the Professional Activity Study (PAS) List A. Developed by the CPHA and currently used extensively by PSROs in setting length-of-stay checkpoints as part of their concurrent review process, the PAS publishes tables summarizing length-of-stay statistics based on primary diagnosis, the presence of additional diagnoses, the presence of any surgeries, and patient age for a large number of major diagnostic categories and subcategories.

A different method proposed by some investigators and termed Disease Staging (Gonnella and Goran, 1975; Gonnella, Louis, and McCord, 1976; Louis and others, 1979; Louis and Spirka, 1979) categorizes any given medical problem into three levels of severity. Patient case mix is defined by considering the severity of a given illness, the manifestation of disease, the cause of the disease, and the organ system affected.

The Patient Management Algorithm methodology developed by Young (1979) is based on the state of the patient at admission rather than the patient's ultimate diagnosis as it appears on the discharge summary. This methodology is based on the premise that physicians diagnose and treat patients according to known symptoms rather than on the basis of a definitive diagnosis, which may remain uncertain for several days after admission. Hence, a better starting point for assessing appropriateness of treatment is the patient's admission status as characterized by presenting symptoms and complaints. This assessment approach is presently being field-tested in ten Veterans Administration hospitals where medical and surgical patients are assigned to one of six levels of care on admission. Assignment is based on evaluations of the patient's needs and on the estimate of the hours of nursing care required. This multilevel care (MLC) project for describing case mix in VA hospitals will provide estimates of the types of patients treated and the relative costs of various types of medical and surgical care (Mulhearn and Eurenius, 1979).

Last but not least among methods for classifying case mix is the Diagnosis-Related Groups (DRGs) approach, developed primarily at Yale New Haven Hospital (Fetter and others, 1976,

1977, 1980; Mills and others, 1976; Thompson, Fetter, and Mross, 1975; Young, Swinkola, and Hutton, 1980). The main objective of this method was to provide definitions of case types, each of which could be expected to receive similar outputs or services from a given hospital. With ICDA standard nomenclature as the basis for classifying diagnoses, 383 final diagnosis-related groups were developed. Each group was defined by a set of the following patient attributes: primary diagnosis, secondary diagnosis, primary surgical procedure, secondary surgical procedure, age, and clinical service area.

Currently, DRGs are being used to compare hospital performance on the basis of such patient care measures as length of stay, costs of admission, and death rates. It is also suggested as an effective mechanism for profile analyses (that is, examinations of the aggregate use of specific interventions) of individual practitioners or institutions because it provides consistent patient class definitions on the basis of which performance in treating similar types of patients can be compared. As is true for the other local coding schemes described, case-mix determinations are presently developed almost exclusively for inpatient care. Nevertheless, there is no reason these methodologies cannot be adapted to a study of ambulatory care data, as Lichtenstein and others associated with the Yale group have advocated.

For quality assurance and cost containment programs, DRG data could be developed to compare one's own institution with other institutions having similar DRGs. For example, mortality/morbidity figures of institution X could be compared with aggregate figures for all institutions for certain diagnosis-related groups; or mortality/morbidity rates for physician A could be compared with aggregate figures for other physicians at the same institution. Similarly, variations in health care outcomes could be compared with variations in treatments given or diagnostic procedures performed for similar DRGs. Likewise, data from individual practitioners or institutions with similar morbidity/mortality figures could be compared on the basis of such variables as days of care or total cost of care. In fact, some institutions are using this method as an internal management instrument, using diagnosis-related groups to obtain hospital data grouped by the following dependent variables: total cost per illness, total days of care per illness, types and amounts of treatments given per illness, types and amounts of diagnostic procedures given per illness, and health outcomes (mortality/morbidity) per illness.

Clearly, many problems of compatibility between national and local data systems remain. However, adoption of uniform diagnostic classification schemes, in conjunction with methods accounting for differences in case mix and severity, may make it possible to provide a uniform data base for quality assurance purposes in hospital care. For example, if an assessment of patients diagnosed as acute myocardial infarction, case-mix type X, can proceed on the assumption that they present the same combination of characteristics in California hospitals as in Pennsylvania, the profession will have taken a giant step toward obtaining comparable information for quality assurance and health services research.

In spite of work by Young on the Patient Management Algorithms, case-mix coding according to patient symptoms in ambulatory care has not progressed as far. Although some investigators (Mushlin and Appel, 1980) are beginning to use patient-reported problem status as one basis for primary care assessment, breakthroughs in this area will probably not occur until some national health insurance program is implemented that requires uniform statistics on ambulatory care in offices and clinics. When that time arrives, the importance of health problem categories adjusted for case mix and severity will be as great in ambulatory care as it is now in hospital care. At the moment, this lack of uniform data continues to impede the development of quality assurance in ambulatory care, and the only present recourse is to national statistics modified for local use through peer judgment or consensus.

## Conclusions

Data classified according to health problems are essential for quality assurance. In a systematic approach to assessment of health care, it is neither possible nor desirable to study all patients or every aspect of care. Consequently, it is essential to have some organizing framework from which to select topics and set priorities. By identifying patient population groups with specific health problems and applying sampling procedures, a limited series of assessments can be made and generalized to a larger population. Consequently, understanding standard health problem nomenclature and coding systems, as well as methods reflecting case mix and severity levels, is a first step toward understanding quality assurance.

This understanding requires the availability of uniformly coded data classified on the basis of health problems. Such data exist at the national level in the form of the International Classification of Diseases, Adapted (ICDA) and the Reason for Visit Classification developed for the NAMCS.

More and more methodologies using ICDA categories are being developed for use at the local level for quality assurance in inpatient settings. Although much remains to be done to develop local classification systems that are compatible with national systems, a sufficient number of schemes now exist that can help quality assurance personnel identify health problems that warrant study.

Although similar systems do not yet exist at the local level for classifying patient symptoms, there is reason to believe that such systems will be developed as quality assurance expands to the ambulatory area and emphasis broadens to include assessment of diagnostic as well as therapeutic skills.

# 5

# Determining Societal Importance of Health Problems

*Mary Lee Ingbar*
*John W. Williamson*

The preceding chapter discussed health problems in a functional and practical framework for establishing quality assurance priorities. As pointed out in the Introduction, four other components must be examined to decide which problems of health care warrant a quality assurance study:

- The importance to society of specific health problems,
- The efficacy of existing health care interventions to prevent, diagnose, cure, or care for these problems,

Some of the research on which this chapter was based was supported by the National Fund for Medical Education through grant number 45/78A sponsored by the American Hospital Supply Corporation.

- The effectiveness and efficiency with which these interventions are applied in actual practice,
- The potential for improving care as currently delivered.

This chapter focuses on the first of these components, the importance to society of specific health problems. Four aspects of this topic are discussed: (1) the determinants of health problem importance, (2) quantifying these determinants, (3) identifying relevant national data, and (4) compiling local information on health problem importance for quality assurance applications.

## Implications for Quality Assurance of Determining the Importance of Health Problems to Society

At present we have no integrated unit of health value that can be used to quantify the burden of health problems on society. Expenditures for health in the United States amounted to $212.2 billion in 1979, almost 10 percent of the gross national product (GNP), and an increase of 12.5 percent over the previous year (when the GNP increased 11.3 percent). This expenditure indicates that Americans value health and are willing to pay to maintain it; what it does not tell us is how to establish the cost to society of health problems themselves. Many attempts have been made to arrive at such determinations, and some of these are described in the following sections. In most of these attempts three factors stand out as the major determinants of health problem importance: (1) the frequency with which health problems occur in a population, (2) the amount of health loss related to these problems, and (3) the economic costs associated with both health and earnings loss and the care provided to prevent, diagnose, and treat them.

*Frequency*, the number of times a health problem occurs in a given population, is equivalent to a measure that epidemiologists use to estimate morbidity in terms of incidence and prevalence. *Health loss* refers to the consequences of a given health problem, whether treated or untreated, including health risk, symptoms, impairment, disability, mortality, and the resulting social disruption in families or communities. *Economic cost* encompasses health care expenditures in the management of health problems as well as other costs consisting of earning loss and opportunity costs caused to individuals and society by morbidity and mortality. Understanding these factors is essential in formulating priorities for quality assurance activity that encompass basic social values. Major emphasis will be given to economic considerations because these aspects are not usually covered elsewhere in medical education curricula.

*Frequency.* The frequency with which health problems occur in the population is obviously an indication of their social importance, particularly when combined with indicators of health loss and economic costs. For example, a frequent problem having moderate or low disability and mortality, such as arthritis, may have equal priority with a condition having low frequency but high health loss, such as malignant melanoma.

Morbidity information has many applications in quality assurance activity aside from indicating social importance. In sampling patients for quality assessment purposes, for example, it is essential to avoid health problems that are so rare that it would take inordinately long to accumulate an adequate sample. At the other extreme, if a problem is widely prevalent, appropriate sampling ratios must be applied to obtain a sample representing a standard time frame, such as six months or one year.

*Health Loss.* The potential health loss associated with a health problem is the second critical component in determining importance. Knowledge of the expected type and extent of health loss associated with a given health problem enables quality assurance personnel not only to derive meaningful standards by which to judge the effectiveness of the care provided but also to select and design appropriate instruments for measuring health outcomes. For example, if care for normal pregnancies is the subject of the quality assessment, data on complications and mortality rates associated with this condition will allow quality assurance personnel to recognize preventable complications, avoidable pain and suffering, and risks of unnecessary operative delivery. Similar data for acute myocardial infarction will enable personnel to recognize preventable losses of longevity and of years of productive life as well as avoidable pain and suffering.

*Economic Cost.* Finally, the economic costs related to a health problem are indicators of its social importance—illustrated by concern about hospital charges is evident in legislative emphasis on utilization review to prevent unnecessary hospital admissions, to reduce length of stay, and to increase appropriate use of ancillary services, among other such economic goals. As noted in Chapter Four, this process has stimulated development of case-mix and severity indices that are becoming a standard element in cost-containment activities around the country.

Another aspect of concern with health care economics involves both the legal costs associated with malpractice litigation and the medical costs associated with the performance of "defensive medicine." In this latter practice, physicians often order costly medical interventions designed less to benefit patients than to protect themselves legally. An entire method of quality assessment, termed *generic screening,* has been developed to identify medical events that carry a high risk of legal action: for example, internal bleeding in patients recovering from surgical procedures, which requires that the patient be rushed back to the hospital; generalized sepsis in patients recently discharged from the hospital that results in emergency readmission; and preventable complications such as pulmonary emboli in patients receiving care for a fracture.

**Illustrations**

Because most health care practitioners are accustomed to establishing health problem priorities in terms of health loss—that is, in terms of associated morbidity and mortality—this determinant of health problems importance does not require detailed illustration. However, economic costs to the individual and society as a determinant of importance are often neglected in local quality assurance planning. One reason is that practitioners typically lack a background in economics and interest in or information on the aggregated economic costs of health care. The following illustrations show how economic costs can be used to identify health problems that warrant a quality assurance study, as well as showing the potential of quality assurance in reducing their total cost to society.

*Bipolar Disorders.* Figure 5.1 shows the overall economic cost to society associated with bipolar disorders (manic depressive illnesses). Expert team estimates reported in a recent study (William-

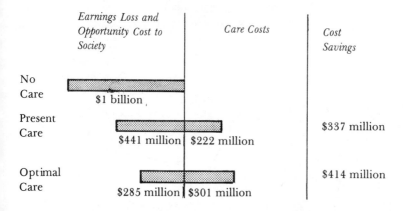

**Figure 5.1. Expert Team Estimates of Economic Cost of Bipolar Disorder, Total Incidence, 1976 (From Williamson, Goldschmidt, and Jilson, 1979).**

son, Goldschmidt, and Jilson, 1979) indicated a potential economic loss of $1 billion associated with bipolar disorders in 1976 if untreated. The components of this loss are quantified in the Figure. Currently available medical treatment probably reduced this loss by $337 million. However, if better methods of managing bipolar disorders were introduced, this net reduction could be enhanced to $414 million at an additional care cost of only $79 million. In part, this potential for reducing the economic cost of bipolar disorders lies in the deficiencies in current care used to treat this health problem. As indicated in Figure 5.2, approximately half of the $22 million spent in 1976 for treatment of these disorders was for care estimated to be either harmful, unnecessary, or of unproven efficacy (Williamson, Goldschmidt, and Jilson, 1979).

*Surgical Procedures.* The potential for reducing a range of surgical expenditures appears to be similar. Rice and Hodgson (1978) report that benign neoplasms account for 55 percent of the amount spent for all neoplasms in office or other visits, 22 percent of the expenditures for hospital care, and 43 percent of those for surgery. If methods were available to improve care for benign neoplasms, perhaps through improved diagnosis, the expenditures associated with this health problem could probably be reduced. The value of second medical opinions before surgery likewise has significant potential for eliminating expenditures related to un-

Total cost: $222 million

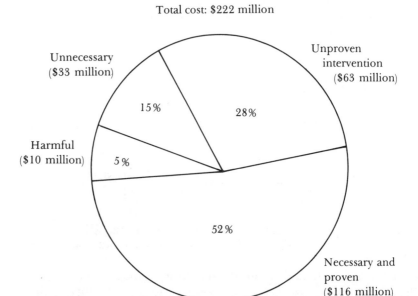

Figure 5.2. Expert Team Estimates of Utility and Cost of Care for
Bipolar Disorder, Total Incidence, 1976 (From Williamson,
Goldschmidt, and Jilson, 1979).

necessary procedures (U.S. Congress, 1977). One study (McCarthy
and Widmer, 1974) measured the impact of second opinions regarding the need for surgery. Overall, in 24 percent of procedures,
the need was not confirmed, although the rate of negative second
opinions varied widely for different procedures. For example, 57
percent of vertebral column surgical recommendations were not
confirmed, compared with only 11 percent of cholecystectomies.

*High-Cost Subpopulations.* Within the past several years a
number of studies have substantiated the proposition that a small
portion of patients consume a major proportion of medical resources in the United States (Birnbaum and others, 1977;
Schroeder, Showstack, and Roberts, 1979; Thibault and others,
1980; Mulley and others, 1980). Studies reported by Zook and
Moore (1980) indicate that in a given year in the United States, 13
percent of patients use as much in care resources as the remaining
87 percent. This suggests, since only one person in ten is admitted
to a hospital in any given year, that as little as 1.3 percent of the U.S.

population accounts for over half the annual consumption of hospital resources. The frequency of repeated hospitalizations of the same person for the same high-cost illness, noted both by Schroeder, Showstack, and Roberts and by Zook and Moore, illustrates the impact of the cost of long-term, chronic diseases on the national medical budget.

Until recently, information on variation in costs for patients with the same illness has not been readily available, particularly for chronic diseases. Illustrative of the necessary information are data from a study of ambulatory services provided under the Universal Medical Care Insurance Program during its first five years in Quebec. Berry and colleagues (1978) reported that patients with hypertension made an average of approximately three and one-half visits to their physicians for treatment of hypertension in each of the five years of the study, 1971–1975. This means that the average annual cost of treating hypertension in ambulatory settings may be thought of as equaling the average price per patient visit multiplied by 3.5. This average cost of hypertension care, however fails to take into account the dispersion in the cost of treatment among different patients. Such variation in costs is illustrated by the Canadian data for a subsample comprising 1,422 women 58–61 years of age. Among this group, 65 percent of the patients visited their doctors no more than three times in one year, whereas almost 10 percent required six or more visits in one year. This small, high-use group thus accounted for 25 percent of the office visits (Berry and others, 1978).

Health problems of specific subpopulations with high frequencies of use or requiring regular high-cost care could, then, also be identified as a priority for quality assurance study because of the high costs involved in their care relative to their numbers.

*Changes in Cost over Time.* Identifying health care cost components that are changing quickly is another way of using an economic approach to identify priorities for quality assurance. By determining how much costs have changed over specific periods of time and what price and/or practice components have shifted, one can consider both the quantitative and qualitative components of changes in practice that may be responsive to quality assurance review. Data from studies of the costs of treating selected episodes of illness conducted by Scitovsky and McCall (1977) in a large group practice in California illustrate how examining changes in cost over time may enable quality assurance personnel to identify those aspects of treatment of illnesses toward which their efforts should be directed. Table 5.1 shows increases in the number of diagnostic and other services rendered in the treatment of selected illnesses for the period 1951–1971, and Table 5.2 shows shifts in the average number of physician visits and the average length of hospital stay per case during the same period. Average length of stay has been reduced for the conditions studied, except for fractures requiring anesthetics, while the number of physician visits increased for most conditions considered, as did the number of laboratory tests and other procedures.

If quality assurance can induce major changes in practice patterns that affect levels of expenditures ordered by providers (for example, by curbing the increase in diagnostic tests where it can be shown that these tests are of little value to outcomes, or by reducing average length of stay), the effects of such changes can be significant in controlling costs. With respect to hospital stays, however, it should be noted that the general reduction in average stays has not been accompanied by a corresponding decrease in hospital costs. On the contrary, a recent staff report of the Council on Wage and Price Stability has stressed that the rise in hospital costs reflects a change in the style or character of the services that hospitals produce and that this change has been induced largely by the growth of insurance (Feldstein and Taylor, 1977). The implication is that increased hospital costs in the face of generally shorter stays reflect neither inefficiency nor unjustified increases in wages or profit margins but, rather, a change in the hospital product toward more complex and expensive care. Although consumers in the aggregate pay the full cost of the expensive care through higher insurance premiums, at the time of illness the choices of the patient (or relatives) and the physician are made in the face of only modest out-of-pocket costs. Feldstein and Taylor argue further that containment of hospital costs may eventually have to come through changing the structure of reimbursement mechanisms rather than merely limiting hospital charges through regulatory processes.

*Aggregate Costs for Diagnostic Tests.* The overall costs of com-

**Table 5.1. Number of Diagnostic and Other Services per Case, Selected Conditions, 1951, 1964, 1971.**

| Type of Service and Condition | 1951 | 1964 | 1971 |
|---|---|---|---|
| Laboratory tests | | | |
| Appendicitis | | | |
| Simple | 4.7 | 7.3 | 9.3 |
| Perforated | 5.3 | 14.5 | 31.0 |
| Maternity care | 4.8 | 11.5 | 13.5 |
| Cancer of the breast | 5.9 | 14.8 | 27.4 |
| Myocardial infarction | N.A. | 37.9 | 48.5 |
| Pneumonia | N.A. | 3.0 | 2.3 |
| Duodenal ulcer | N.A. | 5.4 | 5.4 |
| X rays | | | |
| Cancer of the breast | | | |
| Diagnostic | 0.7 | 2.0 | 2.3 |
| Radiotherapy | 1.7 | 11.0 | 10.6 |
| Forearm fracture | | | |
| Cast only | 2.3 | 2.3 | 2.2 |
| Closed reduction, no | | | |
| general anesthetic | 3.7 | 2.7 | 3.9 |
| Closed reduction, general | | | |
| or regional anesthetic | 2.0 | 5.4 | 6.4 |
| Myocardial infarction | N.A. | 1.3 | 6.3 |
| Pneumonia | N.A. | 2.0 | 1.8 |
| Duodenal ulcer | N.A. | 2.4 | 2.2 |
| Intravenous solutions | | | |
| Appendicitis | | | |
| Simple | 0.1 | 2.4 | 4.6 |
| Perforated | 6.7 | 12.7 | 14.2 |
| Cancer of the breast | 1.0 | 1.7 | 1.7 |
| Myocardial infarction | N.A. | 1.6 | 10.6 |
| Electrocardiograms | | | |
| Myocardial infarction | N.A. | 5.4 | 9.0 |
| Inhalation therapy | | | |
| Myocardial infarction | N.A. | 12.8 | 37.5 |

Source: Scitovsky and McCall (1977, Table 5).

mon diagnostic tests should also be considered for quality assurance study. To identify areas that should have priority, it is necessary to consider not only the unit cost per test but also the number of tests commonly performed. An illustration of the cost implications of this approach comes from a study of charges for common clinical laboratory tests generated by ancillary services

Table 5.2. Average Number of Physician Visits and Average Length of
Hospital Stay per Case, 1951, 1964, 1971.

| Type of Service and Condition | 1951 | 1964 | 1971 |
|---|---|---|---|
| Average number of physician visits | | | |
| Otitis media | 1.8 | 1.7 | 1.9 |
| Appendicitis | | | |
| Simple | 2.9 | 5.6 | 5.5 |
| Perforated | 6.8 | 9.1 | 11.8 |
| Maternity care (obstetrician) | 12.7 | 14.5 | 14.9 |
| Cancer of the breast | | | |
| Surgeons | 12.6 | 13.7 | 12.0 |
| Other MDs | 1.3 | 3.1 | 1.9 |
| Forearm fractures | | | |
| Cast only | 5.3 | 4.5 | 4.4 |
| Closed reduction, no | | | |
| general anesthetic | 6.7 | 6.1 | 7.0 |
| Closed reduction, general | | | |
| or regional anesthetic | 5.8 | 7.9 | 8.1 |
| Myocardial infarction | N.A. | 27.6 | 26.0 |
| Pneumonia | N.A. | 3.0 | 2.6 |
| Duodenal ulcer | N.A. | 4.7 | 3.8 |
| Average days of hospital stay | | | |
| Appendicitis | | | |
| Simple | 4.3 | 4.2 | 3.8 |
| Perforated | 10.8 | 10.7 | 10.1 |
| Maternity care | 4.6 | 3.8 | 2.8 |
| Cancer of the breast | 12.7 | 10.2 | 8.9 |
| Forearm fractures | | | |
| Closed reduction, general | | | |
| or regional anesthetic | | | |
| (all cases) | 0.4 | 1.2 | 0.6 |
| Closed reduction, general | | | |
| or regional anesthetic | | | |
| (hospitalized cases) | 1.0 | 1.2 | 1.4 |
| Myocardial infarction | N.A. | 19.7 | 18.8 |

Source: Scitovsky and McCall (1977, Table 6).

provided to patients in the Ambulatory Care Center of the Beth
Israel Hospital in Boston, Massachusetts, during 1976. Of thirty-six
types of tests provided to these patients, six accounted for over 91
percent of the total charges. Additional studies would be required
to ascertain what proportion of the laboratory's payroll and other
expenditures was associated with these tests.

These illustrations show how consideration of the economic factors associated with health problems can enable quality assurance personnel to establish priorities in areas of health care where improvement can result in better health and economic outcomes. In view of the marked variation in the contribution of various types of service to the aggregate cost for each illness (Scitovsky and McCall, 1977), it is clear that the importance of each type of service with respect to cost containment varies with the nature of the illness.

### Quantifying the Determinants of Importance

Although it is apparent that the factors of health problem frequency, health loss, and economic loss are important considerations for quality assurance and cost containment actions, it is difficult to quantify each of these determinants in terms of societal importance so as to establish priorities for quality assurance applications.

Frequency of health problem occurrence is quantified in terms of the number of persons having a given health condition. These numbers are usually reported as rates, wherein the numerator represents the number having the health problem and the denominator represents a standard measure of the population at risk. Two standard rates are usually applied, incidence and prevalence. Incidence is the number of persons experiencing their initial onset of the specified health problem during the past year per 100,000 base population, for example. Prevalence is the number of persons having the specific health problem during the past year (or whatever time period is specified), regardless of time of onset, per 100,000 base population, for example.

Quantifying health loss and economic costs is far more complex. Figures 5.3 and 5.4 are provided to facilitate understanding of the factors involved and the terminology often found in the literature. Figure 5.3 depicts a medical framework in which health loss and economic costs are related to illness and to health care provided for that illness. Health loss is most conveniently quantified in terms of time units (for example, days, months, years) of a given level of health. For example, years of decreased longevity, the

|  | Health Loss | Economic Cost ($) |
|---|---|---|
| Illness-Related | **A**<br><br>Disability and mortality encompassed by natural history of a health problem, plus intangible costs of pain, suffering, and social dysfunction | **C**<br><br>Productivity loss and opportunity costs of illness (indirect costs) |
| Health-Care-Related | **B**<br><br>Disability and mortality associated with professional management, plus intangible costs of pain, suffering, and social dysfunction | **D**<br><br>Dollar costs of health care (direct costs) |

Each cell implies population data that incorporate the factor of health problem frequency.

**Figure 5.3. Establishing Health Problem Importance: A Medical Framework.**

years of life lost because of the health problem, might be determined by subtracting the age at death from the actuarial life expectancy if the given health problem had not occurred. This method of quantifying mortality is more meaningful than use of simple mortality rates, which indicate only the total number dying per a standard population. In a similar fashion, disability can be quantified in terms of time units at various levels of life function, such as years unable to perform activities of daily living, which include eating, bathing, dressing, and toilet functions; or years unable to perform major life activities, which include fulfillment of one's life goals for a given age period, such as school attendance for children, vocational work for adults, or retirement activities for the elderly. Days or years of symptoms or exposure to high risks of onset of future illness or disability are examples of other time units of health loss or risk of health loss. Economic costs are usually quantified in dollar terms, as will be discussed later in more detail.

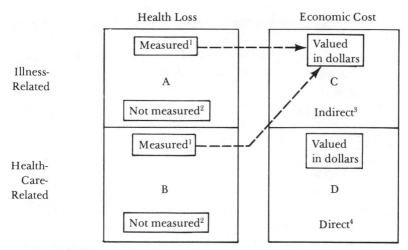

1. Quantifiable as time units (for example, years) of decreased longevity or added disability
2. Sometimes quantified as psychosocial cost of pain and suffering and other subjective factors
3. Quantified as productivity loss to society
4. Quantified as dollar costs/resources devoted to health care

**Figure 5.4. Quantifying Health Problem Importance:
An Economic Framework.**

Thus, in Figure 5.3, Cell A represents health loss as encompassing the risk, symptoms, disability, and mortality that would affect a population with a given health problem, particularly if no formal health care were provided. For example, congestive heart failure, a serious problem often involving extensive disability and early death if untreated, would be quantified in terms of years of decreased longevity or of added disability and symptoms.

Cell B represents the health loss, both preventable and unpreventable, that is related to treatment of a given health problem. Damage to health resulting from medical care is often overlooked, particularly as some of it is not preventable; for example, a mastectomy involves hospitalization, pain and suffering, and some disability. However, much of this type of health loss is in fact preventable. When a radical mastectomy is performed instead of a simple one, considerable disability is produced, often with little or no gain in longevity. The content of this cell would likewise be quantified in terms of years of decreased longevity or added symptoms and disability.

Cell C represents the direct monetary cost of the management of a health problem. This includes preventive, diagnostic, therapeutic, rehabilitative, and long-term care expenditures for procedures, devices, pharmaceuticals, and overall care management, as well as transportation and other personal outlays (Hu and Sandifer, 1981). The content of this cell can be quantified in dollar equivalents.

Cell D represents the indirect costs of illness, such as productivity lost to society, and other types of opportunity costs incurred as a result of morbidity and premature mortality. The content of this cell, like that of Cell C, is usually quantified in dollar equivalents. On the basis of what is often deemed the "human capital" approach, economists in the health field have been attempting to measure the dollar value of these determinants of the importance of a health problem to society. This is difficult, however, because data collected on health loss (Cell A) and on lost productivity and opportunity costs (Cell D) usually combine treated and untreated persons in the population. Figure 5.4 shows which of the components of Figure 5.3 are generally so quantified.

Cells C and D in Figure 5.4 thus represent the measurable costs of health problems—that is, the direct costs of medical management (C) and their indirect costs as constituted by resources lost to society because of premature mortality and morbidity. (Sources of data that provide specific estimates of these costs of illness will be discussed in a later section.) Some of the health loss in Cell A is measured in terms of years—for example, years from death to premorbid life expectancy (death years) and years away from major life activity, such as employment (disability years). Although it is possible to attach a dollar value to these components of health loss, and they indeed form the basis of the indirect costs in Cell D, its other components, such as symptom years, pain and suffering, and risk years, are difficult to value objectively in terms of dollars, as is the loss of life other than in terms of earnings lost.

Equally difficult to quantify is the health loss related to medical care, both preventable and unpreventable (Cell B of Figure 5.4). However, since malpractice awards often attach a dollar value to this facet of health loss (Rosser and Watts, 1975), it should not be ignored. Thus, Cells A and B, with the measurable mortality and morbidity costs removed, represent largely intangible costs of health problems (Pliskin and Taylor, 1977). These have also been described as unmeasured economic costs (Hu and Sandifer, 1981). The difficulty of measuring these costs within the framework of a human capital approach could, at least in theory, be overcome by adopting the "willingness to pay" approach originally proposed by Schelling (1968) and Mishan (1971). This concept would value the entire cost of illness in terms of a subjective consumer response, by establishing how much people would be willing to pay to reduce the probability of death or disease to themselves or others. However, this approach is still in an early stage of development and has been used relatively infrequently—for example, by Acton (1975).

Paringer and Berk (1977), Berk, Paringer, and Mushkin (1978), Banta and Thacker (1979), and Hu and Sandifer (1981) also refer to certain costs (pain and suffering, for example) as being difficult to measure reliably. It is clear, therefore, that the term *cost* is itself ambiguous and subject to many interpretations (see, for example, Hu and Sandifer, 1981). The following will show how some of the costs associated with the components of Figure 5.4 have been measured or estimated to place a value on the overall cost of illness.

*Measuring the Direct Economic Costs of Health Care.* From the economic standpoint, the direct costs of illness are the component of total cost that is most easily measured. They comprise the relative value of the resources expended in the management of the patient, including the value of the time of personnel and of equipment, supplies, and facilities (Cell C of Figure 5.4). The most direct method is to use the prices actually charged for services. These charges can be arrived at in many ways: They may be imposed in an ad hoc, arbitrary fashion; they may be derived from costs in a prior time period in accordance with traditional accounting practices; or they may be designed to be competitive with what others are charging for similar services. Charges may also be established by calculating median charges to assign a weight to each procedure that a physician is likely to perform. This approach, known as the Relative Value Scale (RVS), has been widely used by medical societies

(Delbanco, Meyers, and Segal, 1979; Hsiao and Stason, 1979; Showstack and others, 1979).

   *Measuring the Indirect Economic Costs of Illness and Health Care.* The indirect costs of illness and health care represent an aggregate of several factors that are harder to measure in dollar terms than the direct costs of care. These indirect costs include valuation of morbidity and premature mortality (the measured component of Cell A, Figure 5.4), a valuation of pain and suffering of illness (the remainder of Cell A), and a valuation of both the morbidity/mortality and the pain and suffering associated with health care (Cell B). These aspects will be discussed in terms of present methods of economic valuation. Calculating the economic cost of morbidity and mortality requires information on both the amount of productive time that is lost and the money value to be assigned to this lost output. Both the amount and the value of this loss will vary with conditions in the labor market and with characteristics of the persons who are ill or who die. In most calculations, it is implicitly assumed that work is available for those persons who seek jobs; questions related to employment levels, labor force participation rates, and unemployment measures are usually ignored. In contrast, personal attributes such as sex, age, occupation, productivity, education, and prevailing life expectancies are considered in most of these estimates. For instance, when considering losses from premature mortality, one must remember that although persons aged sixty-five and over account for a relatively large proportion of deaths from certain diseases (for example, almost 60 percent of all deaths from neoplasms in 1975), this age group will account for a much smaller proportion of person-years lost and of lost earnings, a reflection of the lower life expectancy and earning levels of the elderly. Again using deaths from neoplasms as a basis, persons aged forty-five to sixty-four contributed only 35 percent of the deaths in 1974 but 47 percent of the person-years lost and 62 percent of the lost earnings, compared with 36 percent of the person-years lost and 11 percent of the lost earnings for those over sixty-five. Because people in the younger age group have a significant number of productive years remaining and earnings are at a peak, the proportion of lost years and lost earnings is greater than the number of deaths would indicate (Rice and Hodgson, 1978).

Data of this type are now available from tabular presentations of lifetime earnings (Paringer and Berk, 1977).

The indirect costs of morbidity and mortality, as reflected in money values assigned to associated losses, when taken together constitute a substantial portion of the total economic cost of illness. Estimates of the earnings that will be lost from premature mortality, as distinguished from morbidity, are additionally sensitive to a number of factors that reflect expected changes in the levels of earnings in future years. Among these influences is the earning power of money itself, as represented by the interest rate used to convert future income into equivalent present values. The importance of assumptions about interest rates (that is, the so-called discount rate, applied to convert future dollars into present values) is illustrated in Table 5.3. Whereas mortality accounts for 33 percent of indirect costs (earnings loss) if future earnings are discounted at 4 percent, this proposition rises to 45 percent with the assumption of an interest rate of 2.5 percent, and it falls to 26 percent with an interest rate of 10 percent. Thus, the level of costs associated with mortality depends not only on the magnitude of earnings losses suffered as a result of illness but also on the increase in dollar value that would have occurred had that sum been invested at the prevailing interest rate.

The principal limitation of this "human capital" approach is that it values people as though they were machines, using productivity to measure the value of a human life (Acton, 1976). This approach is even dangerous if used as a criterion to determine whether to treat or not to treat. As Acton (1976) points out, it could lead to the conclusion that society should spend no money (or incur no costs) for programs that extend the lives of fatally ill children because these programs would not extend their future earnings.

*Unmeasured Cost of Illness and Care.* There remain the unmeasured, or subjective, costs of illness. These are often described (for example, Abt, 1975) as the social or psychosocial costs of illness to the patient and his or her family and friends, as well as pain and suffering and the loss of well-being (Cell A, Figure 5.4).

As mentioned before, while Acton (1973, 1975) has provided initial methodology for introducing into the concept of the cost of illness subjective evaluations of the amount that people would be

Table 5.3. Percentage Distribution of the Economic Cost of Illness Using
2.5, 4, and 10 Percent Discount Rates, United States, 1975.

| Method of Computing Mortality Losses | Total Economic Costs | Direct Costs | Indirect Costs | |
|---|---|---|---|---|
| | | | Morbidity | Mortality |
| Future earnings discounted at 2.5 percent | 100 | 37 | 18 | 45 |
| Future earnings discounted at 4 percent | 100 | 45 | 22 | 33 |
| Future earnings discounted at 10 percent | 100 | 50 | 24 | 26 |

Source: Berk, Paringer, and Mushkin (1978).

willing to spend to avoid suffering or to save their own life or that of others, the problem is, of course, that personal preferences for risk aversion, saving lives, and improving well-being may vary widely under similar circumstances. Thus, fixed standards of quality assurance may conflict with variable preferences of individuals concerning what they are willing to pay in order to improve or save their lives through medical management. One contribution of an economic analysis of the costs of illness is to expose the need for a more reliable system for determining priorities both in quality assurance and in the delivery of services. The health care system must be flexible enough to correspond to the variety of criteria by which individuals and society as a whole decide how much they are willing to pay for both quality and services in a free market economy. The subjective valuations associated with detection interventions, diagnosis, and treatment are just as difficult to measure precisely as those associated with loss of well-being and pain and suffering due to illness. These losses, nevertheless, must be taken into account when one calculates the benefits and risks to individuals or to populations of a proposed screening program or, for example, an invasive diagnostic procedure. This holds true even when the screening program, diagnostic procedure, or therapeutic intervention is performed with optimum skill and precision.

*Cost of Health Loss from Care.* To all this, one must add a consideration of decreased longevity, disability, and pain and suffering due to untoward and unexpected complications of screening, prevention, diagnosis, or treatment because of neglect, human error, misinterpretations, and other factors. When such mishappenings lead to legal action, the costs of the litigation plus loss of the patient's trust in the professional and the professional's anxiety, worry, and loss of productivity all need to be considered. Because the costs associated with untoward and unexpected complications are difficult to predict, and because one hopes that these occur with minimum frequency, they are seldom if ever calculated. Nevertheless, they do represent real resource utilization and must be reckoned with on a probabilistic basis in the calculation of total cost related to health care.

*Quality Assurance Implications of Economic Framework.* A review of the components of the cost of illness raises vital questions about the relation of quality of care to cost. Poor quality of health care can be seen to have a potential for raising the costs in all categories. For example, poor quality in terms of overdiagnosis or overtreatment can lead to excessive direct health care expenditures even in the absence of untoward events or iatrogenic consequences. Here the principle of "high cost/little benefit" will hold whenever excessive modes of prevention, detection, diagnosis, or treatment are employed. Poor quality in the form of misdiagnosis or mistreatment can increase mortality or morbidity, earnings loss, and therefore the costs of health problems to individuals and to society. Poor quality can also lead to increased pain and suffering and thus increase the total intangible cost of illness.

Quality and cost of health care, therefore, are inexorably interlocked. Generation of higher costs by using more health care resources does not necessarily mean better quality, nor does better quality always imply a need to generate more health care costs. Hence, when investigating the quality of any health care procedure or intervention, one should consider the direct costs of the treatment modality, the indirect costs of the illness in terms of mortality and morbidity if untreated or inadequately treated, and the estimates of pain and suffering attendant on both the treatment and the illness if untreated or inadequately treated. As the approaches already discussed indicate, this type of analysis could be developed either on the national (aggregate) level or on a local (regional, hospital, single group practice) level. It can show which health problems are of sufficient importance to warrant quality assurance studies and which costs are excessive or out of line with aggregated national or regional averages and thus are appropriate subjects for quality assurance scrutiny.

## National Data on Health Problem Importance

The preceding sections have discussed the implications for quality assurance of three determinants of health problem importance—frequency, health loss, and economic costs—as well as some approaches to quantifying these determinants. To conduct a quality assurance study, it is equally necessary to know what types and sources of data on these determinants are available.

*National Frequency Data.* The best sources of data on health problem frequency in the United States are the compilations by the National Center for Health Statistics (NCHS) in its Vital and Health Statistics Series. NCHS conducts ongoing national surveys based on probability sampling of the total population to obtain person interview data *(Health Interview Survey)*, direct physical examination data *(Health Examination Survey)*, hospital discharge abstract data *(Hospital Discharge Survey)*, and physician office data *(National Ambulatory Medical Care Survey)*. The NCHS surveys are particularly well suited for quality assurance purposes because of their sampling methods, their detailed information on the methods used as well as on the reliability and validity of their findings, and their complete glossary of terms. In addition, reprints of the survey encounter forms are provided that indicate the type and depth of questionnaires and other data collection instruments.

Other, less comprehensive national surveys are also available. For example, the Commission on Professional and Hospital Activities (CPHA) surveys provide a range of similar data; however, the CPHA's sources are limited to a sample of hospitals that voluntarily contract with it to compile discharge abstract data. As a result, although the aggregate of the total CPHA file is quite large, it is questionable whether the data can be generalized to the total U.S. hospital population.

The following description of data sources indicates available national statistics on health problem frequency in ambulatory office practice and short-stay hospitals, the two settings of most current quality assurance efforts.

Health problems seen in *ambulatory office practice* are reflected in the data from the *National Ambulatory Medical Care Survey* (NAMCS) of nonfederally employed physicians who are classified by the American Medical Association or the American Osteopathic Association as active in "office-based patient care." (This classification excludes visits to physicians in emergency rooms, hospital clinics, and the like.) The yearly survey, probably the first of its kind to produce valid national data, uses stratified cluster sampling of physicians in office practice and time sampling of the entire year. The following are an illustration of categories of data reported for all physicians and for twenty-five specialty practices: patient characteristics (age/sex/race, whether seen before by a physician, whether seen before for same problem); reason for visit, in patient's words (most important problem, other problems, category of problem); physician diagnoses (for main reason for visit, other current diagnoses, seriousness of main problem); diagnostic/ therapeutic services; disposition of case; and duration of this visit (National Center for Health Statistics, 1978a).

A consideration of health problem frequency in office practice will focus largely on the six physician specialties that deliver most ambulatory care for physical and emotional problems: general and family practice, internal medicine, pediatrics, obstetrics and gynecology, general surgery, and psychiatry. In 1975 these six specialties represented 74.0 percent of all physicians in the United States and provided 77.8 percent of all ambulatory care (National Center for Health Statistics, 1978a). A breakdown by patient age and sex is shown in Table 5.4.

The NCHS also provides data on health problem frequency by *reason for visit*. The most common reasons for visits to all physicians in ambulatory practice for 1974–1976 and associated symptoms are summarized in Table 5.5. Nonsymptomatic visits as defined by the NAMCS classification (National Center for Health Statistics, 1974) constitute the largest single grouping for all physician categories except psychiatry.

Health problem frequency by *diagnostic categories* for ambulatory patients provides a different listing and frequency distribu-

**Table 5.4. Number and Percentage Distribution of Office Visits by Physician Specialty and Patient Age and Sex, United States, 1975.**

| | All Specialties | General and Family Practice | Internal Medicine | Pediatrics | Obstetrics and Gynecology | General Surgery | Psychiatry | All Other Specialties |
|---|---|---|---|---|---|---|---|---|
| Physicians in active ambulatory practice (no. in thousands) | 166.11 | 45.96 | 23.07 | 10.23 | 13.91 | 18.44 | 11.28 | 43.22 |
| All patient visits (annual no. in millions) | 567.60 | 234.66 | 62.12 | 46.68 | 48.08 | 41.29 | 14.81 | 119.96 |
| *Percentage Distribution* | | | | | | | | |
| *Patient Age* | | | | | | | | |
| Under 15 years | 17.4 | 14.4 | 3.3 | 92.7 | 2.2 | 6.3 | 5.1 | |
| 15–24 years | 15.3 | 16.0 | 8.8 | 6.3 | 33.3 | 13.2 | 15.8 | |
| 25–44 years | 25.3 | 24.1 | 21.1 | — | 50.3 | 28.7 | 54.9 | |
| 45–64 years | 25.6 | 27.5 | 37.9 | — | 11.7 | 34.0 | 21.4 | |
| 65 and over | 16.4 | 18.0 | 28.9 | — | 2.4 | 17.8 | 2.8 | |
| *Patient Sex* | | | | | | | | |
| Female | 60.4 | 59.2 | 59.5 | 47.7 | 98.6 | 60.3 | 59.7 | |
| Male | 39.6 | 40.8 | 40.5 | 52.3 | 1.4 | 39.7 | 40.3 | |

*Source:* National Center for Health Statistics (1978a).

**Table 5.5. Patient Reason for Visit and Associated Symptoms in Ambulatory Practice for All Physicians and Six Major Specialties, United States, 1974–1976.**

| Physician Specialty | Total Weekly Visits per M.D. | Nonsymptomatic Visits[a] | Patient Reason for Visit — Common Symptoms | | | | | |
|---|---|---|---|---|---|---|---|---|
| | | | EENT complaints[b] | Visceral complaints[c] | Musculo-skeletal problems[d] | Skin problems[e] | Emotional and vague general complaints[f] | All Other |
| | | | *Percentage Distribution* | | | | | |
| All physicians | 73 | 28.4 | 16.5 | 15.9 | 11.5 | 7.6 | 7.7 | 12.4 |
| Internal medicine | 59 | 24.8 | 11.0 | 20.7 | 13.8 | 3.2 | 13.1 | 13.4 |
| Pediatrics | 97 | 41.1 | 33.3 | 8.3 | 3.1 | 6.6 | 2.3 | 5.3 |
| Obstetrics and gynecology | 72 | 64.0 | 1.4 | 22.2 | 1.4 | 1.0 | 2.5 | 7.5 |
| General surgery | 47 | 35.2 | 6.1 | 19.4 | 13.5 | 10.3 | 4.9 | 10.6 |
| Psychiatry | 29 | 4.8 | 1.1 | 2.8 | 1.5 | 0.3 | 53.7 | 35.8 |
| Family/general practice | 106 | 25.4 | 18.4 | 17.3 | 13.9 | 6.9 | 10.8 | 7.3 |

[a]Well patient: physical examination, insurance examination, "checkup," well-patient services, examination related to normal pregnancy and infancy. Nearly well patient: asymptomatic follow-up of previous illness (medical, surgical aftercare).

[b]Infections and sequelae: sore throat, "cold," earache, sinus trouble, inflamed eye, chills, fever, cough, "flu." Allergy. Impaired vision or hearing.

[c]Chest pain, shortness of breath, "blood pressure." Heartburn, gas, abdominal pain, vomiting, diarrhea. Menstrual cramps, intermenstrual bleeding, discharge. Urinary burning or frequency.

[d]Pain, swelling, injury of head, neck, back, upper and lower limbs.

[e]"Acne," pimples, warts, allergy, minor wounds and lacerations.

[f]Anxiety, restlessness, depression, fatigue, "tired blood," loneliness, sexual problem.

*Note:* Data represent a three-year cumulative total of 1.733 billion office visits.

*Source:* National Center for Health Statistics (1979a).

Table 5.6. Ranks and Percentages of Office Visits for the Twenty-Five
Most Frequent Diagnoses Made by Physicians, United States, 1975.

| Rank | Principal Diagnosis | Percentage |
|------|---------------------|------------|
| 1 | Medical or special examination | 7.2 |
| 2 | Medical and surgical aftercare | 4.7 |
| 3 | Essential benign hypertension | 4.0 |
| 4 | Prenatal care | 3.7 |
| 5 | Acute respiratory infection, site unspecified | 2.6 |
| 6 | Neuroses | 2.4 |
| 7 | Chronic ischemic heart disease | 2.2 |
| 8 | Otitis media | 1.7 |
| 9 | Diabetes mellitus | 1.7 |
| 10 | Eczema and dermatitis | 1.7 |
| 11 | Acute pharyngitis | 1.5 |
| 12 | Refractive errors | 1.4 |
| 13 | Hay fever | 1.4 |
| 14 | Obesity | 1.3 |
| 15 | Bronchitis, unqualified | 1.2 |
| 16 | Observation, without need for further medical care | 1.2 |
| 17 | Acute tonsillitis | 1.1 |
| 18 | Sinusitis, bursitis | 1.1 |
| 19 | Influenza, unqualified | 1.0 |
| 20 | Cystitis | 1.0 |
| 21 | Diseases of sebaceous glands | 1.0 |
| 22 | Osteoarthritis | 1.0 |
| 23 | Arthritis, unspecified | 0.9 |
| 24 | Inoculations and vaccinations | 0.9 |
| 25 | Asthma | 0.8 |
| | Total | 48.7 |

Source: National Center for Health Statistics (1978a, Table 20).

tion; it represents a classification of health problems as seen from
the physician's point of view. Table 5.6 ranks twenty-five diagnoses
associated with all office visits to physicians in order of frequency.
These diagnoses, which reflect ICDA subcategories, accounted for
nearly half of the 576.6 million office visits in 1975. A similar listing
of specific diagnoses related to each practice specialty is available in
various publications of the National Center for Health Statistics.
Table 5.7 uses the same data base to show the number of visits and
percentage of total visits associated with fourteen of the eighteen
major ICDA categories and the most frequent subcodes, which

**Table 5.7. Number and Percentage Distribution of Office Visits by Selected Principal Diagnoses, United States, 1975.**

| Principal Diagnosis and ICDA Category | Visits (in Thousands) | Percentage of Total |
|---|---|---|
| Infective and parasitic diseases | 22,747 | 4.0 |
| Neoplasms | 13,332 | 2.3 |
| Endocrine, nutritional, and metabolic diseases<br>Diabetes mellitus (9,671)<br>Obesity (7,569) | 24,177 | 4.3 |
| Mental disorders<br>Neuroses (13,641) | 25,061 | 4.4 |
| Diseases of the nervous system and sense organs<br>Diseases and conditions of the eye (20,185)<br>Refractive errors (8,169)<br>Otitis media (9,899) | 44,941 | 7.9 |
| Diseases of the circulatory system<br>Essential benign hypertension (22,824)<br>Chronic ischemic heart disease (12,513) | 56,358 | 9.9 |
| Diseases of the respiratory system<br>Acute respiratory infections (except influenza) (37,599)<br>Influenza (6,123)<br>Hay fever (7,675) | 80,125 | 14.1 |
| Diseases of the digestive system | 20,061 | 3.5 |
| Diseases of the genitourinary system<br>Diseases of male genital organs (4,381)<br>Diseases of female genital organs (19,852) | 37,626 | 6.6 |
| Diseases of the skin and subcutaneous tissue | 28,564 | 5.0 |
| Diseases of the musculoskeletal system<br>Arthritis and rheumatism (17,765) | 32,732 | 5.8 |
| Symptoms and ill-defined conditions | 26,177 | 4.6 |
| Accidents, poisoning, and violence<br>Fracture (6,858)<br>Dislocation, sprain (14,374)<br>Lacerations (6,935) | 40,893 | 7.2 |
| Special conditions and examinations without sickness | 100,787 | 17.8 |

Table 5.7. Number and Percentage Distribution of Office Visits by
Selected Principal Diagnoses, United, 1975, Cont'd.

| | | |
|---|---|---|
| Medical and special examinations (40,863) | | |
| Prenatal care (20,851) | | |
| Medical and surgical aftercare (26,782) | | |
| Other diseases | 14,019 | 2.5 |
| Total | 567,600 | 100.0 |

Source: National Center for Health Statistics (1978a, Table 21).

account for almost all principal diagnoses made for patients seen in office practice in 1975. Diagnoses listed under "Special Conditions and Examinations Without Sickness" account for nearly one out of five diagnoses; "Diseases of the Respiratory System" for one out of seven; and "Diseases of the Circulatory System" for one out of ten. Similar data are available for a range of other categories—for example, by physician specialty, by age and sex of the patient, and by whether the problem is new or old.

The data on reasons for visits and associated symptoms and diagnoses for ambulatory patient care provide a nationwide overview of the frequency of health problems seen in this setting. Similar overviews of the most frequent health problems treated in *short-stay hospitals* are available in terms of discharge diagnoses.

The most accurate source of data on hospital discharges is again provided by the National Center for Health Statistics in its annual hospital discharge survey of a national sample of short-stay hospitals. In 1975, there were 34,043,000 discharges in the United States (National Center for Health Statistics, 1978b). These data are available for a range of patient characteristics (see Table 5.8 for the age/sex distribution of these patients) and by ICDA-based categories showing, for example, both first-listed and all other diagnoses, length of stay, hospital deaths, and hospital characteristics.

Table 5.9 shows the frequency among 27,535,000 short-stay hospital discharges (81 percent of the United States total) of health problems grouped according to the major body systems (including pregnancy and childbirth). These data illustrate well that four out of five short-stay hospital discharges in this country and most physician time spent on hospitalized patients involved only thirty

Table 5.8. Short-Stay Hospital Discharges by Age and Sex,
United States, 1975.

| Patient Age | Discharges (in Thousands) | Patient Sex | Discharges (in Thousands) |
|---|---|---|---|
| Under 15 years | 3,826 | | |
| 15–44 years | 14,171 | Female | 20,524 |
| 45–64 years | 8,391 | Male | 13,519 |
| 65 years and over | 7,654 | | |
| Total | 34,043[a] | Total | 34,043 |

[a]Items do not add to total because of rounding.
*Source:* National Center for Health Statistics (1978b).

diagnostic categories out of the 10,000 four-digit categories listed in the International Classification of Diseases, Adapted (ICDA). This finding certainly supports the old maxim of differential diagnosis, "Common problems are common."

It is important to recognize that the seven groupings in Table 5.9 represent a summary of the major categories of the ICDA. Standard ICDA etiological categories such as "Infective and Parasitic Diseases," "Neoplasms," and "Accidents, Poisoning, and Violence" were eliminated and related to body systems as much as possible. For example, "Diarrheal Diseases," traditionally listed with "Infective and Parasitic Diseases," were incorporated into "Diseases of the Digestive System." Table 5.10 provides the standard display by first-listed diagnoses according to ICDA categories.

In summary, these data on reasons for visits, associated symptoms and diagnoses, and hospital discharges illustrate how a measure of the overall frequency of a health problem can be obtained for office and short-stay hospital practice. Comparable data on the institutionalized population requiring long-term care, for example, are available from other NCHS publications series. Such data, in conjunction with the more specific estimates of health loss and economic costs derived from them, are one of the bases for determining the importance to society of particular conditions and the human effort and resources spent on their medical management.

Table 5.9. Short-Stay Hospital Discharges[a]
by Selected Common Diagnoses,[b] United States, 1975—
Special Tabulation by Body System.

|  |  | Discharges (in Thousands) |
| --- | --- | --- |
| Diseases of the digestive system |  | 5,036 |
| Inflammatory disease, lower gastrointestinal: enteritis, appendicitis, colitis | 900 |  |
| Hernias, inguinal and others | 842 |  |
| Inflammatory disease, upper gastrointestinal: peptic ulcer | 701 |  |
| Cholelithiasis | 468 |  |
| Inflammatory disease of liver, gall bladder, bile ducts, and pancreas | 420 |  |
| All other | 1,705 |  |
| Diseases of the circulatory system |  | 4,666 |
| Chronic ischemic heart diseases | 1,442 |  |
| Cerebrovascular disease | 608 |  |
| Acute myocardial infarction | 390 |  |
| Hypertensive heart disease | 301 |  |
| Congestive heart failure | 253 |  |
| All other | 1,672 |  |
| Diseases of the genitourinary system |  | 4,407 |
| Urinary tract infections | 682 |  |
| Menstrual disorders, intermenstrual bleeding | 582 |  |
| Malignant neoplasms (including breast) | 572 |  |
| Inflammation, infection of female organs | 488 |  |
| Uterine fibromyomas, prolapse | 486 |  |
| All other | 1,597 |  |
| Pregnancy and childbirth |  | 4,365 |
| Delivery without mention of complications | 2,345 |  |
| Delivery with complications | 790 |  |
| Abortion | 487 |  |

**Table 5.9. Short-Stay Hospital Discharges[a]
by Selected Common Diagnoses,[b] United States, 1975—
Special Tabulation by Body System, Cont'd.**

| | | |
|---|---|---|
| Congenital anomalies | 334 | |
| All other (including other complications of pregnancy) | 409 | |
| Diseases of the respiratory system | | 3,675 |
| Pneumonia, all forms | 715 | |
| Hypertrophy of tonsils and adenoids | 702 | |
| Chronic obstructive lung disease: bronchitis, asthma, and emphysema | 523 | |
| Upper respiratory infections and flu | 465 | |
| Acute bronchitis, bronchiolitis | 252 | |
| All other | 1,018 | |
| Problems of the musculoskeletal system | | 3,471 |
| Fractures | 1,156 | |
| Arthritis, synovitis, bursitis | 672 | |
| Sprains/strains and dislocations | 513 | |
| Vertebrogenic pain and displaced disc | 499 | |
| All other | 631 | |
| Diseases of the nervous system and sense organs | | 1,915 |
| Infections of eye, ear, and mastoid | 596 | |
| Intracranial injury and head wounds | 477 | |
| Cataract | 333 | |
| Diseases of central nervous system | 330 | |
| All other | 179 | |
| Total selected diagnoses | | 27,535 |
| All other diagnoses | | 6,508 |
| Total | | 34,043 |

[a]National Center for Health Statistics (1978b).

[b]Adapted from National Center for Health Statistics (1967), consolidating common health conditions into seven basic categories by systems.

Table 5.10. Short-Stay Hospital Discharges by ICDA Category of
First-Listed Diagnosis, United States, 1975.

| ICDA Category of First-Listed Diagnosis | Discharges (in Thousands) |
|---|---|
| Infective and parasitic diseases | 829 |
| Neoplasms | 2,353 |
| Endocrine, nutritional, and metabolic diseases | 887 |
| Diseases of the blood and blood-forming organs | 294 |
| Mental disorders | 1,494 |
| Diseases of the nervous system and sense organs | 1,438 |
| Diseases of the circulatory system | 4,418 |
| Diseases of the respiratory system | 3,393 |
| Diseases of the digestive system | 4,260 |
| Diseases of the genitourinary system | 3,480 |
| Complications of pregnancy, childbirth, and the puerperium | 4,031 |
| Diseases of the skin and subcutaneous tissue | 549 |
| Diseases of the musculoskeletal system and connective tissue | 1,704 |
| Congenital anomalies | 334 |
| Certain causes of perinatal morbidity and mortality | 20 |
| Symptoms and ill-defined conditions | 603 |
| Accidents, poisonings, and violence | 3,562 |
| Other diseases | 396 |
| Total | 34,043[a] |

[a]Items do not add to total because of rounding.
Source: National Center for Health Statistics (1978b, Table 1).

*National Health Loss Data.* Here we include types and sources
of data for two major health loss categories: mortality and disability. As yet, no nationally generalizable measures of symptom days
or years and time spent at higher than average risk are available.

Of all vital and health statistics, *mortality* data are the most
complete and accurate; certainly they have been collected longest.
Again, the National Center for Health Statistics provides the most

comprehensive data *(Vital Statistics of the United States II: Mortality)*. Detailed diagnostic-specific listings are shown for ICDA three-digit-code categories. In addition, general and infant mortality data are available in Vital and Health Statistics Series 3 *(Analytic Studies)*, reporting trend data; Series 20 *(Data on Mortality)*; and Series 22 *(Data from the National Natality and Mortality Surveys)*. In these data, the unit of observation is number of deaths in a given year.

A more useful computation for quality assurance is in terms of "years of life lost per death." Table 5.11 compares the absolute number of deaths, potential years of life lost per death (on the assumption that current life expectancy at death would have applied to all 1974 decedents in each age category underlying these estimates), and national total for years of life lost, by sixteen major ICDA categories. For example, although diseases of the circulatory system lead as causes of death and of total life years lost, they rank last in average life years lost per death. Neoplasms are the second most frequent cause of death but rank third for total life years lost and fifth in average life years lost per death; the latter category is headed by congenital anomalies.

Although NCHS data on *disability* are extensive, they still lack diagnostic-specific tabulations comparable to those for mortality data. Detailed disability data related to acute conditions (Vital Health Statistics Series 10, *Data from the Health Interview Survey*) summarize types of disability (days of restricted activity and of bed disability; days lost from school and from work for twelve disease categories) for rural and urban areas and U.S. census regions, for each month of the year, and for selected sociodemographic characteristics. Chronic condition data are classified by thirty diagnostic-specific conditions and various levels of activity limitations in addition to the standard sociodemographic variables. The total burden of acute and chronic disability is shown by selected diagnostic categories. More detail on diagnostic-specific disability is available on *Public Use Statistical Tapes*, as are specific compilations in Series 10 on time lost from work among the currently employed, types of injuries, and associated disability; reasons for hospitalization by annual number of hospital episodes and days; disability among persons in the labor force; and length of convalescence after surgery.

Table 5.11. Number of Deaths, Potential Years of Life Lost per Death,
and Years of Life Lost by Disease Category of the Underlying
Cause of Death, United States, 1974.

| ICDA Category | Deaths | Potential Years of Life Lost per Death[a] | Potential Years of Life Lost[a], National Total |
|---|---|---|---|
| Infective and parasitic diseases | 15,722 | 26.9 | 423,000 |
| Neoplasms | 365,532 | 16.1 | 5,875,000 |
| Endocrine, nutritional, and metabolic diseases | 45,688 | 15.1 | 692,000 |
| Diseases of the blood and blood-forming organs | 5,354 | 20.6 | 111,000 |
| Mental disorders | 9,603 | 24.9 | 239,000 |
| Diseases of the nervous system and sense organs | 17,356 | 27.7 | 482,000 |
| Diseases of the circulatory system | 1,028,575 | 11.7 | 12,006,000 |
| Diseases of the respiratory system | 109,303 | 15.3 | 1,677,000 |
| Diseases of the digestive system | 73,195 | 19.1 | 1,398,000 |
| Diseases of the genitourinary system | 26,068 | 13.4 | 351,000 |
| Pregnancy, childbirth, and the puerperium | 462 | 46.7 | 22,000 |
| Diseases of the skin and subcutaneous tissue | 2,097 | 14.7 | 31,000 |
| Diseases of the musculoskeletal system and connective tissue | 5,045 | 17.8 | 89,000 |
| Congenital anomalies | 13,526 | 62.9 | 849,000 |
| Accidents, poisonings, and violence | 156,931 | 35.8 | 5,623,000 |
| Other | 59,931 | 49.4 | 2,961,000 |
| Total | 1,934,388 | 17.0 | 32,829,000 |

[a]It is assumed that current life expectancy at death would have applied to all 1974 decedents in each age category underlying these estimates.

Source: Rice, Feldman, and White (1976, Tables 1 and 2).

Table 5.12 illustrates some of the health loss data needed to estimate the indirect cost of illness, again using the sixteen major ICDA diagnostic categories, as well as the distribution over these categories of chronic conditions limiting or causing loss of major life activity and bed days caused by health conditions. Table 5.13 shows a similar distribution for inpatient days in short-stay hospitals and nursing homes and other long-term care facilities. These data, taken from an astute summary of the current burden of illness in the United States by Rice, Feldman, and White (1976), illustrate well the significance of measuring the health loss caused by various diseases and conditions and determining their relative importance for the allocation of resources and for setting priorities for quality assurance and cost containment. In particular, and as mentioned previously in this chapter, it is important not only to establish absolute frequency data but to examine which health problems cause the largest losses in health, productivity, and functional ability, both for the individual and for society as a whole.

*National Data on Economic Costs of Health Problems.* Aggregated data on total national health expenditures (direct measures of diagnostic and treatment costs) are among the earliest statistics related to health for which the government assumed responsibility. Data published in the *Social Security Bulletin,* a monthly publication of the Social Security Administration, show both type of expenditure and source of funds. Such data dramatically illustrate the economic importance of the health industry to both the national economy and the population at large. For 1977, for instance, the total of $163 billion spent on health care (Gibson and Fisher, 1978) amounted to 8.8 percent of the gross national product. Nearly 90 percent of these expenditures went for personal health care; the remainder was spent for research, for construction of medical care facilities, and for those aspects of health services and supplies associated with administration and government health activities. In fiscal year 1979, expenditures for health care had reached nearly 10 percent of the gross national product. Data on the shares of these expenditures borne by the individual, third-party payers, and employers are now being collected in the National Medical Care Expenditure Survey (NMCES) being undertaken by the National Center for Health Statistics.

Table 5.12. Percentage Distribution of Work Loss Days, of Chronic
Conditions Causing Major Activity Limitation, and of Bed Days
by Disease Category, United States, 1974.

| ICDA Category | Work Loss Days[a] | Chronic Conditions Causing Limitation of Major Life Activity[b] | Condition Bed Days[c] |
|---|---|---|---|
| Infective and parasitic diseases | 4.6 | 0.7 | 5.2 |
| Neoplasms | 2.2 | 2.3 | 3.8 |
| Endocrine, nutritional, and metabolic diseases | 1.4 | 3.8 | 2.4 |
| Diseases of the blood and blood-forming organs | 0.4 | 0.8 | 0.8 |
| Mental disorders | 2.9 | 3.7 | 2.7 |
| Diseases of the nervous system and sense organs | 3.0 | 5.4 | 3.9 |
| Diseases of the circulatory system | 8.2 | 23.2 | 13.1 |
| Diseases of the respiratory system | 29.3 | 7.6 | 28.5 |
| Diseases of the digestive system | 8.1 | 5.4 | 6.5 |
| Diseases of the genitourinary system | 5.2 | 2.1 | 4.7 |
| Pregnancy, childbirth, and the puerperium | 0.6 | — | 1.3 |
| Diseases of the skin and subcutaneous tissue | 1.3 | 0.9 | 0.9 |
| Diseases of the musculoskeletal system and connective tissue | 5.4 | 14.7 | 6.8 |
| Congenital anomalies | 0.1 | 1.7 | 0.5 |
| Accidents, poisonings, and violence | 18.2 | 4.2 | 8.8 |
| Other | 9.0 | 23.4 | 10.0 |
| Total | 100.0 | 100.0 | 100.0 |

[a]As percentage of 461,489,000 total work loss days (including counts due to multiple conditions). Work loss days are counted only for those currently employed.
[b]As percentage of 33,694,000 conditions (including counts due to multiple conditions).
[c]As percentage of 1,783,034,000 bed days (including counts due to multiple conditions).

Source: Rice, Feldman, and White (1976, Tables 6 and 8).

In the past, national expenditure data have not been disease-specific, nor have they attempted to measure, on a regular basis, indirect as well as direct costs of illness. All these costs should be measured, however, if cost data are to be used in identifying areas of emphasis in quality assurance. As pointed out before, several studies have established a methodology for measuring indirect costs in terms of the loss in earning capacity associated with illness and premature death. These studies have also extended the measurement of direct costs by estimating the costs of services provided and resources expended for medical care by disease category.

Following on the pioneering efforts represented by the early studies of Rice (1966) and updated ten years later by Cooper and Rice (1976), the Public Services Laboratory of Georgetown University, under Mushkin's direction, completed a major study of the cost of illness by disease category. Estimates were derived for both direct health services costs and indirect costs of morbidity and mortality in eighteen major ICDA categories (Berk, Paringer, and Mushkin, 1978; Berk, 1977a, 1977b; Mushkin and others, 1978; Paringer and Berk, 1977). In Table 5.14 (derived from Mushkin's Georgetown data as summarized by Rice, Feldman, and White, 1976), the impact of these costs on what was described as total economic costs of illness in Figure 5.4 is evident; for fiscal year 1975, indirect costs related to morbidity and mortality accounted for 59 percent of the total economic cost, 35 percent of the total being associated with the costs of mortality and 24 percent being attributable to the loss of earnings associated with morbidity. The concepts underlying these calculations were described in an early classic study by Mushkin and d'A. Collings (1959), which raised the question of the impact of the economic costs of disease and injury on the use, distribution, and availability of economic resources.

### Local Data on Health Problem Importance

The preceding national statistics are based on sampling methods that permit generalizing the data on the entire U.S. population. Although these data are subdivided only by geographic region and urban/rural areas and cannot be applied directly at the

Table 5.13. Distribution of Inpatient Days by Disease Category of Diagnosis According to Type of Health Care Facility, United States, 1974.

| ICDA Category | Short-Stay Hospitals | | Nursing Homes | | Other Long-Term Care Facilities | |
|---|---|---|---|---|---|---|
| | Number (in Thousands) | Percentage | Number (in Thousands) | Percentage | Number (in Thousands) | Percentage |
| Infective and parasitic diseases | 5,301 | 2.1 | — | — | — | — |
| Neoplasms | 24,301 | 9.5 | 9,344 | 2.4 | 2,386 | 1.1 |
| Endocrine, nutritional, and metabolic diseases | 8,663 | 3.4 | 17,557 | 4.5 | — | — |
| Diseases of the blood and blood-forming organs | 2,207 | 0.9 | 2,774 | 0.7 | — | — |
| Mental disorders | 15,248 | 6.0 | 42,267 | 10.8 | 201,713 | 89.8 |
| Diseases of the nervous system and sense organs | 8,990 | 3.5 | 23,433 | 6.0 | 7,901 | 3.5 |
| Diseases of the circulatory system | 47,598 | 18.6 | 164,360 | 41.9 | — | — |
| Diseases of the respiratory system | 19,548 | 7.6 | 8,103 | 2.1 | — | — |
| Diseases of the digestive system | 32,084 | 12.5 | 7,482 | 1.9 | — | — |

| | | | | | | |
|---|---|---|---|---|---|---|
| Diseases of the genitourinary system | 21,272 | 8.3 | 5,694 | 1.5 | — | — |
| Pregnancy, childbirth, and the puerperium | 14,970 | 5.9 | — | — | 1,798 | 0.8 |
| Diseases of the skin and subcutaneous tissue | 3,848 | 1.5 | 2,190 | 0.6 | — | — |
| Diseases of the musculoskeletal system and connective tissue | 16,024 | 6.3 | 26,682 | 6.8 | 1,287 | 0.6 |
| Congenital anomalies | 2,212 | 0.9 | 1,132 | 0.3 | 1,287 | 0.6 |
| Accidents, poisonings, and violence | 28,865 | 11.3 | 17,994 | 4.6 | 1,287 | 0.6 |
| Other | 4,477 | 1.8 | 62,962 | 16.1 | 6,853 | 3.1 |
| Total | 255,688[a] | 100.0 | 391,974 | 100.0 | 224,512 | 100.0 |

[a]Items do not add to total because of rounding.

Source: Rice, Feldman, and White (1976, Table 4).

**Table 5.14. Percentage Distribution of Direct, Indirect, and Total Economic Costs of Illness by Disease Category of Diagnosis, United States, 1975.**

| | Direct Costs[a] | Indirect Costs | | Total Costs | |
|---|---|---|---|---|---|
| ICDA Category | (Percentage) | Morbidity (Percentage) | Mortality[b] (Percentage) | Percentage | Amount (in Millions) |
| Infective and parasitic diseases | 2.0 | 2.7 | 1.2 | 1.9 | $4,648 |
| Neoplasms | 5.3 | 1.9 | 18.2 | 9.1 | 22,358 |
| Endocrine, nutritional, and metabolic diseases | 3.4 | 2.9 | 1.9 | 2.7 | 6,731 |
| Diseases of the blood and blood-forming organs | 0.7 | 0.5 | 0.3 | 0.5 | 1,255 |
| Mental disorders | 9.5 | 15.1 | 1.2 | 7.8 | 19,187 |
| Diseases of the nervous system and sense organs | 7.5 | 9.9 | 1.6 | 5.9 | 14,566 |
| Diseases of the circulatory system | 16.1 | 15.1 | 29.2 | 20.6 | 50,408 |
| Diseases of the respiratory system | 7.6 | 14.8 | 4.1 | 8.1 | 19,752 |
| Diseases of the digestive system | 14.7 | 5.9 | 5.5 | 9.3 | 22,803 |
| Diseases of the genitourinary system | 5.6 | 3.1 | 1.0 | 3.3 | 8,205 |
| Pregnancy, childbirth, and the puerperium | 3.4 | 0.3 | 0.1 | 1.5 | 3,660 |
| Diseases of the skin and subcutaneous tissue | 2.1 | 0.7 | 0.1 | 1.1 | 2,594 |
| Diseases of the musculoskeletal system and connective tissue | 5.2 | 12.7 | 0.3 | 5.2 | 12,717 |
| Congenital anomalies | 0.4 | 0.8 | 1.8 | 1.0 | 2,500 |
| Accidents, poisonings, and violence | 6.9 | 9.8 | 26.9 | 14.8 | 36,196 |
| Other | 9.6 | 3.8 | 6.6 | 7.2 | 17,565 |
| Total dollars (in millions) | 99,374 | 57,846 | 87,926 | | 245,145 |
| Total percentage | 100.0 | 100.0 | 100.0 | 100.0 | |

[a] Personal health care expenditures allocated to diagnoses.
[b] Based on a 4 percent discount rate.

*Source:* Rice, Feldman, and White (1976, Tables 11 and 12).

local level, they can be used as a starting point for developing local data for quality assurance purposes.

*Local Frequency Data.* The error tolerance in most quality assurance priority decisions is such that raw national data can generally be used to obtain relative frequency rates. Most ambulatory care and hospital discharge data provide breakdowns according to age and sex and allow local application at any point on the spectrum. For example, if priorities for quality assurance topics for pediatric practice are being developed, it is possible to refer to national data tables for the relevant age groups.

One alternative is to modify national data according to known epidemiological trends. If a certain area usually has an exceptionally high prevalence of rheumatic fever, national statistics might be applied with necessary modifications for streptococcal and rheumatoid heart disease. In addition, for studies involving hospital discharge statistics, a great deal of local data is already available. Most hospitals have their own tabulations on discharges, particularly if they use computerized services such as the Professional Activities Study of the CPHA. For private office practice and clinics, however, there are no comparable local compilations at this time.

Another approach to determining health problem frequency at the local level is to rely on the judgment of those participating in quality assurance priority setting. Experience has shown that the aggregate group judgment of local providers can be fairly accurate, albeit intuitive, and generally indicates quite well which health problems are of such low frequency in a particular setting as to exclude them from study. If there is doubt, it is a relatively simple matter to conduct a brief prevalence check of several hundred consecutive clinic visits, for example, to determine the frequency of a given health problem among patients' reasons for visit or diagnoses. This procedure can be used even in hospitals where discharge statistics are not available. Sampling of complications such as congestive failure in hypertensive patients may well require such a procedure.

Informal consultation with a local subspecialist is another practical way of checking local prevalence rates. If a certain type of valvular heart disease is rarely seen by local cardiologists, the local prevalence may indeed be low. Here the use of specialists is required, however, because primary practitioners may miss certain health problems despite high prevalence. In this instance, a quality assurance study to measure diagnostic false negatives might well be considered.

*Local Health Loss Data.* National data are readily available regarding the prevalence of symptoms, loss of work days, institution days, restriction of activities of daily living (eating, bathing, dressing), and bed days by age and sex. Tabulations by diagnostic-specific categories are, in general, available only on public-use tapes from the National Center for Health Statistics.

The exception to this usual paucity of detailed diagnostic breakdowns is mortality data, which are available not only nationally but by three-digit ICDA codes for states and counties. If a quality assurance team is concerned with determinations of relative mortality, accurate data are available in vital statistics publications at these levels. Here it should be noted that errors may exist in coding, as well as in coding conventions regarding the major cause of death, when data are drawn from death certificates that contain multiple diagnoses.

*Local Economic Costs Data.* Aggregate data on national health care resource expenditures are now available monthly through the *Social Security Bulletin;* population survey data will be provided by NMCES. Periodic tabulations of expenditures for a given year are available through reports or special studies (Berk, Paringer, and Mushkin, 1978; Berk, 1977a, 1977b; Mushkin and others, 1978; Paringer and Berk, 1977).

Such aggregated data, however, are of limited usefulness to those involved in local/regional quality assurance and cost containment studies. Until recently, no local or regional interinstitutional data on health care expenditures were available that were disease- or health-problem-specific. The only diagnostic-specific data available for comparisons among institutions were utilization data on hospital stays collected for PSRO utilization review and by the Commission on Professional and Hospital Activities (CPHA).

Recent trends promoted by state hospital rate-setting review boards, and more recently by the Health Care Financing Administrations (HCFA), reflect efforts to develop equitable reimbursement policies for hospitals participating in Medicare/Medicaid programs by means of case mix and related indicators. The purpose of these approaches has been to consider reimbursement in the light of the complexity or severity of cases (case mix) rather than the average days of hospitalization, as discussed in detail in Chapter Four. The best known of these, the Diagnosis-Related Groups (DRGs) approach, for example, can yield an overview of services provided by the hospital to patients grouped according to primary diagnosis, secondary diagnosis, primary surgical procedure, secondary surgical procedure, age, and clinical service area.

## Conclusions

To ensure the relevance of quality assurance efforts in a given setting, an awareness of the importance to society of topics selected for study is essential. Determining which health problems are of sufficient importance for study requires knowledge of their frequency, the amount of health loss involved, and their economic costs. I have discussed various methods of and approaches to establishing health problem importance in these terms, with particular emphasis on aspects of direct and indirect economic costs. Sources of national and local data have been suggested that will be useful to quality assurance personnel in deciding which problems warrant study. Once the importance of the problem has thus been established, the next considerations are (1) the efficacy, effectiveness, and efficiency of care interventions related to the problem and (2) the potential for improving current levels of performance. These latter factors are discussed in Chapters Six through Eight.

## Suggested Projects

1. The following are the ten most frequently studied audit topics in U.S. short-stay hospitals for fulfilling PSRO quality assurance requirements:

| | |
|---|---|
| myocardial infarction | pneumonia |
| appendectomy | cholecystectomy |
| hysterectomy | diabetes mellitus |
| hip fracture | Caesarean section |
| tonsillectomy and adenoidectomy | gastroenteritis |

a.  Have students estimate the probable disability for a patient with one of these problems if no professional medical care were given. Estimate the health loss of this illness in terms of morbidity and mortality. Assign patient characteristics (age, sex, occupation) to arrive at indirect economic costs.

b.  Have students estimate the degree of disability that could be prevented by the best care currently available and project in terms of added years and added years of productive life the indirect costs saved by providing treatment. Assign patient characteristics (age, sex, occupation) to arrive at indirect cost savings.

2.  Have students estimate the direct costs of treating one of the ten problems with no complications. Provide a list of procedures and services associated with care of this problem.

# Documenting Efficacy of Health Care Technology

*Daniel M. Barr*
*John W. Williamson*

꙼꙼꙼꙼꙼꙼꙼꙼꙼꙼꙼꙼꙼꙼꙼꙼꙼꙼꙼꙼꙼꙼

In addition to understanding how health problems and their importance can be used as a framework for establishing quality assurance priorities, one needs points of reference for assessing the quality of care. Knowing the extent of the benefit that can realistically be expected from given health care interventions depends on knowing their efficacy—that is, what benefit can be expected under ideal conditions of use. Efficacy, then, is a precondition for determining effectiveness of clinical performance. Further, since most interventions involve some risk of harm, one should be familiar with the safety of various medical procedures before attempting to assess the quality of care.

Health services researchers currently distinguish between the efficacy of interventions and the effectiveness and efficiency with which they are used. Historically, such distinctions were not consistently made. What Codman (1916) called efficiency in his classic studies is now generally termed effectiveness; Cochrane (1972) used *efficacy* and *effectiveness* interchangeably. To avoid ambiguities, the following definitions are used in this text:

- *Efficacy* is the ability of an intervention or procedure to produce the intended benefit to a defined population under ideal conditions of use.
- *Effectiveness* is the extent of benefit that is being achieved under usual conditions of care.
- *Efficiency* is the extent to which that benefit is achieved with a minimum of unnecessary expenditure of resources.

Determining the efficacy of health care requires clinical research. Such studies are designed to estimate the true potential of interventions for achieving the desired outcomes of care and to establish evidence of a causal relationship between care and its outcomes. Determining health care effectiveness requires quality assurance and evaluation studies. Such studies presume the existence of a causal relationship between the intervention and the outcome; their purpose is to estimate the extent of benefit achieved and to determine to what degree provider, patient, and institutional variables affect the outcome. Determining efficiency requires studies conducted within the framework of health care assessment to examine the costs or resources expended to achieve a given benefit.

In the foregoing definitions, four terms require elaboration: *interventions, conditions of use, outcome,* and *benefit.*

1. *Health care interventions* are preventive, screening, diagnostic, therapeutic, or other management procedures used to cure or ameliorate a particular health problem or to respond to a health care need. Some interventions (for example, serum cholesterol determinations used for screening those at risk for coronary atherosclerosis) are single, discrete procedures; others (for example, coronary artery surgery, a therapeutic intervention for patients with partly occluded arteries) involve multiple, complex procedures. Complex interventions or those that combine two or more

interventions, as in coronary care units for acute myocardial infarction patients, are often termed *management interventions*.

2. *Conditions of use* refers to the situation in which the intervention is used. Whereas definitions of *interventions* and *benefit* apply equally to both efficacy and effectiveness of care, the meaning of *conditions of use* differs. For example, in efficacy studies, *conditions of use* refers to ideal clinical situations in which the variables that affect the delivery of care are carefully controlled: Physicians are highly skilled, knowledgeable, and experienced in the intervention tested; medication is carefully administered, and a range of controls is used to determine its effect; and the relevant characteristics of patients receiving care are known. When applied to effectiveness, *conditions of use* refers to care given in average, nonexperimental practice settings where these and other variables affecting health care delivery cannot be carefully controlled.

3. *Health care outcomes* are those characteristics of patients, health problems, providers, or the care process that result from care interventions as measured at one point in time. They may be uncertain (tentative outcomes) or conclusive (final outcomes). This definition goes beyond the unduly restrictive, traditional meaning of *outcome*—namely, patient health outcomes. Although it includes such outcomes as increased longevity (a patient health outcome), it implies that care outcomes may also be economic (for example, increased or decreased societal expenditures for health care) or legal (for example, malpractice suits). Outcomes can be measured at different points in time; immediate outcomes are those measured minutes or days after the intervention; intermediate outcomes, weeks or months later; and long-term outcomes, years later. Studies to measure outcomes must specify what outcome of what process is measured at what point in time.

4. *Health care benefits* are the desired outcomes of care. Although it is possible to identify many benefits of health care, the three highlighted in this text are improved health and both tangible and intangible societal and economic benefits. Health care benefits can be measured or assessed by means of evaluation studies that incorporate an objective element (measurement of a desired outcome), a causal assumption (attribution of the measured outcome to the care provided), and a subjective element (attach-

ment of positive or negative value to the measured outcome). In determining whether benefit has been achieved, one must take into account the value attached to the outcome by the population affected. For example, although birth control measures may produce the desired outcome of controlling population size, this outcome will not be considered a benefit among a population that places a positive value on fecundity, particularly a preindustrial society that values having many children so that enough may survive into adulthood to ensure the continuance of families.

This chapter addresses the issue of finding and interpreting scientific evidence of efficacy. It also distinguishes among the types of evidence needed to demonstrate efficacy for different types of care (that is, diagnostic, therapeutic, and preventive) and provides sources to be used in obtaining such evidence for the purpose of quality assurance and care evaluation.

### Efficacy and Its Implications for Quality Assurance

The extent to which an intervention achieves the desired outcome under ideal conditions of use determines its efficacy. In an ideal world, there would be no doubt about the efficacy of interventions being used to provide care. However, many, if not most, interventions have never been studied in a systematic way to determine and document their efficacy, and numerous procedures are being used which do not work as claimed or whose efficacy is uncertain. The current concern to document efficacy is of relatively recent origin. There is as yet no overall system for assessing the efficacy of new or old procedures; nor, with the possible exception of drugs and medical devices, is there a systematic process for identifying which interventions should be studied. In fact, the informality of the process by which interventions are selected for efficacy study has fostered interest in new therapeutic procedures, while studies of existing procedures and of care related to prevention, diagnosis, rehabilitation, and management have been neglected. This situation is further complicated by the lack of a synthesis of study results. Even when studies have been conducted, there is no generally accepted interpretive mechanism for weighing them and providing an integrated judgment; hence the authority of the interpreting individual or group usually prevails. Given these difficulties, it is not surprising that physicians, faced with the need to help a patient, do what they think is best on the basis of their perception of the efficacy of a particular intervention and their experience.

The quality assurance team, however, must conduct a search for documented evidence of efficacy. The team does not *establish* efficacy of the intervention; that is, it does not create controlled conditions of use, apply the intervention to a particular health problem, and measure the benefit achieved. Rather, its task is to find prior evidence that the intervention is efficacious and to use this evidence as a basis for designing a study of health care effectiveness in the local setting.

The information gained in this search for documentation of efficacy serves several purposes. First, identifying the degree of benefit that can be expected from an intervention under ideal conditions of use provides a standard against which to measure the effectiveness of the intervention under normal conditions. Second, verifying that a particular intervention is efficacious for the health problem under study eliminates the possibility that unsatisfactory outcomes of care are due to the use of an inappropriate intervention; conversely, evidence that a particular intervention is of doubtful efficacy may indicate that the intervention itself should be examined as a possible source of the problem. Finally, because properly documented evidence of efficacy includes information on the patient population for which the intervention has been tested, it enables quality assurance personnel to assess whether the intervention is being used on appropriate subjects.

All this implies that the quality assurance team must be familiar with studies that document efficacy and must be able to interpret these studies in terms of their scope and their reliability and validity.

*Understanding the Scope of Efficacy Studies.* In reading reports of an efficacy study for a particular intervention, one must carefully note four components: the type of health problem to which the intervention is applied, the conditions of use, the characteristics of the study population, and the benefits achieved by the intervention.

The *health problem* is the disease or condition for which the intervention is being tested. It may be a disease, symptom, syndrome, or other health care need. One intervention may be used for a variety of problems. For example, hysterectomies are surgical interventions used for treatment of premalignant states and localized cancers, descent or prolapse of the uterus, or obstetric catastrophes and as prophylactic measures to prevent later cancer or pregnancy (Office of Technology Assessment, 1978). An efficacy report on hysterectomies, therefore, should specify which of these diseases/conditions was the subject of study. Even if hysterectomies were shown to be efficacious for one of these problems (for example, localized cancers), one cannot assume they are necessarily efficacious for the other conditions. Moreover, if a particular intervention is shown to be efficacious at one stage of an illness, one cannot conclude that it would be efficacious at a different stage. For example, a total hysterectomy might be lifesaving for a Stage I cervical carcinoma but only palliative for Stage IV of the same problem. Therefore, in reading an efficacy study report, one must note the health problem and/or the stage of the problem for which the intervention was applied.

*Conditions of use* must be noted to ensure that the providers, the use of the intervention, and the population to which it was delivered were carefully selected and controlled. To determine that the outcome is directly related to the intervention, the conditions of use must be standardized and replicable. Otherwise the outcomes may be associated with differences in the variables of care. Controlling the conditions of use not only helps establish a direct causal relationship between the intervention and the outcome but also provides a standard against which to evaluate the use of the intervention in an average setting (that is, its effectiveness).

The *study population* describes specific characteristics of patients on whom the effect of the intervention is being reported. The effect of an intervention varies, for instance, with such characteristics as patient age, sex, and disease stage. Even if an intervention has been determined to be efficacious for patients of a certain age, sex, and disease stage, it cannot automatically be assumed that the intervention will be efficacious when applied to a patient population that has different characteristics. For example, in the Veterans Administration study of antihypertensive agents, the study population was originally composed of men under sixty-five years of age with diastolic blood pressure above 105 mm Hg (Veterans Administration, 1970). The study did not include females, and its initial report did not evaluate patients with diastolic blood pressure in the 90–105 range. Although it may seem logical to assume that the agents studied will work for both sexes, this assumption cannot be made on the basis of this study. Furthermore, without additional study, it would not be reasonable to assume that antihypertensive agents reduce risk sufficiently to make their use worthwhile in patients with diastolic blood pressures in the 90–105 range. Noting the scope of a study, then, requires identifying the characteristics of the patient population for whom the intervention was used.

The *benefit* of an intervention lies in the achievement of the desired outcome. A positive effect on levels of mortality or morbidity is one possible benefit but not the only one. Palliation and improved psychosocial functioning are also beneficial outcomes. Moreover, benefits may not directly relate to the health status of the recipients of care. Although reports of efficacy of therapeutic interventions show a direct relationship between the therapy and improved health of the patient, reports on diagnostic interventions may refer to an entirely different type of benefit. For example, the benefits of an efficacious diagnostic intervention may be defined in technical terms (its reliable performance and the accuracy of diagnostic information) independent of its intended therapeutic benefit (affecting the planning and delivery of therapy and contributing to improved patient care). It is important to note exactly which benefit obtained by the intervention is being reported.

*Understanding the Study Design in an Efficacy Research Report.* Once the foregoing components of the study report have been noted, it is necessary to observe whether the study design was a valid test of the relationship between the intervention and the outcome. Certain frequently used study designs are more appropriate to one kind of intervention than another.

1. *Diagnostic interventions and validation designs.* Diagnostic interventions are used to confirm the presence or absence of disease. Although such clinical activities as history taking and physical

examinations are considered diagnostic interventions, the term is most commonly associated with diagnostic tests whose technical accuracy is determined by a validation design. This type of study compares the results of a particular diagnostic test with those obtained from an existing procedure accepted as a clearly more valid indicator of disease—for example, coronary angiography compared with autopsy. A perfect test administered to fifty diseased and fifty well persons will produce fifty true positives (with the disease), fifty true negatives (without the disease), and no false positives or false negatives. There are no perfect tests, however. Tests vary in their sensitivity, or in how well they pick up the disease; in their specificity, or in how much they avoid negative diagnoses; in predictive value, or in how often positive test results truly indicate that the patient has the disease; and in efficiency, or in how often positive or negative results are truly positive or negative. Often the predictive value of a test is considered the measure of its accuracy, particularly in clinical practice. However, all four characteristics must be evaluated to determine the efficacy of a diagnostic test. Figure 6.1 illustrates the way diagnostic efficacy is measured.

2. *Therapeutic interventions and clinical trials.* The efficacy of therapeutic interventions is usually determined by their benefit to the patient. A perfect treatment will benefit all those who require and receive it. However, to determine whether the outcome of treatment is the effect of the intervention and not of some other cause, controlled clinical trials (Figure 6.2) are used. In these trials the benefit of the intervention under study is compared with that of a placebo or an alternative treatment in terms of alleviation of symptoms, control of disease progression, increased length of survival, decreased morbidity, or cure. The types of trial used to assess therapeutic efficacy as well as safety differ according to the intervention and include the following:

- *Trial:* The simultaneous comparison of two or more treatments, one of which may be a placebo, to determine the relative benefit of the treatments.
- *Sequential trial:* A trial whose conduct at any stage depends on the results so far obtained; usually the results influence only the number of observations made.

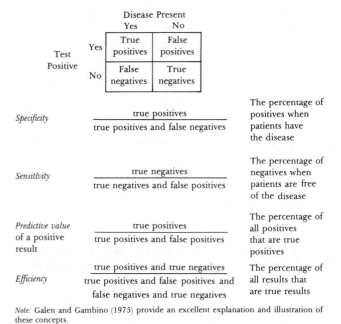

The percentage of

*Specificity*     $\dfrac{\text{true positives}}{\text{true positives and false negatives}}$     positives when patients have the disease

*Sensitivity*     $\dfrac{\text{true negatives}}{\text{true negatives and false positives}}$     The percentage of negatives when patients are free of the disease

*Predictive value* of a positive result     $\dfrac{\text{true positives}}{\text{true positives and false positives}}$     The percentage of all positives that are true positives

*Efficiency*     $\dfrac{\text{true positives and true negatives}}{\text{true positives and false positives and} \atop \text{false negatives and true negatives}}$     The percentage of all results that are true results

*Note:* Galen and Gambino (1975) provide an excellent explanation and illustration of these concepts.

**Figure 6.1. Validation Design Used to Determine the Diagnostic Value of a Test, and Associated Measures.**

- *Controlled trial:* An experimental method in which subjects are assigned, according to predetermined rules, either to an experimental group, which receives the intervention, or to a control group, which receives a standard treatment or placebo.
- *Randomized, controlled trial:* Subjects in a controlled trial are randomly assigned to experimental and control groups.
- *Double-blind, randomized, controlled trial:* A randomized, controlled trial in which both subjects and clinical evaluators are unaware of the specific treatment identities—that is, who receives and who does not receive treatment.

In judging *efficacy,* the definition of therapeutic benefit and the type of trial depend on the objective of the intervention. For example, use of decongestant antihistamine combination drugs is intended to provide palliation of rhinitis; lung resection for carcinoma is intended to cure this condition. Thus, it would be appro-

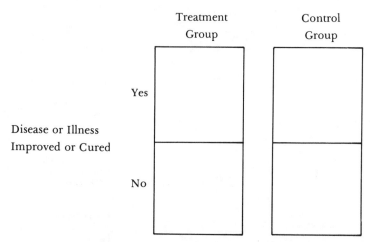

**Figure 6.2. Controlled Clinical Trial Design Used to Determine the Therapeutic Value of a Preventive, Curative, Rehabilitative, or Management Procedure.**

priate to assess the therapeutic efficacy of a drug used to relieve rhinitis by a double-blind, randomized clinical trial, whereas the efficacy of a surgical intervention is more often assessed by means of a randomized controlled trial. The benefit of surgery in this case may be compared with outcomes when no treatment or, more likely, another treatment, such as radiation therapy, was provided.

   In addition to noting how the efficacy of the therapy was assessed, one must also take note of reported evidence of its *safety*. Safety is determined in relation to the degree of risk associated with the intervention. Risks include adverse reactions, side effects, expected reactions, and idiosyncratic reactions. Because many interventions carry risks, it is important to decide what level of risk is acceptable. This is often determined by the severity of the medical problem, the characteristics of the population, or the conditions of use. For example, certain cancer chemotherapies, though efficacious as treatment, may produce bone marrow suppression. Given the severity of the disease, this may be considered an acceptable risk, virtually a side effect or an expected reaction; hence the intervention would be considered safe. However, if bone marrow suppression resulted from an anti-inflammatory drug used in treating acute tendonitis, a disease of much less severity, the intervention would be considered unsafe, as it produced an adverse reaction more severe than the condition being treated. Similarly, phenylbutazone, a nonsteroidal drug used for acute inflammatory conditions such as tendonitis, would be unsafe for patient populations with recent ulcer or congestive heart failure histories, because this drug reactivates peptic ulcers and increases intravascular volume.

Although evidence of safety is important, such information may not be available in published reports. It is often difficult to complete studies of adverse reactions before introducing a new therapy, because large population sizes and long induction times are required. To avoid this difficulty, multicenter studies are often used to increase the size of the study population, or a sequential trial design is employed to obtain a sufficient number from which to infer statistical significance, thus avoiding some ethical problems and reducing trial costs. Some adverse reactions, however, such as thromboembolism resulting from birth control pills, or cancer of the uterus resulting from conjugated estrogens used for menopausal symptoms, cannot be determined without studying large populations over a long period; hence, the safety of these interventions cannot be easily or quickly evaluated.

3. *Preventive interventions and case-control designs.* Preventive interventions are used to reduce risk attributable to a habit, life activity, environmental influence, or health care intervention. A study to estimate the efficacy of preventive interventions must document the relationship between such characteristics and the risk. The extent of risk associated with various behaviors has been studied extensively by epidemiologists and others. The study designs used to establish risk vary but generally are similar to the case-control design (Figure 6.3). The case-control design is used to determine the relative risk of illness, disease, or death in persons with a characteristic hypothesized to be detrimental to health, compared with those with a lower level of the characteristic or those without it. The case-control design may be used in prospective studies, which follow subjects forward over time while they are exposed to various levels of the health-impairing characteristic, or it may be used in retrospective studies, which examine the effect of past exposure on present health status. Retrospective studies using the case-control design have provided estimates of the risk of car-

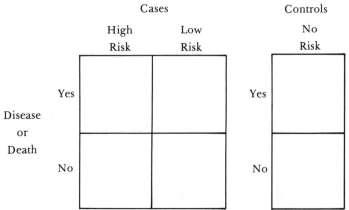

**Figure 6.3. Case-Control Design Used to Document Relative Risk Before Disease Onset.**

cinoma of the uterus associated with use of conjugated estrogens for menopausal symptoms, of death and disease associated with cigarette smoking, and of general thrombosis associated with use of oral contraceptives.

Once it has been established that risk is attributable to certain behaviors, environmental influences, habits, or health care interventions, it is necessary to note evidence of the efficacy of the preventive interventions intended to reduce risk. The ability of an intervention to reduce risk is the major measure of efficacy for preventive medicine. Study designs used to determine the efficacy of preventive measures are similar to clinical trials used for evaluating the efficacy of therapeutic interventions. Because it is difficult to assess the effect of risk reduction on health outcomes, however, reduction in the purportedly noxious characteristic is sometimes used as a measure of the efficacy of the preventive intervention. The following terms are associated with studies of preventive interventions:

- *Relative risk:* Rate of disease in a group exposed to the risk divided by the rate of disease in a nonexposed group.
- *Attributable risk:* Rate of disease in an exposed group that can be attributed to the exposure. Assuming the courses of diseases other than the one under examination had equal effect on the exposed and nonexposed groups, the rate of disease among

nonexposed persons is subtracted from the rate among those exposed.

- *Cohort studies:* The group or groups of persons to be studied are defined in terms of characteristics appearing before the detection of the disease under study and observed over a period of time to determine the frequency of the disease among them.
- *Cross-sectional studies:* Characteristics being compared are present in the cases and controls at the time of the study.
- *Retrospective studies:* Characteristics being compared are sought by data collection regarding past events (using medical records, patient and/or physician interviews, and the like).
- *Prospective studies:* Characteristics being compared are planned for future data collection (using direct observation or other, indirect methods).

Lilienfeld (1976) and MacMahon and Pugh (1970) are useful references for further understanding of these concepts.

In summary, in conducting a search for documented research evidence on efficacy, the quality assurance team needs to be familiar with the processes described above to assess the credibility of the studies it reviews. The design of the study, the precise nature of the results, and the authority of the authors must all be taken into consideration when the team is evaluating the studies. Gifford and Feinstein (1969) have provided an excellent illustration of how to review such studies critically.

### Data on Efficacy

To those who regularly search for efficacy studies, it seems that the frequency of such studies is inversely related to the frequency and importance of the problem to which the intervention is a response. Generally there will be fewer controlled studies of interventions for important, common problems than for relatively unimportant but rare conditions. This observation is less true for drugs, devices, and laboratory tests than for history and physical examinations, operations, and special diagnostic and therapeutic procedures.

Evidence on the frequency of use of various study designs in clinical research is available. During the period 1946–1976, "Cross-sectional studies increased from 25 to 44 percent [of 612 randomly selected articles from three general medical journals], cohort studies declined from 59 to 34 percent, and clinical trials increased from 13 to 21 percent of articles. . . . Randomized controlled trials comprised 5 percent of articles published in 1976 and were not represented thirty years before" (Fletcher and Fletcher, 1979).

Some feel that government regulation of drugs has caused lags in availability of efficacious agents. Others argue that the lag in introduction of new drugs is due to lack of basic science support and associated slowing of research in fields ripe for discoveries of practical value, such as immunology. Awareness of the lack of efficacy data or judgments for commonly used drugs led to a review of many agents in the 1960s by an authoritative group in cooperation with the Food and Drug Administration. A parallel review process is clearly needed for many current common interventions. Efforts in this direction, combined with quality assurance studies, are being conducted for laboratory tests, and third-party payers are insisting on similar reviews for high-cost special procedures. Interest in efficacy among surgeons is certainly high (Bunker, Barnes, and Mosteller, 1977), but there is a debate about the role, ethics, and value of controlled surgical trials.

The most deficient single area for efficacy studies is interventions used in a primary care environment. There are at least three reasons. Until the 1960s, primary care had low priority within academic institutions. Although its importance is now recognized, how it will fare in view of the current and continuing resource scarcity is uncertain. Once, the situation was that there were no academics to conduct studies in this environment. Now there are people but insufficient resources to conduct the needed studies. Primary care differs from the usually more specialized circumstances of specialists. Disease prevalence is thought to be less in primary care populations. When prevalence is low, the specificity of diagnostic tests is lessened. Consequently, a diagnostic procedure that is efficacious for a specialist's circumstance may lack efficacy in a general primary care situation. Add to this the considerable load of psychosocial problems and of undifferentiated complaints (which perhaps are diagnosed only half the time in the sense of a disease classification), and one can appreciate the need for diagnostic, therapeutic, and management efficacy studies in relation to this practice environment. Finally, the efficacy of periodic health assessment for well persons as part of primary care is also not well documented (Breslow and Somers, 1977).

Perhaps one day there will be a handbook that will provide all necessary data on the efficacy of health care interventions used in community practice. The National Center for Health Care Technology (NCHCT) could have performed the function of collecting such data for health care practitioners, rating them in terms of scientific validity, and then indexing this information for ready access by researchers, practitioners, and consumers, analogous to epidemiological tables produced by NCHS. However, as NCHCT is no longer funded and no other national source of efficacy data exists, quality assurance personnel must obtain information on efficacy from two sources: research literature and consensual expert groups.

*Research Literature.* Research literature is the most desirable source of information in terms of scientific validity; however, because clinical research required to establish efficacy is inadequately funded, not enough studies are conducted to meet the need for efficacy data. An overview of the major funding sources for such studies indicates that less than 5 percent of federal biomedical research funds was expended for such purposes as clinical trials in 1975–1976 (National Center for Health Statistics, 1978c). Furthermore, unless replicated controlled clinical trials or diagnostic validation studies are identified, the data in most published research reports are difficult to interpret for quality assurance teams who lack research or statistical expertise. In addition, even if reported data are indeed valid, they may not be generalizable to the local population. Hence, research literature should be read and interpreted according to the points of reference outlines in the first section of this chapter. Appendix B of this text provides a detailed example of the documentation yielded by a comprehensive literature search on the efficacy of selected common interventions for one major health problem, coronary artery disease.

*Consensual Group Judgment.* When a literature search produces insufficient or conflicting documentation of efficacy, a useful resource for quality assurance purposes is consensual group judgment. Health science information developed by such methods both by the federal government and by the private sector is now widely considered our most valid and credible source of efficacy data.

1. *Expert consensus groups funded by the federal government.* The task of assessing a field of literature, screening it for content relevance and scientific validity, and synthesizing from it generalizable findings for community application can be accomplished by expert consensus. In the federal government, such consensual group data are being provided by the Food and Drug Administration, the National Institutes of Health, the National Center for Health Services Research, and the Health Standards and Quality Bureau. The following describes the type of data available from these sources and the approaches used to generate them.

The classic model for illustrating expert consensus as a source of efficacy data is the Drug Efficacy Study Implementation Project (DESI) of the Bureau of Drugs of the Food and Drug Administration (FDA). In 1928 the FDA was authorized to review the safety of new drugs to be marketed. In 1962 Congress required review of efficacy as well as safety and asked the National Research Council of the National Academy of Sciences (NAS/NRC) to assist the FDA in review of over 3,500 prescription drug formulations first marketed between 1928 and 1962. The results of efficacy reviews of manufactured drugs marketed after 1962 were thus supplemented by this retrospective evaluation of older products.

In essence, the FDA, with the NAS/NRC, appoints a team of national experts on methods of pharmaceutical, biochemical, and clinical research and biostatistics. For any group of drugs studied, the scientific literature, including relevant unpublished material, is reviewed and the resulting information compiled for team review. Team members may be assigned to report on aspects within their expertise. The entire team meets periodically to arrive at consensus regarding the efficacy of each drug, for a specified use, rated on a scale from (1) ineffective, (2) possibly effective, (3) probably effective, to (4) effective. Theoretically, drugs without adequate evidence of efficacy are to be removed from the market. Actually, such action is usually delayed pending appeals or final administrative proceedings. Consequently, it is the practitioner's responsibility to be aware of the FDA efficacy team classification of products. This information is available in the *FDA Interim Index to Evaluations Published in the Federal Register for NAS/NRC Reviewed Prescription Drugs.*

The *National Institutes of Health* have organized technical consensus development to provide an additional source of efficacy information. Teams of national experts on a given medical technology are asked to agree on five issues: the clinical significance of new research findings; the adequacy of efforts to validate efficacy and safety; the need to identify cost, ethical, or other social impact as points for caution; the need for feasibility demonstrations in community settings; and whether research results are phrased for easy understanding and acceptance by health practitioners.

One of the first teams organized was the Committee on Detection, Evaluation, and Treatment of High Blood Pressure. This group, representative of a wide range of professional organizations (including the American Medical Association, the American College of Cardiology, the American College of Physicians, and the American Heart Association), formulated recommendations on the diagnosis and therapeutic management of hypertension that have become widely accepted in the medical community today. Another group, the Committee on Breast Cancer Screening, which included experts in radiology, medical oncology, surgery, and general medicine, as well as representatives of the clergy, the legal profession, and the public, made recommendations on such matters as which risk groups should continue to undergo periodic screening, the appropriate radiation dose for treatment, and the need for additional research.

Although the *National Center for Health Services Research* (NCHSR) concentrates more on cost effectiveness and cost-benefit studies and demonstrations of technological innovations studied in actual health care delivery settings, it has funded occasional technical consensus projects—for example, the American College of Cardiology conference report on optimal electrocardiography. (See the NCHSR *Research Summary Series* for such reports.)

Using the standards set by the *Health Standards and Quality Bureau* in its criteria and standards development process, the Professional Standards Review Organization (PSRO) develops consensus regarding the appropriate use of medical technologies. The American Medical Association Screening Criteria for quality assessment use were developed in this way, cosponsored by the American College of Physicians and in collaboration with other professional specialty societies and university hospitals. Although most of these criteria sets focus on the medical necessity for hospitalizing patients with given health problems, some criteria sets include indications for the effective use of drugs, devices, and procedures.

2. *Private sector expert consensus groups.* Within the private sector as well, expert consensus groups for developing efficacy data are being used by professional medical associations, such as the American College of Physicians, the American Society for Testing and Materials (ASTM), the Association for Advancement of Medical Instrumentation (AAMI), and the Alliance for Engineering in Medicine and Biology.

Although most evaluation of efficacy and safety of medical technologies conducted by professional associations is part of the federally funded programs just described, the associations themselves directly sponsor and fund several such projects. For example, the American Academy of Pediatrics develops recommendations on immunization practices and, under a contract with the National Center for Health Services Research, has developed consensual criteria for evaluation of ambulatory child health care. The American Public Health Association periodically compiles a list of efficacious preventive and therapeutic procedures for infectious diseases. A consensual efficacy report on such questionable practices as lumbodorsal sympathectomy, uterine suspension, and basal metabolic rate determinations was completed for Blue Cross by the Council of Medical Specialty Societies, the American College of Surgeons, and the American College of Physicians.

The American Society for Testing and Materials is the largest source of voluntary consensus standards development in this country. It mainly covers devices such as implantable mechanisms and prosthetics. The Association for the Advancement of Medical Instrumentation has developed a consensus forum that includes health care professionals, manufacturers of medical devices, and government representatives to establish basic performance and user information requirements. The Alliance for Engineering in Medicine and Biology concentrates on medical technologies such as ultrasonic diagnosis, and its reports are intended to increase practitioners' awareness of the importance of considering both the type and the validity of efficacy and safety information related to technologies they plan to use in their own practice.

3. *Local peer-group consensus.* At present, most efficacy decisions required from quality assurance teams to set standards, develop criteria, and establish priorities must be made without the benefit of research literature or reports from expert groups. Hospitals can rarely afford to organize groups of national or regional experts for quality assurance purposes, and implicit judgments of individual local practitioners are not sufficient to document scientific validity. Therefore, where national efficacy data are lacking, the quality assurance team will have to rely on teams of local peers for efficacy decisions of acceptable validity and applicability. Using structured group judgment techniques to elicit experiential and intuitive judgments on efficacy and safety can minimize individual bias. A growing body of research literature shows the validity of using such groups for improving decisions made under conditions of uncertainty (see also Chapter Nine).

**The Search for Documentation of Efficacy: General Principles**

The principles relating to the concept and documentation of efficacy for quality assurance purposes can be summarized in the following basic rules.

*Search the Literature.* In addition to the literature sources mentioned under "Data on Efficacy," earlier in this chapter, computerized data bases may serve as a starting point for an information search. Textbooks provide a basic understanding of the interventions used for common and important problems, and computerized data bases supply references to recent reviews of common interventions. Criteria lists developed by various organizations (for example, the AMA and PSROs) and journals that regularly review the essentials of care for given problems are also useful sources of information for broad searches. For focused searches on particular interventions used for a given indication, manual searches of recent reviews and reference lists of good sources are often valuable. However, these literature sources often do not provide full answers to specific efficacy questions about broad problem areas, such as coronary artery disease. Therefore, they must be supplemented by other sources of information.

*Examine the Scope and Design of Reported Studies.* For the reasons mentioned earlier, it is often difficult to find conclusive, concordant documentation of the efficacy of health care interventions. When documented studies are found, they should be scrutinized to ensure that their scope corresponds to the particular needs of the quality assurance team. Further, to ascertain the relevance and validity of the study in establishing a relationship between intervention and outcomes, the study design should be carefully examined. The material is relevant when the topic searched is central to the article being examined and when this article applies to medical practice. Validity refers to information maturity and methodological and analytic aspects of the study reviewed.

Uncontrolled studies, case reports, editorials, reviews, and commentary are not conclusive evidence of efficacy. They may report "experience with" an intervention, but one should recognize that their conclusions are tentative and subject to more definitive work. For some interventions, efficacy has not been and may never be satisfactorily studied. Some of these may be interesting historical interventions of little current relevance that only provide a context for present technologies. Others may be interventions whose efficacy is manifest, such as casts for forearm fractures (Office of Technology Assessment, 1978). When efficacy is manifest and not controversial, there is little difficulty in accepting the fact that the intervention works; when efficacy is manifest but controversial, there remains a problem to be solved that may be insoluble. For example, to some physicians, the efficacy of tonsillectomies to reduce the incidence of respiratory illness episodes in children with six or more bouts of pharyngitis or otitis media a year is established. To others, it is not. The studies needed to settle the issue probably cannot be done (Carden, 1978); therefore, the efficacy of tonsillectomies for this health problem may never be documented.

*Obtain Information from National or Local Experts or Peers.* After becoming familiar with the literature, one can consult national or local experts. Several expert consensus groups were mentioned earlier in this chapter as sources of information. In addition, experts are often found among the faculty of academic medical centers. These persons may in fact be national experts or at least would be able to identify such experts. Finally, if peers will be affected by the results of a study or will affect the results, their opinions and judgments should be sought.

*Describe the Results of the Search.* It is useful to record the result in terms of the amount and quality of the evidence identified (Figure 6.4). First, the intervention is described; then its relation to the problem for which it is used is specified, as are the outcomes studied and the population of concern. The evidence from the review is examined to see whether efficacy is manifest or not manifest. If not manifest, one then notes whether the evidence has been studied or not studied. If studied, the evidence is described according to its location on two continua—sparse versus plentiful and conflicting versus concordant. If not studied, efficacy status as under study, not under study, or unknown is stated. Then substantive statements about the efficacy of the intervention can be offered, as indicated in Appendix B.

*Use the Information for Developing the Quality Assurance Plan.* Information from the efficacy studies can be used to suggest the maximum expected benefit and to develop minimum or maximum standards for care.

The scope of the problems on which the team is asked to make judgments may range from the specific to the general. The team may need to address a specific task, such as setting criteria and standards for V intervention used in W problem for population X for a study to be conducted on patients seen during Y time period at Z hospital, clinic, or office. A more general task would be to develop for quality assurance/cost containment studies a list of topics reflecting significant age groups (infants, children, adolescents, young adults, middle aged, elderly) and sex characteristics as well as important aspects of care provided (prevention, diagnosis, treatment, rehabilitation, and management). This list would be based on the best available data on frequency of hospital discharges

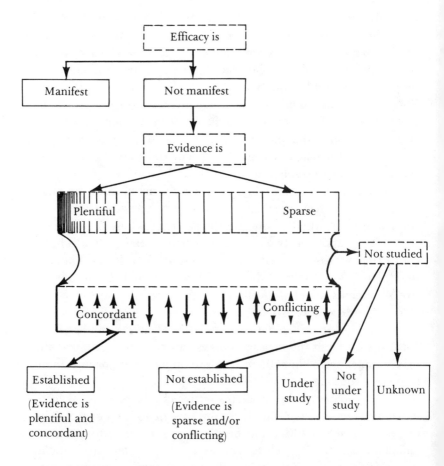

*Note:* Cochrane (1972) and the Office of Technology Assessment (1978) are two readable texts on the subject of efficacy.

**Figure 6.4. The Scope of an Efficacy Search and its Product:
Classification of Efficacy in Relation to the State of the
Health Sciences Literature.**

or ambulatory visits in the nation (see Chapter Five) and the efficacy of primary care interventions.

## Conclusions

Examining the efficacy of interventions requires determining whether a particular health care intervention works for a given health problem in a given population under ideal conditions of use. Despite the importance of efficacy both in clinical practice and in quality assurance, there are many areas where no valid documentation can be found. For example, FDA guidelines require manufacturers to supply evidence of efficacy for drugs manufactured after 1962 and all medical devices (that is, any physical items such as instruments, machines, implants, and reagents). Yet the safeguards that are intended by requiring manufacturers to supply evidence of efficacy may not be as stringent as needed. In fact, some may wonder about the possibility of bias when a company's financial status may depend on the results of such tests. Even worse is the current status of evaluating the efficacy and safety of medical and surgical procedures, such as surgical operations, that require skilled application of any combination of drugs, devices, and provider abilities. No present legislation requires such procedures to be subject to systematic study or consensus evaluation.

Nevertheless, the quality assurance team must conduct a search for studies that document the efficacy of the interventions in question in the practice setting in order to focus its efforts on areas where care can be improved or costs reduced. This is a difficult task, given the number of interventions that may be involved in managing a single health problem and the lack of documented evidence for many interventions. To tackle this problem, searches for documented evidence in the literature must be augmented by the resources of expert and peer groups. Structured consensual group assessment, incorporating the most relevant and valid scientific literature in the review process, may be the most meaningful current source of efficacy and safety information. The information from either source serves as the basis for developing standards and criteria used to evaluate the effectiveness and efficiency of the health care provided and to guide the team in designing its improvement action. Because of the importance to quality assurance of establishing the efficacy of the health care interventions being used, this search for documented evidence must be part of any quality assurance effort.

### Suggested Projects

(*Note:* See also Appendix B)

1.  The following are the ten most frequently studied audit topics in U.S. short-stay hospitals for fulfilling PSRO quality assurance requirements: myocardial infarction, appendectomy, hysterectomy, hip fracture, tonsillectomy and adenoidectomy, pneumonia, cholecystectomy, diabetes mellitus, Caesarean section, and gastroenteritis.
    a.  Have students give documented proof that efficacious diagnostic and therapeutic interventions exist for these problems. (1) What percentage of false positives and false negatives has been documented to occur in diagnostic validation studies conducted by expert diagnosticians under ideal conditions of use? (2) For which problems can one find reports of controlled clinical trials of therapeutic interventions? (*Caution:* One documented study, if not replicated, does not necessarily suffice.)
    b.  Divide class into groups of five or fewer. Consider the general purpose, methods, and analytical design of (1) a controlled clinical trial to establish efficacy of the coronary bypass surgical procedure; (2) a quality assurance study of patient health outcomes of coronary bypass surgery.

        •  What are the similarities and differences?
        •  What evidence of attribution of health outcomes to therapy is acceptable in the research study? In the quality assurance study?
        •  What evidence is available for either?
        •  Record and compare the conclusions of the different groups.

    c.  Assign one member from each student group to a team

for completing a brief literature review of coronary bypass surgery in terms of both scientific evidence of efficacy and quality assurance considerations. Give copies of especially relevant articles to each group for study and then reconsider each of the above questions.

*See:* Bunker, J. P., Barnes, B. A., and Mosteller, F. *Costs, Risks, and Benefits of Surgery,* Chapter 21. New York: Oxford University Press, 1977.

Takaro, T., and others. "Veterans Administration Cooperative Randomized Study of Surgery for Coronary Arterial Occlusive Disease." *Circulation,* 1975, *54* (Supplement 3), 107.

Selden, R., and others. "Medical Versus Surgical Therapy for Acute Coronary Insufficiency." *New England Journal of Medicine,* 1975, *293,* 1329–1333.

2.   Assuming that studies exist that give documented evidence of the survival rate for coronary artery bypass surgery, ask students to provide the minimum expected survival rate (that is, the percentage below which care would be regarded as inadequate or unacceptable and thus warranting a quality assurance review) for patients with single isolated left anterior descending (LAD) coronary artery lesions of 50 percent (diameter) or more with the following associated conditions:

|   |   | *Two Years* *Percentage of* *Survivors* | *Five Years* *Percentage of* *Survivors* |
|---|---|---|---|
| 1. | None | _____ | _____ |
| 2. | Poor left ventricular function | _____ | _____ |
| 3. | Poor distal runoff | _____ | _____ |
| 4. | Dominant LAD artery | _____ | _____ |
| 5. | #2, 3, 4 together | _____ | _____ |

# Establishing Effectiveness and Efficiency of Current Health Care

*Jay Noren*

The basic concern of quality assurance is the effectiveness and efficiency of health care provided in the community under usual conditions of practice. Using a health problem approach, Chapters Five and Six have shown how to develop priorities for quality assurance planning that center on those problems most important to society (because of their frequency, potential health loss, or economic costs) and encompass health care interventions whose efficacy is reasonably well documented. This chapter discusses means of identifying (1) the extent to which the potential benefit of care considered achievable is actually being achieved in the community and (2) the extent to which such benefit is *not* being achieved, so as to enable quality assurance personnel to formulate targets for improvement.

If assessment methods are to be useful in determining the effectiveness and efficiency of health care, they must provide both reliable measurements and an acceptable standard against which such measurements can be compared to indicate the quality of current performance. When people think of quality assurance, this assessment process usually comes to mind, although, as has been stressed before, assessment is but one of several tasks of a quality assurance system.

The first section of this chapter discusses the quality assurance implications of assessing the effectiveness and efficiency of care. The next section develops theoretical considerations, with particular emphasis on differentiating efficacy, effectiveness, and efficiency and on understanding the strengths and limitations of various current quality assessment methods. The last section outlines the sources of data reporting assessment of current health care and briefly considers methods and references for local application of effectiveness and efficiency assessments.

## Health Care Effectiveness and Efficiency: Implications for Quality Assurance

The Institute of Medicine (1974) expresses the relationship of effectiveness and efficiency to quality assurance as follows: "The primary goal of a quality assurance system would be to make health care more effective in bettering the health status and satisfaction of a population, within the resources which the society and individuals have chosen to spend for that care." Here the effectiveness of care is defined in terms of health and satisfaction outcomes; quality assurance is seen as a means of improving these outcomes and increasing the benefits of care. The requirement that outcomes be achieved within the limits of the resources available for care indicates that a review of the costs associated with health care and the efficiency of the use of resources is likewise an essential and implicit part of quality assurance.

Hiatt (1975) adds a temporal factor to the concern about the effectiveness and efficiency of the health care system with his idea of the "medical commons." He draws an analogy between the total resources available for health care and a common pasture shared by the cattle of several herdsmen. Just as overgrazing the common pasture to maximize each herdsman's cattle production in the short run will ruin all herdsmen in the long run, so too will overuse of health care resources in the short run deplete the resources available for the future. Hiatt describes three kinds of current medical practice that could endanger the medical commons in the long run: (1) doing everything possible for the individual patient regardless of risks or benefits to society at large; (2) expending resources on health care interventions that benefit neither the individual nor society; and (3) applying highly technological medical interventions to attempt to cure conditions that could have been prevented by less costly approaches.

The first practice, caring for the individual patient no matter what the expense, could contribute to overutilization of resources to benefit the few with high needs, thus decreasing the resources available for the many. Using procedures of no or unproven efficacy, a second type of medical practice, endangers the medical commons by expending resources on procedures of insufficiently documented benefit that might otherwise have been allocated to better health care interventions. Like gastric freezing for peptic ulcers, lobotomy for mental disorders, or internal mammary artery ligation for angina, all once common procedures, several unproven current practices fall into this category. Studies by Mather and others (1976) in England have questioned whether hospital treatment of myocardial infarction is more effective than home care. Coronary artery bypass surgery, whose effectiveness and efficiency continues to be debated, is another example.

The third medical practice, allocating resources involving high levels of technology to treatment of preventable diseases, may be less effective and efficient than developing or using preventive procedures or interventions. It is almost generally accepted now that a significant portion of dental decay can be prevented by water fluoridation. Occupational illness and injury may likewise be reduced by promoting changes in behavior, eliminating environmental pollutants, and controlling health hazards at the workplace. Furthermore, as was noted with regard to the economic aspects of health problems (see Chapter Five), overtreatment and overutilization, mistreatment and misdiagnosis, and inappropriate utilization can lead not only to unnecessary increases in the direct costs of health problems to individuals and to society but also to increases in the indirect costs. Each of these types of medical practice, therefore, is an appropriate target for effectiveness and efficiency evaluations.

Several current methods of quality assurance seek to identify aspects of inefficient or ineffective care with a view to eliminating or reducing the dangers and costs of inappropriate utilization or overutilization or of care of unproven benefit. The following section reviews these techniques and summarizes their advantages and disadvantages.

### Theoretical Considerations in Assessing Effectiveness and Efficiency

Three aspects often cause confusion among those learning about the field of quality assurance. The first is the need to develop a working understanding of the different connotations of efficacy, effectiveness, and efficiency of care (see also Chapter Six) and on how to measure them in relation to one another. The second relates to the profusion of quality assessment methods currently being applied to meet quality assurance regulations and requirements. Acronyms and brand names abound for methods of different applications and varying strengths and weaknesses. The third aspect involves issues concerning current national quality assurance programs and their requirements regarding health care quality assessment.

*Distinguishing Among Efficacy, Effectiveness, and Efficiency.* No matter what the approach or technique used in conducting quality assurance, the underlying assumption is that it is possible, however crudely, to specify and eventually quantify the benefits of care being achieved in actual practice and to compare these with hypothetical benefits of other conditions of care, ranging from "no professional care" to "optimum care." The following graphic displays (Williamson, 1978) illustrate how efficacy, effectiveness, efficiency, and achievable improvement might be so specified. Assuming that it is possible to quantify health outcomes, as has been attempted in recent cost-benefit studies, one can use a scale that represents units of health ranging from 0 to 100. The amount of health achieved under different conditions of health care will then indicate how the potential for improvement in care outcomes can be identified.

Figure 7.1 quantifies outcomes in terms of health units resulting under varying conditions of care for a given patient population (here, patients having congestive heart failure). If patients in this population received no professional medical care, they might achieve a health outcome of 25 units. However, given currently optimum care, using such interventions as digitalis, they might gain an additional 45 units of health (up to 70 units), which represents the benefit limit of current treatment—that is, its efficacy. Note that this gain still does not represent perfect health (let us say, 90 units), which might be considered attained if these patients had no health disability whatever until the day of their death.

Since the health outcome under currently optimum care is 45 units beyond the outcome of no health care (70 − 25 = 45 units), compared with a possible 65 additional units achievable by theoretically perfect care (90 − 25 = 65 units), the relative efficacy of health care can be expressed as a rate or percentage of perfect health:

$$45/65 \times 100 = 69 \text{ percent}$$

The additionally postulated 20 units of health—that is, 31 percent of 65—represent the improvement that could be attained if a breakthrough in biomedical research permitted prevention or total cure of congestive heart failure. This 31 percent, or 20 units of health, is the target of clinical research.

Figure 7.2 quantifies health outcomes for the same patient population resulting from care provided under usual conditions in the community. Again, without professional care these patients might achieve a health outcome of 25 units. If they received care under usual conditions of current practice, they might achieve an additional 27 units of health out of the 45 units that could be achieved under optimum conditions of care. These 27 units represent the level of effectiveness of current treatment. The shortfall of 18 units from the outcomes of optimum care might be accounted for by such factors as poor patient compliance (for example, failure to take digitalis and avoid sodium in the diet) or untimeliness of care. Thus, it should be possible to gain an additional 27 units of

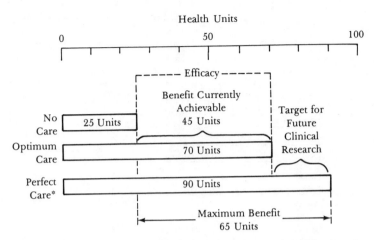

*A theoretical construct that assumes complete care eliminating all disability through remainder of average life expectancy.

**Figure 7.1. Efficacy of Health Care Intervention: An Approach to Quantifying Achievable Benefit. Adapted from Williamson (1978).**

health by current care as compared with no care. In relative terms, this would be expressed as percentage of optimally achievable benefit, or

$$27/45 \times 100 = 60 \text{ percent}$$

The additional 18 units of health—that is, 40 percent of 45— represent the extent of improvement that would be achieved if current performance were changed to meet optimum levels. This improvement potential is the target of quality assurance.

Figure 7.3 addresses the aspect of costs involved—that is, the efficiency of care. In this illustration, we assume that the health benefit for this patient population (that is, those with congestive heart failure) was achieved at a cost of $90,000. If $30,000 of this cost resulted from unnecessary care (for example, avoidable hospital days), then care under usual conditions of effectiveness could have been rendered for an optimum cost of $60,000. This optimum cost of necessary care ($60,000) represents efficiency in absolute units. It can be expressed in relative terms, as a percentage of present costs:

$$\$60,000/\$90,000 \times 100 = 67 \text{ percent}$$

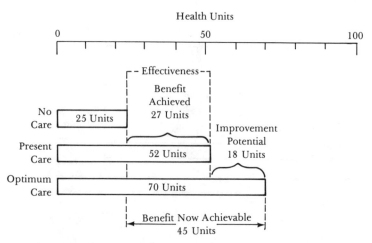

Figure 7.2. Effectiveness of Health Care: An Approach to Quantifying Improvement Potential. Adapted from Williamson (1978).

The possible 33 percent improvement in the cost of health care will be the target of cost containment efforts in quality assurance studies.

  *Current Methods for Evaluating Effectiveness and Efficiency.* Current methods for assessing both the effectiveness and efficiency of care are still being developed and do not permit a precise quantification of targets as suggested in the foregoing. They must be examined critically, therefore, and adapted to local needs and particular improvement programs. For practical reasons, regulatory agencies such as the PSRO have encouraged the use of assessment methods that could draw on available data, particularly the medical record. As a result, utilization review, intended to determine the appropriateness of hospital admissions and length of stay (that is, efficiency), was among the first methods to be implemented widely. Subsequent efforts to measure effectiveness relied on chart audits that used explicit criteria developed primarily to assess care processes of organic medical problems. It was soon discovered that the results of these assessments could vary widely, depending on the particular method used (Brook, 1974). It is now becoming apparent that more valid results can be obtained by using a problem-based approach and by adapting data collection methods to the problem

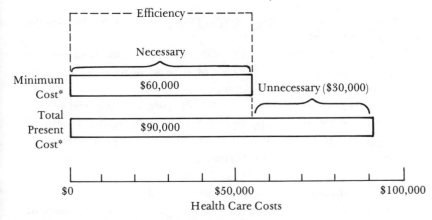

*To achieve 27 health benefit units depicted in Figure 7.2.

**Figure 7.3. Efficiency of Health Care: An Approach to Determining Cost Effectiveness. Adapted from Williamson (1978).**

being assessed. In fact, this approach, long advocated by some investigators (Brown, 1973; Williamson, Alexander, and Miller, 1968), forms the basis of the new quality assurance standard approved by the Joint Commission on Accreditation of Hospitals in April 1979. It is also being proposed in guidelines for future PSRO activities and will undoubtedly lead to an adaptation of currently available methods and the development of new ones.

1. *General approaches.* The four most commonly used general approaches to assessing effectiveness and efficiency of care are medical audit, interview, observation, and utilization review.

*Medical audit* based on either implicit or explicit criteria is an assessment of medical care using process data from medical records. In an implicit criteria audit, physicians review the entire patient record and make summary judgments of whether the process of care is acceptable. In an explicit criteria audit, criteria for acceptable care are predetermined, and nonphysicians then review medical records to ascertain whether the care rendered has met those criteria.

The *interview* approach relies on the judgment of outside reviewers. Survey sampling through direct interview has not been used as widely as medical audit. When employed as an assessment method, it usually focuses on patients, although it can also be applied to providers.

*Direct observation* as well relies on the judgment of outside reviewers. It assesses the process of care as it actually occurs or retrospectively through videotapes and films.

*Utilization review* examines claims forms or medical record abstracts to determine appropriateness of admissions, length of stay, and amount of ancillary services consumed. Explicit empirical criteria (the "average" performance in practice) are used for screening according to these parameters, with follow-up implicit review by physicians for cases of noncompliance.

Table 7.1 summarizes the advantages and disadvantages of each of these general approaches.

2. *Specific assessment techniques.* A range of assessment techniques have been developed and are being used in a variety of settings for conducting studies of effectiveness and efficiency. These techniques are briefly described in alphabetical order; a source of additional information is noted at the end of each description.

*Bi-cycle* is an assessment technique that uses medical audits of patient care to determine physician needs for continuing medical education. As its name suggests, this is a twofold process, involving (1) selection of those clinical problems having the highest priority for attention as reflected in the amount of disability caused and (2) assessment of how well actual practice complies with predetermined performance criteria for these high-priority problems. Discrepancy between criteria and actual practice highlights the target area for continuing medical education. After physicians have completed their continuing education programs, a reassessment is done to see whether care has improved (Brown, 1973; Brown and Fleisher, 1971).

*The Comprehensive Quality Assurance System* (CQAS), a method developed by the Kaiser-Permanente Medical Centers in northern California, begins with review by two practitioners of a small sample of charts to identify problem areas in patient care. The results of this screening review are presented to a quality assurance committee, which selects the most significant problems for further assessment. The committee then sets standards for selected problem areas. The chart review that follows determines compliance with the predetermined standards. Charts indicating noncompliance are reviewed by a physician, who judges whether the problem truly represents unacceptable quality (ineffectiveness or inefficiency). For true problems, corrective action is taken and a reaudit follows (Rubin and Kellogg, 1977).

*Concurrent Quality Assurance* (CQA), developed by Private Initiative in PSRO (PIPSRO), examines individual diagnoses for which a panel of experts has determined three categories of process criteria: (1) diagnostic criteria; (2) documentation criteria stipulating information that should be entered in the medical record on comorbidity, predisposing factors, severity, and complications; and (3) treatment criteria, stipulating efficacious and contraindicated treatment. Additionally, immediate outcome data are prominently posted in the charts of all participating patients. Adherence to criteria is assessed concurrently by nonphysician review coordinators (Sanazaro and Worth, 1978).

*Criteria Mapping* uses a decision tree to analyze the effectiveness and efficiency of physician decision making for a particular clinical problem. The decision tree is basically a diagram of the numerous sequential decisions that must be made for a given clinical problem, including the alternatives at each step in that process. Criteria of performance are predetermined for each step (or "node") in the decision tree, and compliance with these criteria is assessed at each decision node. Thus, this method should be suited to provide insight into the quality of clinical judgment. The method has not been applied widely as yet but has much potential for further development (Kaplan and Greenfield, 1978).

*Educational Patient Care Audit,* developed by the California Medical Association/California Hospital Association (CMA/CHA), is a retrospective review of the medical record to discern compliance with predetermined criteria. An important feature of this method is that the practitioners being evaluated are required to ratify the predetermined criteria. Additionally, these practitioners must set a "threshold for action," a minimum percentage of charts that must meet the predetermined medical record criteria in order for care to be considered acceptable. If results fall below this threshold, corrective action must be taken. This system has been

**Table 7.1. General Approaches to Quality Assessment.**

| Type | | Advantages | Disadvantages |
|---|---|---|---|
| I. Medical Audit | | | |
| A. In General | | 1. Medical records are accessible. <br> 2. Patient confidentiality can be reasonably maintained. | 1. Accessible records are often illegible and voluminous though incomplete, owing to physician charting behavior rather than actual patient care. <br> 2. Personal interaction between physician and patient is usually not recorded in the chart. <br> 3. Scope of review is restricted to organic medical diseases. |
| B. Implicit Criteria Audit | | 1. A wide range of patient problems can be included. <br> 2. Multiple factors in patient care can be considered. | 1. Judgment is subjective. <br> 2. Disagreement among judges is frequent because of this subjectivity. <br> 3. The method is expensive. |
| C. Explicit Criteria Audit | | 1. Review can be done by nonphysicians after standards have been developed. <br> 2. Standards can be readily applied to multiple institutions and providers. <br> 3. The method can be adapted to computers. | 1. It is difficult to develop agreed-upon standards. <br> 2. New standards must be created for each condition. <br> 3. Compliance with standards could become an incentive to practice cookbook or laundry-list medical care. |

| | Method | Advantages | Disadvantages |
|---|---|---|---|
| II. | Interview | 1. It provides an opportunity to sample from individual opinions of both providers and consumers.<br>2. It has the potential to address patient satisfaction with care.<br>3. It includes a broad range of factors beyond the organic disease focus of medical audit. | 1. Response rate to questionnaires is often low.<br>2. Identifying a representative population to interview is difficult.<br>3. The method is somewhat costly. |
| III. | Direct Observation | 1. Assessment of such factors as provider/patient interaction is possible.<br>2. Multiple parameters of care can be assessed.<br>3. It provides the only means to evaluate directly certain technical skills (for example, surgical procedures and psychotherapy). | 1. This method is extremely costly because of the necessity for trained observers.<br>2. Potential for observer bias is great.<br>3. The validity of the results is open to question because provider and patient may behave artificially when observed. |
| IV. | Utilization Review | 1. The methodology is simple.<br>2. It can be standardized across multiple institutions and/or providers.<br>3. It provides a screening method for determination of problem areas. | 1. Criteria are quite crude, with more emphasis on cost control than on quality.<br>2. The approach applies only to hospital care.<br>3. Use of empirical standards tends to perpetuate the status quo. |

made available to many institutions in California (California Medical Assocation/California Hospital Association, 1975).

*Generic Screening* assesses the number and severity of potentially compensable events that could be attributed to medical management. Compensable events include hospital-incurred trauma, adverse drug reactions, readmission, and death. Judgment of compensability is based on twenty-three generic criteria that can be applied across all diagnoses and clinical problems. This technique originated with the California Medical Insurance Feasibility Study (Mills, 1977).

*Health Accounting* is a problem-oriented quality assurance strategy that uses a combination of methods, such as medical record review, patient survey, and patient reexamination or testing, depending on the problem assessed. In a five-stage approach, quality assurance personnel must formulate priorities for study topics, conduct an initial assessment to verify that high-priority problems exist that are likely to encompass achievable health care benefits not being achieved, make a definitive assessment to identify correctable deficiencies of care and formulate an improvement plan, implement the plan, and reassess outcomes to determine whether improvement has been achieved and to document its extent. In Stages 1 and 2 of this process, a group of local experts estimates how well current health care practice is attaining potentially achievable benefits. The group assigns scores, or "ABNA" ratings (achievable benefit not achieved), to individual health care problems, higher ratings indicating greater disparity between benefits actually achieved and the potential for such achievement. Thus, the higher the ABNA rating, the greater the justification for devoting quality assurance efforts to the problem (Williamson, 1978; Williamson and others, 1975).

*The Performance Evaluation Procedure* (PEP) is a retrospective, outcome-based method using patient records to identify problem areas. Developed in the early 1970s by the Joint Commission on Accreditation of Hospitals, it focuses on such parameters of inpatient care as validation of diagnosis, justification for admission, justification for surgery or special procedures, discharge outcomes, complications, length of stay, and charges. It also includes some critical process criteria (Joint Commission on Accreditation of

Hospitals, 1974). The commission has recently revised its quality assurance requirements and has adopted a new standard that requires participating hospitals to organize a comprehensive quality assurance program, develop a written plan for quality assurance activities, use a problem-focused approach for review and evaluation of patient care and clinical performance, conduct an annual reassessment of the program, and document improvement in patient care and clinical performance (Joint Commission on Accreditation of Hospitals, 1979, 1980).

*The Problem Status Index/Outcome* (PSI) is a technique used to measure ambulatory care outcomes from the patient's perspective. The method uses questionnaires sent to patients at a predetermined time following contact with a health care provider for a particular clinical problem. It assesses frequency and severity of symptoms and limitation of activity compared with the expected result following acceptable health care. PSI also correlates the observed outcome to process information from the medical record (Mushlin, 1974; Mushlin and Appel, 1978).

*Quality Assurance Monitor* (QAM), a continuous monitoring technique for surveillance of patient care to determine priority problem areas requiring more detailed study, was developed by the Commission on Professional and Hospital Activities as a service available to hospitals. In each hospital, hospitalwide, departmentwide, and diagnosis-specific or surgery-specific groups are examined. Each monitored hospital receives a "priority for investigation" listing indicating areas in which the hospital's performance is substandard compared with that of other hospitals of its type (Lowe, 1977a, 1977b).

*Sentinel Health Events* is a technique that provides a negative index of health in terms of three types of events: unnecessary disease, unnecessary disability, and untimely death. Its focus is on preventable or treatable medical conditions, and the measure used is the incidence of these three general types of events (Rutstein, Berenberg, and Chalmers, 1976).

*Staging,* an outcome-based system for assessing ambulatory care, separates health problems into three levels of severity: (1) condition with no complications or minimal severity, (2) local complications or moderate severity, and (3) systemic complications or maximal severity. The patient's stage on entering the health care system is determined, and change in stage over time is measured. The method provides insight into factors related both to the effectiveness and efficiency of medical care and to its accessibility. The former are revealed by the degree of change in stage associated with medical care experience, and accessibility is assessed by the stage at first entrance into the system; for example, a high stage of severity at this time may indicate unacceptable accessibility. The distribution of stages for the patient population being studied can be compared against standards for comparable populations (Gonnella and others, 1977).

The *Tracer Conditions* method evaluates both process and outcome for a small number of specific common health problems and assumes that care provided for these problems is representative of care in general. The tracer condition must meet six criteria: It must have functional impact; it must be diagnostically well defined; it must have high prevalence; it must be amenable to medical care; it must be characterized by a clear understanding of prevention, diagnosis, treatment, and rehabilitation; and effects of nonmedical factors must be well understood. The criteria used to assess quality of care for the tracer condition are set at a minimum acceptable level; they focus on pragmatic rather than sophisticated technological care, are subject to periodic revision, and apply to the population at large rather than to individuals (Kessner, Kalk, and Singer, 1973).

*Current National Quality Assurance Systems.* Two national systems predominate in the quality assurance field at present. One is sponsored by the voluntary sector—namely, the Joint Commission on Accreditation of Hospitals. The other is sponsored by the government—namely, the Professional Standards Review Organization (PSRO).

1. *Joint Commission on Accreditation of Hospitals.* The following description of the historical evolution of the JCAH's quality assurance program is abstracted from the *Program on Hospital Accreditation Standards* (Joint Commission on Accreditation of Hospitals, 1976) and the *QA Guide* (Joint Commission on Accreditation of Hospitals, 1980).

The Joint Commission on Accreditation of Hospitals is a

voluntary, nongovernmental organization that, since its incorporation in 1951, has established standards for the operation of hospitals and other health-related facilities and services and conducted survey and accreditation programs to promote high quality of care in all respects, in order to ensure that patients receive the optimal benefits that medical science has to offer. It emphasizes organization and administration of functions for efficient care of the patient. A major goal is to recognize compliance with standards by the issuance of certificates of accreditation.

The governing body of the JCAH, the Board of Commissioners, consists of twenty persons appointed by its four member organizations—the American College of Physicians, the American College of Surgeons, the American Hospital Association, and the American Medical Association.

JCAH accreditation is considered a voluntary process and is not the same as certification or licensure by state or local authorities. However, accreditation has come to be recognized as a benchmark of quality and is used by some regulatory agencies as one criterion for granting certification and licensure, by some insurance agencies as a condition for honoring reimbursement claims, and by some educational accrediting committees of professional organizations.

In 1966 the Board of Commissioners voted "to review, reevaluate, and rewrite the hospital accreditation standards and their supplemental interpretations to attain two objectives: (1) to raise and strengthen the standards from their present level of minimum essential to the level of optimal achievable and to assure their suitability to the modern state of the art; (2) to simplify and clarify the language of standards and interpretations to remove all possible ambiguities and misunderstandings." The standards underwent extensive revision, resulting in the 1970 *Accreditation Manual for Hospitals.* In revising the standards, the JCAH became increasingly aware of the evolving changes in the organizational structure of hospitals. To keep pace with new demands, the JCAH has recognized various means of reviewing and evaluating care. In 1972 it developed an audit methodology to assist hospitals in an objective review and evaluation of patient care and established a requirement for medical audits, and in 1974 it specified the number of audits to be performed (Joint Commission on Accreditation of Hospitals, 1974).

Although the establishment of such numerical requirements was initially seen as an overwhelming task involving extensive paperwork, health care professionals responded favorably. They recognized the value of reviewing the quality of patient care, if not the value of conducting extensive audits. However, during the period of questioning that typically accompanies any new procedure or requirement, both the JCAH and the health care professionals evaluating care began to realize that medical audit requirements are self-limiting, in that adherence to numerical requirements limits the amount and scope of care evaluated. In addition, emphasis on broad diagnosis-based review encouraged hospitals to focus only on diagnostic topics rather than on identified or potential problems in patient care or clinical performance. Other quality assessment and quality-related activities (for example, review of nursing care and support services; tissue, antibiotic, and blood utilization review; delineation of clinical privileges; and monitoring of clinical practice) were not coordinated with audit activities or recognized as part of an overall quality assurance program.

Hence, as hospitals attempted to evaluate care and meet requirements, survey findings indicated that patient care and clinical performance had not improved to the extent expected, despite some impressive results in the evaluation and improvement of care. In some cases, changes in patient care and clinical performance were not in proportion to the amount of time and the costs invested in audit activity. Accordingly, a wider perspective that would take into account all hospital activities contributing to patient care was sought.

These factors were important considerations in the JCAH decision to eliminate the numerical audit requirement as of April 1979 and to revise substantially its approach to quality assurance requirements. The new and more dynamic problem-based quality assurance standard for hospitals is designed to help health care professionals develop a more sophisticated, comprehensive approach to quality assurance activities. The standard, effective for accreditation decision purposes on January 1, 1981, "emphasizes the value of a coordinated, hospitalwide quality assurance program; allows greater flexibility in approaches to problem identification, assessment, and resolution; emphasizes the importance of focusing quality assurance activity on problems whose resolution will have a significant impact in patient care and outcomes; emphasizes the importance of focusing quality assurance activity on areas where demonstrable problem resolution is possible; and discourages the use of quality assurance studies only for the purpose of documenting high-quality care" (Joint Commission on Accreditation of Hospitals, 1980, p. xi).

   2. *Professional Standards Review Organizations.* The Professional Standards Review organizations (PSROs) were created in response to cost overruns in the Medicare and Medicaid programs. In the early 1960s, the federal government had made a major commitment to provide monetary reimbursement for health care to the aged and the poor. To assure the quality of this care, the medical necessity of hospitalizations, of length of hospital stay, and of professional services given was to be monitored through a system of utilization review by physician staff committees in hospitals and claims review by organizations managing the payments—that is, fiscal intermediaries.

   By 1972 it was estimated that the cost overrun of this federal hospital insurance program would be more than $240 billion over a twenty-five-year period. This skyrocketing of costs has been attributed to both the increasing cost per unit of care and the increasing number of services provided to each beneficiary. Evidence subsequently compiled indicated also that a significant proportion of this care was likely to have been medically unnecessary and/or inappropriate. Congress, therefore, passed an amendment to the Social Security Act that was enacted in October 1972 and established a more comprehensive system of quality assurance to monitor the services purchased by government, the Professional Standards Review Organization (Goran, 1979).

   The program is responsible for ensuring that federally reimbursed health care is medically necessary, is of a quality that meets professional standards, and is provided at the most economical level consistent with those standards. To achieve these goals, the nation has been divided geographically into 203 PSRO areas. In theory, each area would develop an independent organization, called a PSRO, to monitor federally reimbursed care within its own geographical boundaries. Some PSROs cover a state, others only a part of a large city, depending on population density. Major emphasis was initially given to review of short-stay hospital care, with subsequent expansion to include ambulatory and long-term care in, for example, nursing homes and psychiatric hospitals. Three review component functions are mandated (Dobson and others, 1978; Goran and others, 1975).

Concurrent review is designed to certify the necessity, appropriateness, and quality of services rendered during a hospital episode. In practice, the medical chart is reviewed, usually by a nurse-coordinator who determines whether certain diagnostic-specific screening criteria have been met justifying the hospital admission (admissions certification) or, for patients previously admitted, whether continued hospital care is required (continued stay review). If the admission or continued stay does not meet criteria, a physician reviewer must judge the case. If the review physician's decision is contested, a designated peer review committee must decide; a final option in extreme cases is a state or national hearing. This process determines whether fiscal reimbursement will be given to the hospital and the attending physician for the care rendered to a particular patient.

Medical Care Evaluation (MCE) studies assess in depth the quality of health care services in terms of appropriateness and timeliness. These studies focus on the care given to aggregate groups of patients—for example, those having a common health problem. Explicit criteria that go into greater depth than the screening criteria of concurrent review are developed and applied. Deficiencies noted become the target for improvement actions to assure higher quality of care. Local physician teams participate in developing quality criteria. A set number of such studies must be completed each year for an institution to remain eligible for fiscal reimbursement.

Profile analysis is a retrospective analysis of data compiled on aggregate patient populations within a given area or institution. Patterns of services, such as the number and type of x rays ordered, are examined and compared with norms derived from previous practice or from data for the community as a whole. A standard data set is used to permit the development of utilization data as indicators of problems of care or utilization patterns. This data approach to quality assessment has received recent emphasis. Marked discrepancy from usual practice would trigger a "focused review," such as an MCE study. If deficiencies are then identified, corrective action is required.

It is clear from the foregoing that, with the exception of Health Accounting, the Problem Status Index, and the standards recently advocated by the Joint Commission on Accreditation of Hospitals, which permit a more dynamic approach, current methods of evaluating effectiveness and efficiency focus heavily on those aspects of care that can be identified in some form in the health care record. Consequently, the emphasis in these assessments is on aspects of management that are usually recorded, such as a laboratory test ordered or the therapeutic regimen prescribed. Evaluation of clinical judgment or decision making, of motor skills in the conduct of physical examinations or surgical procedures, or of psychosocial skills such as the ability to perceive nonverbal cues in patient interviews, is beyond the scope of these methods of assessment. Yet all these factors influence the quality of care. To evaluate these processes, one must turn to other techniques, such as observation of surgical performance and use of simulated patient management problems, which have considerable potential for quality assurance.

Despite the limitations of many of these current methods, they have provided both national and local data that are useful for conducting studies of efficiency and effectiveness in actual practice. These data sources will now be reviewed.

### Data Sources

As for efficacy data, there is no "Handbook of Health Care Effectiveness and Efficiency" that would compile data on current levels of performance. Nor are there national assessment surveys yielding data comparable to those of the National Center for Health Statistics on the magnitude of health problems, levels of health, and health care resources and their utilization and costs. The Health Care Financing Administration is beginning to request reliable and valid procedures for measuring efficiency of national short-stay hospital utilization. If such a procedure can be designed and implemented, it will be the first ongoing national quality evaluation survey ever conducted in this country in the field of health care. Meanwhile, quality assurance personnel must rely on data collected from isolated national or local studies.

*National and Regional Studies.* The most extensive study of health care effectiveness and efficiency to date is that of the Office of Policy, Planning, and Research of the Health Care Financing Administration, conducted in response to the congressional mandate to the secretary of the Department of Health and Human Services (formerly DHEW) to provide annual evaluative reports to Congress regarding the accomplishments of national PSRO programs.

The 1978 and 1979 evaluations focused on the Medicare utilization study, which attempted to measure the impact of the PSRO program on days of hospital care and hospital discharges per 1,000 Medicare enrollees and on average length of stay. Essentially, the study was designed to obtain utilization statistics from hospitals in the approximately 100 active geographical PSRO districts and to compare these statistics with similar data from roughly 100 inactive districts. However, because of numerous methodological problems in the evaluation design, these findings must be interpreted very cautiously. PSRO had a statistically significant impact as measured by reduced total days of care in 1977, but overall statistical significance was lost when data for the period 1974–1978 were analyzed. The Northeast showed a significant reduction in total days of stay, but a significant increase was found in the South. Despite these limitations, this first attempt at a national assessment of health care efficiency is noteworthy and promises more concerted efforts to devise reliable and valid methods of obtaining efficiency data.

There also are many efforts to measure and collect data on effectiveness. Many local PSROs have conducted areawide medical care audits, which consist in applying an agreed set of criteria in a chart-review assessment of care for an entire community. All PSRO hospitals in the area are expected to participate in these studies, so that the results will permit a representative evaluation of the effectiveness of care for that region. Topics such as adult pneumonia, one-unit blood transfusions, and cholecystectomies are being evaluated.

Recently, several PSROs throughout the United States have joined together in an areawide study of Caesarean sections. Because it is estimated that nearly one in five deliveries in the United States today is by operative intervention, this is a timely topic. Although the results of this study will not be generalizable outside the participating PSRO districts, it should generate a considerable body of interesting data on the effectiveness of this important aspect of obstetrical practice and will allow for comparisons among different regions of the United States. This type of study is analogous to the multiuniversity controlled clinical trials producing efficacy data, although it differs from them in both purpose and rigor.

*Local Studies.* By far the majority of studies of effectiveness or efficiency of health care have been conducted as isolated local endeavors. In the PSRO program alone, several thousands of such completed investigations are on record. During 1975–1977, for example, 15,546 medical care audits were recorded as having been completed through the initial chart-audit phase. Twenty topics accounted for 6,557, or 42 percent, of these quality assurance studies (Table 7.2). Table 7.3 lists the most frequently audited topics classified as medical, surgical, and administrative or miscellaneous interventions. These studies, which revealed a significant improvement in terms of unmet criteria on initial audit that were met on final audit, are of interest because they represent the bulk of the assessments of health care effectiveness and efficiency performed during 1975–1977. However, the data cannot be aggregated nationally, since topic definitions differ radically, criteria vary in content and quality, and the completion rate for initial audits, let alone reaudits, varied enormously from hospital to hospital and from PSRO to PSRO. What is important to recognize is the fact that, throughout the country, all hospitals managing Medicare/Medicaid patients have been required to evaluate the care provided by this means since 1976, and all hospitals that wished to be certified by the JCAH have likewise had to complete such audits. Although most of the results of these studies are not available outside the respective

Table 7.2. Twenty Most Frequently Initially Audited
Topic Categories, PSRO, 1975–1977.

| Topic Category | Number of Audits | Percentage of 15,546 Audits |
|---|---|---|
| Myocardial infarction | 721 | 4.64 |
| Pneumonia | 586 | 3.77 |
| Medicinal agents | 537 | 3.45 |
| Cholecystectomy | 448 | 2.88 |
| Appendectomy | 405 | 2.60 |
| Diabetes mellitus | 373 | 2.40 |
| Hysterectomy, abdominal | 361 | 2.32 |
| Cesarean section | 361 | 2.32 |
| Hip fracture | 321 | 2.06 |
| Tonsillectomy and adenoidectomy | 314 | 2.02 |
| Gastroenteritis | 308 | 1.98 |
| Cerebrovascular accident | 286 | 1.84 |
| Congestive heart failure | 266 | 1.71 |
| Normal delivery | 232 | 1.49 |
| Emergency room | 203 | 1.31 |
| Transurethral resection | 201 | 1.29 |
| Urinary tract infection | 193 | 1.24 |
| Hypertension | 185 | 1.19 |
| Pulmonary embolism | 135 | 0.87 |
| Cancer of colon | 121 | 0.78 |
| Total | 6,557 | 42.16 |

Source: Office of Research, Demonstration and Statistics (1980).

hospitals, practicing physicians can obtain results of such audits in their own hospitals. These evaluative data on local medical practice might provide meaningful insights as well as important information for identifying future topics for quality assurance efforts.

Finally, an impressive number of such studies of health care effectiveness and efficiency have been of sufficient quality to be published in the medical literature. Various universities have departments or research centers specializing in health services research, and many of these investigations were carefully designed and provided valid data about the current quality of health care. Many hospital and clinical staff members, though not researchers, have completed studies that have passed the review of refereed journals.

Table 7.3. Ten Most Frequently Audited Topic
Categories in Medical, Surgical, and Administrative
and Miscellaneous Classifications, PSRO 1975–1977.

| Topic Category | Rank |
|---|---|
| *Medical* | |
| Myocardial infarction | 1 |
| Pneumonia | 2 |
| Diabetes mellitus | 3 |
| Medicinal agents | 4 |
| Gastroenteritis | 5 |
| Cerebrovascular accident | 6 |
| Peptic and duodenal ulcers | 7 |
| Congestive heart failure | 8 |
| Urinary tract infection | 9 |
| Hypertension | 10 |
| *Surgical* | |
| Cholecystectomy | 1 |
| Appendectomy | 2 |
| Hysterectomy, abdominal | 3 |
| Cesarean section | 4 |
| Tonsillectomy and adenoidectomy | 5 |
| Hip fracture | 6 |
| Transurethral resection | 7 |
| Normal delivery | 8 |
| Herniorrhaphy | 9 |
| Cataract extraction | 10 |
| *Administrative and Miscellaneous* | |
| Emergency room | 1 |
| Blood usage and transfusions | 2 |
| Admissions, discharges, and transfers | 3 |
| Respiratory therapy | 4 |
| Intensive care units, CCU, PICU, and so on | 5 |
| Physical and related therapies | 6 |
| Patient/medical records | 7 |
| Surgical service (pre- and postoperative; recovery room) | 7 |
| Urological procedures, including indwelling catheters | 8 |
| Nursing procedures and care | 8 |

*Source:* Office of Research, Demonstration and
Statistics (1980).

## Identifying Information on Assessing the Effectiveness and Efficiency of Health Care

Finding sources of quality assurance data or methods in the literature nonetheless offers a challenge. It is important to recognize that to meet this information need, the strategies of search will be different from those for the efficacy literature. A major difference is that traditional indexes, such as MEDLARS or the *Index Medicus,* should be given relatively low priority in terms of effort. These sources, though of exceptional value in locating biomedical research, are often lacking in descriptors for most quality assurance needs and exclude much of the literature that provides relevant content. Many valuable data and methods are reported in other than journal form by such sources as the National Center for Health Statistics, the PSRO transmittals, and the *Bulletin* of the Joint Commission on Accreditation of Hospitals and similar publications not indexed by the National Library of Medicine in MEDLARS. Two sources are available, however, that contain much of this literature: Williamson (1977) for literature before 1976 and the index of the National Health Standards and Quality Information Clearinghouse for literature of 1976 and later.

*Literature Before 1976.* The bibliographic guide to quality assurance before 1976 (Williamson, 1977) is an extensive compilation of literature related to quality assurance for the period from 1900 to 1976. It provides citations and abstracts for over 3,500 articles, each coded to indicate its relevance to the assessment of effectiveness and efficiency of health care and the improvement of health. Detailed, indexed descriptors identify the patient population, the health problem, the type of health care provider, and the care interaction assessed (for example, diagnostic or therapeutic), as well as quality assurance content in terms of assessment mechanisms or improvement modalities. This concept-coding method of indexing (also adopted by the National Health Standards and Quality Information Clearinghouse) makes it possible to search combinations of codes delineating the concept that is the search target. For example, outcome assessment studies of diagnostic performance by general practitioners in a short-stay community hospital treating geriatric patients suspected of having neoplastic disease can be found by a combination of codes indicating type of study, provider, setting, and patients, as well as health problem. If the reader's main emphasis in this search is on the effectiveness of diagnostic care, an additional code can be added; this applies also if emphasis is on efficiency.

It is estimated that over 75 percent of the studies cited in Williamson (1977) would not be accessible through traditional indexes of medical literature. The main reason is that most of the quality assurance terms coded in this bibliography did not come into use until after the early 1970s. Further, it requires expert quality assurance knowledge to recognize relevant articles that were written in traditional research terms, such as the "observer error" studies of the 1950s and 1960s, which provide examples of classic diagnostic validation investigations. For example, Garland's 1960 study indicated the level of agreement and accuracy that can be achieved under ideal conditions (efficacy) and documented that, in reading chest films, the average radiologist will miss 25 percent of known lesions, regardless of the size or configuration of the lesion. This and similar observer-error studies can have important implications for designing quality assessment projects.

Although the structure of this bibliography requires some time from the reader in becoming adept at using the coding system, many relevant articles can be identified to facilitate not only the assessment of the effectiveness and efficiency of health care but most other quality assurance functions as well.

*Literature of 1976 and Later.* The National Health Standards and Quality Information Clearinghouse provides the only ongoing reference index to the quality assurance literature, including that of cost containment. The clearinghouse covers the traditional biomedical literature in MEDLARS/MEDLINE as well as numerous unpublished sources, such as the information transmittals of the national PSRO program. Even pertinent information published in the Federal Register and the lay press (for example, the *Wall Street Journal*) is indexed, as is much important information related to quality assurance regulations and policy. An example is the recent changes in the quality assurance requirements of the Joint Commission on Accreditation of Hospitals described earlier (Joint Commission on Accreditation of Hospitals, 1979, 1980). An invaluable aspect of this clearinghouse is that it provides access to such information long before it will be available in traditional medical journals. The search base has recently been augmented to provide access to literature on long-term care that was previously difficult to locate. Additionally, the coding index provides ready access to the jargon terms of quality assurance. (As much as one might decry its excessive use, jargon will always be a part of a specialized field, especially one that is growing as rapidly as quality assurance. As pointed out by Evans and Evans in their *Dictionary of Contemporary American Usage,* such terms of a trade or a profession are as respectable as the group that uses them.)

To obtain access to this clearinghouse, one should ask to be put on its mailing list and to receive the monthly *Information Bulletin,* together with annual collations of coded and indexed citations. Copies are also often available in the offices of local PSROs, university libraries, and, possibly, local hospital libraries. The monthly bulletins provide complete abstracts of all articles indexed, and special searches can be requested from the clearinghouse staff.

Among additional valuable references useful as a starting point for understanding effectiveness and efficiency evaluations are Donabedian (1980), Dobson and others (1978), Institute of Medicine (1974, 1976), Greene (1976), and Goran and others (1975).

## Conclusions

This chapter has presented a brief overview of methods for assessing effectiveness and efficiency of health care. In conducting such an assessment it is essential to follow four simple steps: (1) state the problem, (2) search for background information, (3) choose an appropriate evaluation method, and (4) analyze and interpret the results.

In stating the problem it is essential to specify the health service that is being evaluated for effectiveness/efficiency and the desired outcome to be achieved under the actual conditions in which the health care intervention has been applied. The health service will typically be one or a combination of diagnostic, therapeutic, or preventive interventions. The outcome must be carefully defined, including its measurement parameters and time frame. Outcome parameters may take the form of traditional health status measures, such as mortality or morbidity, or they may include other, less traditional benefits, such as patient or provider satisfaction.

By conducting a literature review of at least modest proportions, the quality assurance personnel will acquire basic information on prevalence of the health care problem of concern and associated costs. Available data sources related to the problem of concern must be reviewed, and choices among those sources must be made on the basis of their feasibility, reliability, and validity. This chapter discussed potentially useful data sources on health problems. After reviewing background information, quality assurance personnel must choose a method for conducting the evaluation. This chapter also described several methods that can be used, as well as references for additional information on each method.

# Achieving Improved Health Care Performance and Outcomes

*William F. Jessee*

ᚤᚤᚤᚤᚤᚤᚤᚤᚤᚤᚤᚤᚤᚤᚤᚤᚤᚤᚤᚤᚤᚤᚤᚤ

The concepts and types of information described in the preceding chapters provide the basis for identifying problems in the delivery of health care, setting quality assurance and cost containment priorities, and identifying areas for improvement. One other set of principles must be understood if quality assurance and cost containment is to be effective. These principles relate to ways of planning and implementing changes in both individual behavior and organizational functioning. As noted in Chapter Seven, effectiveness and efficiency measurements indicate what benefits are actually being achieved by the health care provided. The gap between these benefits and those that could reasonably be achieved, the "improvement potential," is the area that improvement planning addresses. To improve outcomes of health care, the improvement plan and the approaches used to implement it must be based on proven and effective ways of producing change.

The concepts of efficacy, effectiveness, and efficiency are closely allied to principles of clinical medicine and research. Improvement planning and implementation, however, must draw heavily on the fields of adult education, industrial engineering, systems analysis, and organizational development. These fields, derived in part from the behavioral sciences, adapt knowledge on how individuals change into approaches to changing organizations and systems. They require an understanding of how professionals define themselves and how this self-definition affects functioning and change, how various components or subgroups within an organization interact, and how changes in organizations actually occur.

In considering improvements in health care, it is important to recognize the dynamic tension that exists in any health care encounter among the three principal interacting components: patient, practitioner, and organization. Taken together, these interacting components may be viewed as a system to which the concepts of, and techniques for, change can be applied. At any point in time, the patient's health status is influenced by the process of care (whether preventive or curative) provided by the practitioner, by the patient's own attitudes and behaviors, and by such organizational variables as equipment, personnel, policies, and procedures. When problems in quality of care (for example, less than optimal achievable patient health status) are identified, change must take into account not only the role of the practitioner but also those of the patient and organization. However, attention to problem identification and verification alone, without equal attention to the skills needed to *solve* such problems, is destined to produce frustration and to reduce the impact of any quality assurance efforts to improve health care (Williamson, Alexander, and Miller, 1967; Jessee, 1977a). This chapter therefore examines the characteristics of each of the components of the health care encounter that affect health status and have an impact on improvement planning and suggests practical approaches to achieving improvement.

A Theory of Planned Change: Implications
for Quality Assurance

The process of achieving improvement through quality assurance is analogous to that of planned change. As defined by
Schein (1972), planned change involves learning new ideas and
concepts, new attitudes and skills, and new patterns of behavior. It
can be divided into three stages: (1) unfreezing, or unlearning
present ways of doing things; (2) developing new beliefs, values,
and behavior patterns; and (3) refreezing, or stabilizing and integrating new beliefs, attitudes, values, and behavior patterns.
Theories of planned change can be applied to both individuals and
organizations; hence they are appropriate to a discussion of change
in the health care system, which encompasses both.

*The Change Agent.* This model of planned change, based on
principles adapted from organizational development, implies the
presence of a change agent who, for the most part, is external to
the system. The competencies of the change agent, as identified by
Bennis (1969), are conceptual diagnostic knowledge, familiarity
with the theories and methods of organizational change, knowledge of sources of help, and awareness of the ethical and evaluative
functions of the change agent's role. The change agent must be
able to identify the problem and the individuals or subsystems affected by the problem, assess their readiness to change, communicate and share information with the members of the subsystem or
system, and provide necessary and appropriate education (Beckhard, 1969).

*The Change Process.* Schein (1972) maintains that no change
will occur unless the members of the system feel that it is safe to
give up old responses and try something new. The change agent
must therefore create a balance between, on the one hand, introducing disconfirming forces that arouse discomfort, threat, or tension and, on the other, creating sufficient psychological safety to
permit motivation for, rather than resistance to, change. Schein
also points out that once motivation to change has been created, the
system or person will need new sources of information to assist in
developing new attitudes or responses. This seeking of new infor-

mation may take the form of selecting a model with which to identify or of scanning several sources from which ideas can be culled to formulate a package that fits the unique situation. The "refreezing," or stabilizing and integrating, of the new responses requires that the change fit both the personality of the individual and the social system to which he or she belongs (Schein, 1972).

*Application to Quality Assurance.* Although Schein's model and processes were originally developed and applied in the context of changing professional education, they illustrate principles that can be adapted to quality assurance. For example, a quality assurance team composed of members of a health care institution who assume a new or additional role within the institution can legitimately be considered an entity or "change agent" in itself. The quality assurance team must have many of the competencies of the change agent, including ability to assess the care being provided and to diagnose the problems affecting health, satisfaction, or economic outcomes; familiarity with information resources that can clarify the nature of the problem; knowledge of methods and approaches that can be used to correct the problem; and ability to involve providers, patients, and institutional administrators in seeking or implementing solutions.

Bennis (1969) also identifies steps to be taken by the change agent. He or she must identify the appropriate point of entry into the organization, diagnose interdependencies within the system, involve those who will be affected by the change in goal setting and planning, obtain voluntary commitment of participants, and select approaches to achieving change that are congruent with the goals and values of the institution or organization. Translating these steps into the quality assurance and cost containment field means that the team must be able to identify the clinical department, clinical subgroup, or patient population to whom the improvement actions are to be directed; enlist the cooperation of key staff in setting standards or developing criteria; obtain support of department chiefs or chief administrators as well as of those who will be affected by the improvement activities; and adopt procedures that are compatible with the goal of improving patient care.

With this conceptual framework in mind, it is now possible

to examine ways these theories of change can be applied to improving provider performance, patient compliance, and organizational functioning.

### Improving Provider Performance

Of major importance in achieving improvement in health care or a reduction in cost without a concomitant reduction in quality is the ability to effect change in the performance of health care providers. However, a series of attitudes and characteristics common to most professionals must be recognized before a particular improvement action can be designed and implemented.

*Factors Affecting Provider Behavior.* Health care providers share many characteristics common to all professionals. As summarized by Schein (1972), these include control of a specialized body of knowledge acquired by prolonged education and training; exercise of a high degree of autonomy in making judgments and decisions on behalf of clients; assumption of a detached, neutral attitude toward clients; cultivation of a relationship based on mutual trust; a strong orientation toward service; and a position of power and status in one's area of professional expertise.

These characteristics are means by which professionals define themselves. At the same time, they are factors that change agents must recognize in selecting approaches to achieve improvement. For example, if improvement in patient care is to be achieved, a high level of collaboration is frequently required among health care providers, quality assurance team, and administrative staff. Given the tendency of professionals to operate autonomously, the quality assurance team may have to include techniques for promoting collaboration in its improvement planning. One approach to fostering a sense of collaboration is to involve the providers in setting standards and criteria for quality assurance and cost containment at the outset of a study. In this way, they would be better prepared for accepting the results of the initial assessment of the quality of care and for participating in the improvement actions. Similarly, recognition that professionals have a high degree of service orientation may mean that the improvement planner can appeal to their altruism to motivate them to change their behavior, particularly if providers are convinced that better-quality patient care will result.

*Techniques for Achieving Improvement in Provider Behavior.* Some fundamental understanding of the principles of human psychology and adult education is important to planning improvement of provider performance. One of the primary adult education principles is that adults learn when they perceive a benefit to themselves in doing so (Knox, 1977). Therefore, identifying a reward system for persons in whom behavior change is desired can be a critical prerequisite to effecting change.

A corollary of Knox's principle is that people will learn what they need to know. One technique widely advocated for improving professional competence is continuing medical education (CME). During the past ten years, the frequency of requirements mandating specific hours of continuing medical education as a prerequisite for physician relicensure has risen dramatically. Yet there is little evidence that mandatory continuing medical education is associated with increased physician competence (Bertram and Brooks-Bertram, 1977; Jessee, 1977b), except when a problem of patient care is related to lack of knowledge. For example, Ogilvie and Ruedy (1972) described a significant improvement in the care of patients receiving digitalis preparations immediately after an intensive CME program on digitalis therapy at a hospital in Montreal. In their original paper stressing a cyclic concept linking patient care evaluation and continuing medical education, Williamson, Alexander, and Miller (1967) described a classic example in which continuing education programs produced improved care in terms of response to unexpected laboratory test abnormalities (see also Chapter Ten). Building on this work, Brown and Uhl (1970) reported several additional instances of effecting change. Laxdal and colleagues (1978) also reported significant improvement in physician prescribing practices after an intensive, problem-oriented CME program over a one-year period.

MacDonald (1975) has described the favorable impact of a "computer reminder" system, using algorithms to assure adequate evaluation and follow-up of outpatients under treatment for diabetes mellitus. Such approaches to modifying physicians' behavior are important tools to be incorporated into plans and activities for achieving improvement in physicial performance.

All these approaches to practitioner behavioral change assume that the individual is responsive to altruistic rewards for change or can be motivated by appeals to self-interest or self-improvement. However, it is also important to recognize financial motives, which may conflict with altruistic goals. For this reason, it is appropriate to consider a variety of available sanctions that can be used in improving provider performance:

• Mandatory preadmission review of elective hospital admissions.
• Mandatory consultation or surgical assistance for certain diagnoses or procedures.
• Reduction, modification, or suspension of hospital privileges.
• Sanctions under the PSRO law, such as recoupment of Medicare/Medicaid payments, removal from participation in Medicare/Medicaid, or fines.
• Denial of insurance payment for inappropriate, unnecessary, or poor-quality services.
• Suspension or revocation of licensure.

Clearly, the legal and economic consequences of these approaches require that they be used only where appeals to other motives for change have failed. In addition, according legal due process to the person concerned is critical. Nonetheless, this range of sanctions is an important part of the repertoire of change tactics available to the health care system and of quality assurance and cost containment.

### Improving Patient Compliance

Because patient behavior and attitudes are important determinants of health care outcomes, particularly with regard to compliance with therapeutic or preventive regimens, improvement planners should understand some of the forces that shape this behavior and apply techniques that are successful in modifying it.

*Factors Affecting Patient Compliance.* Becker and Maiman

(1975), in their "health beliefs" model, postulate that patient preventive health behavior is controlled by (1) the individual's perceived susceptibility to health problems and perception of their severity; (2) the individual's assessment of the "benefits" of the proposed health action as opposed to its "costs," whether economic, physical, or psychological; and (3) cues to action, either internal or external, which interact with predisposing perceptions to produce the health action. In addition, Becker and Maiman point out that patient compliance is shaped by (1) predisposing factors such as motivation, value of illness threat reduction, and probability that compliant behavior will reduce the perceived threat; (2) modifying factors such as age, sex, race, attitudes about health care, access, and economic status; and (3) enabling factors such as prior experience with illness or treatment and social pressures.

To improve compliance, it is necessary to recognize how these factors operate to shape health beliefs, how radically these beliefs may differ in different patients, and how to modify beliefs in such a way as to improve patient compliance. Knowledge of these factors and health beliefs, as well as of demographic and psychosocial characteristics of the patient population involved in the quality assurance effort, is the basis for selecting appropriate techniques to improve compliance.

*Techniques for Achieving Improvement.* Brook, Williams, and Avery (1976) note that skills in modifying patient beliefs and compliance behavior become increasingly important as medical technology nears the limits of its potential for improving care and it becomes necessary to seek other ways to achieve additional improvement in health status.

There is a rather extensive body of research on techniques for modifying patient behavior by altering particular patient perceptions and beliefs. For example, increasing the perceived (subjective) level of vulnerability has been shown to be effective in increasing patient compliance with practitioner recommendations in such areas as cancer screening (Flach, 1960; Fink, Shapiro, and Lewison, 1968; Kegeles, 1969; Haefner and Kirscht, 1970), tuberculosis (Hochbaum, 1958), and heart disease (Haefner and Kirscht, 1970). Becker, Drachman, and Kirscht (1974) also have reported increased compliance with oral treatment regimens among mothers who believed their children susceptible to recurrence of otitis media. Similarly, patient estimates of the seriousness of an illness are consistently predictive of compliance with the prescribed medical regimen (Becker and Maiman, 1975).

Because these techniques are based on theories of behavior modification, however, it is important that those planning to use them recognize some of the problems associated with this approach. Chief among them is the need to take into account the values and interests of those whose behavior is being modified. Therefore, in developing improvement actions that rely on behavior modification techniques, it is essential for the quality assurance team to determine what patients value and to ensure that these values are given priority over any institutional or social goal.

Other techniques for improving patient compliance rely on adult learning principles similar to those applying to practitioners. These include recognizing that learning takes place when the learner perceives a need to know something and that learning is more effective when the learner participates in planning the educational process and when the process is adapted to accommodate learners' individual differences and prior knowledge. For example, patient ownership of the medical record can improve patient self-sufficiency and physician/patient relationships (Bouchard and Tufo, 1977; Tufo and others, 1979). Starfield (1978), in a study to test the efficacy of joint goal setting by practitioners and patients, noted a higher level of concordance and better coordination of care than were achieved through traditional means of continuity. These and other studies on patient education, life-style modification, and patient self-care provide many suggestions for approaches to improving compliance and patient satisfaction. They are invaluable sources to the quality assurance team in planning approaches to achieve improvement.

## Improving Organizational Functioning

Many of those involved in quality assurance and cost containment acknowledge that a substantial proportion of identified problems in patient care require improvements in the administration or structure of the health care institution. Effective planning to improve organizational functioning and obtain more effective and efficient patient care can incorporate the theories and techniques for effecting change in individuals. These theories can be supplemented by those derived from the relatively new fields of organizational psychology and systems analysis and from the broad concepts of organizational development discussed earlier in this chapter. A thorough discussion of these theories, particularly as applied to health care services, would require a text in itself. However, it is useful for the purpose of this discussion to point out some characteristics of organizations that might profitably be considered when attempting improvement in organizational functioning and to explore techniques that bear further investigation.

*Factors Affecting Organizational Functioning.* Schein (1970) defines an organization as "the rational coordination of the activities of a number of people for the achievement of some common explicit purpose or goal, through division of labor and function, and through a hierarchy of authority and responsibility." Implied in this definition are characteristics of an organization that must be taken into account when attempting to change organizational functioning. For example, it is necessary to understand the individual diversity, the types of subgroups and subsystems, the interactions among subgroups, the interdependency of human and technological factors, and the levels of authority that constitute any given organization. Because of their complexity, organizations often seem resistant to change. This particularly applies to hospitals, which are among the most complex organizations in any industry from the point of view of operating time, personnel, and levels of authority. Hospitals operate twenty-four hours a day, seven days a week; hospital personnel range from the most highly skilled professionals to the unskilled, all with critical responsibilities for the success or failure of care; the organizational structure is such that medical staff and administration function as equals but with overlapping areas of responsibility, both answering to a board of trustees that may know little or nothing of the technical aspects of the institution's operation. Hospitals have been described as having "diverse goals, diffuse authority, low task interdependence, [and] few performance measures" (Weisbord, 1976), all of which contribute to the difficulty of effecting organizational change.

Despite these and other problems associated with bringing about changes in a hospital setting, the principles and methods of organizational development can provide important information for those attempting to achieve improvement. A strategy designed to encourage change in "the beliefs, attitudes, values, and structures of organizations so that they can better adapt to new technologies, markets, and the dizzying rate of change itself" (Bennis, 1969), organizational development has been successfully used in the hospital industry (Drexler, Yenney, and Hohman, 1977a; Weisbord, 1974; Lawrence, Weisbord, and Charms, 1974). Furthermore, many of the concepts used in this approach are already known to the quality assurance "change agent" because they derived from the behavioral sciences (for example, Gestalt, transactional analysis, normative reeducation, interpersonal and group dynamics) and are included in the medical school curriculum.

*Techniques for Achieving Organizational Improvement.* Conflict management is one aspect of organizational development that is particularly valuable to the quality assurance change agent. Lawrence and Lorsch (1969) have written extensively on the relation between an organization's ability to manage conflict situations constructively and its efficiency, productivity, and product quality. The most productive organizations are those in which managers (or change agents) are able clearly to differentiate the positions of the parties to a conflict and then proceed to integrate the various points of view into an acceptable compromise to which all parties can commit themselves. Drexler, Yenney, and Hohman (1977b), describe four basic styles of conflict management: autocratic, democratic, laissez faire, and pantisocratic.

*Autocratic (low differentiation, low integration).* This unilateral style of decision making rests on the concept that the manager exercises unquestioned authority. Although this style of conflict management works well in the military, in more complex organizations it creates a win/lose situation that stifles diverse, creative approaches to solving problems. It is also likely to produce resentment and ill will, impairing the productivity of the organization.

*Democratic (high differentiation, low integration).* This is another win/lose style of conflict management. It tends to be counterproductive because the losers on any given decision spend their energies preparing for the next skirmish rather than working to carry out the decision of the majority. Organizations that use this form of conflict management divert much of their time and energy to engaging in political intrigues, soliciting votes, and preparing for the constant battles that characterize their operation.

*Laissez faire (low differentiation, high integration).* This approach is characterized by behavior patterns of smoothing over, avoidance, or presumed ignorance of the presence of conflict. Health care institutions often use laissez faire conflict management because they often equate professionalism with the ability to be rational, unemotional, and always in control of a situation. Whenever conflict threatens, it is smoothed over (or integrated) without providing an opportunity for differences to become fully explicated. In this approach, the conflict is often not actually solved but merely "put away," and it frequently erupts again at some future, usually unpropitious time. Organizations that engage in this type of conflict management are often characterized by low morale, high incidence of psychogenic illness among employees, rapid turnover of personnel, and low productivity. Since this mode of conflict management is often dominant in health care institutions, it is especially important for those concerned with improving organizational functioning to be aware of its effects.

*Pantisocratic (high differentiation, high integration).* This approach is the most productive style of conflict management. It legitimizes open differences of opinion and uses those differences in creative problem solving. It fosters the cooperation, collaboration, and commitment that are essential to effective teamwork, in that all personnel involved in the decision-making process contribute to the final decision. Organizations using this style of conflict management are likely to have higher morale, lower turnover, less illness, and higher productivity than those using another dominant mode of conflict resolution.

By targeting their efforts toward producing a style of conflict management that promotes collaboration and cooperation among the members of an institution, quality assurance change agents have a greater chance of success in improving organizational functioning.

## Minimizing Resistance to Change

*Factors Contributing to Resistance.* In planning and implementing improvement through quality assurance activities, those involved as change agents (that is, the quality assurance team) should recognize that their attempts to change provider, patient, or organizational behavior may be perceived as an attack on individual self-worth. Festinger (1957) coined the term *cognitive dissonance* to describe the tension state created by an external threat to one's ego. Those who experience this state normally react by taking steps to reduce it through rationalization or other evasive actions intended to preserve a favorable self-image.

For example, the chairman of a hospital medical audit committee may inform a provider through a formal written communication that his or her practice of routinely transfusing cholecystectomy patients with one unit of blood postoperatively poses an unnecessary risk of hepatitis and is inconsistent with standards of acceptable medical practice. This communication will undoubtedly create cognitive dissonance in the provider. To reduce this tension, the provider may deny the data ("I never give single-unit transfusions"), minimize its importance ("There is no objective evidence of increased risk"), or personalize the conflict ("The chairman of that committee envies me and has been out to get me since he took over the audit committee.") These reactions may indeed preserve the provider's self-esteem, but they will do little to improve the problem of care. Therefore, the quality assurance team acting as a change agent needs to select an approach to achieving improvement that will not provoke resistant behavior.

*Seven Suggestions for Promoting Change.* To avoid the type of defensive behavior just described and to achieve the desired changes in provider performance, patient compliance, or institutional effectiveness, seven simple rules can be applied. These are modifications of "change rules" originally formulated by Richard E. Thompson.

*Be sure of the facts.* Before a change is initiated, change agents must be sure that their data are accurate and that they have complete information on the problem. Acquiring accurate and complete information is a critical first step in the change process, since errors can so undermine the credibility of the change agent that he or she becomes totally ineffective. For instance, a medical audit finding that weights are not recorded on infants seen in the emergency room for gastroenteritis clearly indicates the existence of a patient care problem. However, attempts to remedy the problem by providing physician or nurse education would not only fail but be detrimental to the entire quality assurance program if the cause of the problem were found to be the lack of a baby scale in the emergency room. Consideration of all possible alternative causes may require collection of additional data or additional analysis of available data as a prerequisite to effective change programs (see also Chapter Ten).

*Take appropriate action.* Appropriate action increases the likelihood of change instead of provoking additional resistance. In deciding what constitutes appropriate action, change agents should use the concept of cognitive dissonance, whether the change activity is directed toward an individual or an organizational unit. Approaches that increase tension or cognitive dissonance are more likely to stimulate rationalization and opposition to change than are approaches that make the point clearly but minimize the threat to the individual or collective ego. For instance, in a quality assurance study of treatment of pediatric asthma, if physicians failed to comply with the agreed criterion that arterial blood gases should be taken at least once for each patient, two strategies for changing provider behavior could be attempted.

The first strategy, autocratic in approach, would be to send a letter to physicians who failed to comply with the criterion. The letter, signed by the medical audit chairman and marked "Personal and Confidential," would note the failure to meet the criteria set by the department of pediatrics. It would go on to inform the provider that this was unacceptable practice and that compliance would be expected in the future. The letter would conclude by stating that the provider's practice in this area would be monitored during the next six months and that failure to meet the criterion during this time could constitute grounds for modification of practice privileges. This approach is likely to produce hostility, defensiveness, and a conviction that "they" (that is, the medical audit committee) are wrong, resulting in no change in provider behavior.

An alternative strategy, more in keeping with a pantisocratic approach to conflict management, would involve an informal personal meeting between the medical audit chairman and each noncomplying physician. This approach would allow the chairman to present the findings of the study with regard to the physician's behavior and to explain why taking blood gases was considered important. It would also give the chairman an opportunity to elicit an opinion from the noncomplying physician on the ordering of arterial blood gases to improve management of asthmatic children. In adopting this approach, the committee chairman might learn that, as a result of many years of treating such children, the physician had developed a personal set of criteria that took into consideration the trauma to the patient and the expense of blood gases. This approach would likely lead to a productive discussion of substantive patient care issues and to modification in both the behavior of the noncomplying physician (increased use of arterial blood gases) and that of the rest of the staff (greater discrimination in determining for what patients the use of arterial blood gases is appropriate).

*State the problem specifically.* If the problem is not clearly understood, it is difficult for any individual or organization to respond positively to the change initiative. Failure to be specific and direct in identifying the problem can produce anxiety and resistance. Therefore, a direct statement of the problem, including its severity and the potential consequences of leaving it unresolved, is essential.

*State the desired solution.* Not only must the problem statement be specific, but the solution desired by the change agent should also be clearly stated. Too often, individuals or organizational units are told only, "You have a problem—fix it." A specific possible solution, in operational or behavioral terms, is more likely to produce the type of change envisioned by the change agent. For this reason, it is important to give careful consideration to alternative solutions and to be able to suggest the desired alternatives before initiating the change. Some problems may be insoluble, given the constraints of currently available facilities and resources. In such cases, reflecting on possible solutions might lead the change agent to conclude that it would be inappropriate to focus on the identified problem at that time.

*Be prepared to answer the "So what?" question.* Before initiating the change activity, careful thought must be given to what the consequences would be if the individual (or unit) who is the focus of the change effort continued with the present behavior. If the present behavior has no adverse impact on patient care, risk, or resource utilization, it is probably not worth the cost (in both human and economic terms) to attempt the change. For instance, if one physician routinely uses intramuscular penicillin for otitis media, while the majority of his colleagues use oral amoxicillin, the change agent must consider carefully the consequences of permitting the first physician to remain "out of compliance" with the behavior of his peers. If no adverse consequences (patient outcomes, exposure to risk of injury, or unacceptably high cost) are evident, then it may not be appropriate to seek change. Medical practice and health care delivery are sufficiently diverse to allow for a number of acceptable approaches to patient management. Attempts to force rigid compliance with a single approach are likely to meet with failure unless one mode of care has clear advantages over another.

*Don't force the issue.* Excessive zeal in trying to make the point that change is required may produce the same type of cognitive dissonance as an authoritarian change strategy. The harder the change agent pushes to make the point or to elicit an admission of responsibility, the harder the object of the change activity will resist. For this reason, the change agent must control the normal human tendency to force the issue. Stating the problem clearly and describing the desired change fully implies belief in the principle of "rational man" (that is, when informed of a problem and its solution, a "rational man" will take action to correct the problem). Although this may not always prove true, for the most part adults will modify their behavior when they perceive some personal advantage accruing from the change. People are much more likely to conclude that change is in their best interests if allowed to consider the issue, weigh the advantages and disadvantages of change, and reach their own conclusion concerning the desired behavior. Forcing the issue often results in a further determination by the individual or the organization *not* to change, as a demonstration of power, and it is counterproductive to the objective of improving care.

*Use concurrent monitoring to ensure that new behavior is maintained.* Behavior within organizations (such as hospitals) is often determined as much by convenience, administrative procedures, and habit as by the knowledge and skills of people within the organization. To ensure that improved behavior is maintained, therefore, it is important to establish mechanisms for concurrent monitoring of the performance of the individual or organizational unit. This monitoring also serves to protect patients against adverse consequences if the undesirable behavior should persist. For example, if failure to record daily weights on patients with congestive heart failure is found to be the patient care problem and appropriate action is initiated, the review coordinator might engage in concurrent monitoring of this aspect of nursing performance until it is evident that the problem has been corrected and a new behavior integrated.

## Conclusions

Knowledge of theories and techniques to encourage change in both individuals and organizations is as critical to quality assurance as is an understanding of more clinically related concepts, such as frequency of health problems and efficacy, effectiveness, and efficiency of interventions. The most accurate diagnosis of a health care problem and the most valid assessment of the factors contributing to it will not produce the desired improvement unless effective techniques for changing individual and organizational behavior can be applied.

The most useful sources of information to guide those concerned with quality assurance and cost containment are found in the literature on organizational development, planned change, systems analysis, adult learning theory, and the behavioral sciences. By incorporating theories and techniques from these fields into quality assurance improvement planning, change agents will strengthen the potential for success of the quality assurance effort.

The body of knowledge and skills used in managing change is like that of the highly specialized field of neuroendocrinology: not all physicians need in-depth knowledge of the field, but an understanding of its rudiments is an important part of physician competence. Similarly, to be an effective physician and an effective member of the quality assurance team, one must be able to diagnose the organizational problem and know where and when to contact a subspecialist who can treat that problem if health care improvement is to be achieved.

### Suggested Projects

1.  Have a small number of students interested in adult education read Knox (1977).
2.  Give students copies of two of the university hospital medical audits and ask them to review the improvement actions recommended under the "Action" column in Section 3 of the audit forms. Have students critique the improvement actions recommended by the hospital medical audit committee in light of the principles presented in this chapter and the assigned reading.
3.  Have a group of students review quality assurance literature to identify reported examples of successful improvement programs developed in response to deficiencies in care. Discuss the validity of these actions.
4.  Assign the article by Bertram and Brooks-Bertram (1977) evaluating the impact of continuing medical education. Have students indicate what evidence they would require to evaluate quality assurance improvement actions involving continuing education.

# Applying Clinical Problem Solving to Quality Assurance and Cost Containment: A Five-Stage Approach

*John W. Williamson*

ᴊᴇᴊᴇᴊᴇᴊᴇᴊᴇᴊᴇᴊᴇᴊᴇᴊᴇᴊᴇᴊᴇᴊᴇᴊᴇᴊᴇᴊᴇᴊᴇᴊᴇᴊᴇ

The stages of quality assurance are, in principle, parallel to the steps a physician takes in the clinical management of a patient, both in the types of information and in the decision-making process required. Both are problem-solving processes in which particular actions are performed in a logical sequence. When a patient presents with a health problem, the physician follows five basic steps. First the patient's history is taken and a physical examination made, to develop a problem list and test preliminary hypotheses about known or suspected problems. Second, laboratory tests and special procedures are performed to obtain more objective clinical evidence to verify the most serious suspected problem. Third, differential diagnoses are formulated and additional data elicited to identify the most likely cause of the problem and to provide a framework for planning therapy. Fourth, the therapeutic plan is implemented. Fifth, follow-up assessment evaluates the treatment provided and becomes the basis for planning further action; where necessary, this implies recycling to previous stages.

Quality assurance and cost containment studies involve similar stages and require comparable types of information. Here, however, the "patient" is an aggregate of both patients and providers in a medical setting (a hospital or office, for example); the "provider" is the quality assurance team. This group must proceed similarly to the clinician. First, by questioning personnel and examining data, the team develops a list of problems that appear to require attention. Second, the team takes direct measurements to obtain additional information to confirm the most serious suspected problem. Third, to lay the groundwork for therapeutic or remedial action, it obtains more definitive data on probable causes of the problem and other management considerations to formulate a plan of improvement action. Fourth, it implements this plan. Fifth and finally, it reassesses the outcome of the plan to determine whether and what extent the desired improvement was in fact obtained. Here, it may be necessary to go back to earlier stages. Figure 9.1 illustrates this five-stage cycle.

A major point in this analogy is that a quality assurance study must not be limited to rigid techniques for verifying narrowly defined problems. Instead, it should be a flexible process in which problems are identified and traced back to their roots, whether these are behavioral or organizational or whether they lie in the limitation of medical interventions. Students must understand that each of the five stages is concerned with obtaining, assessing, and communicating information. The expected and foreseeable problem need not be the real one; its probable cause need not be its actual cause; and the object of assessment and improvement should not be narrowly defined. Further, students should not assume that recognition of a problem and of ways of alleviating it constitutes a lasting solution.

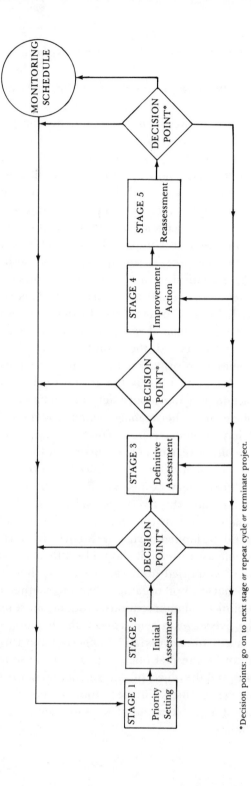

*Decision points: go on to next stage *or* repeat cycle *or* terminate project.

**Figure 9.1. Quality Assurance Cycle for a Problem-Oriented System.**

## Stage 1: Selecting Topics and Setting Priorities

The first and critical stage in a quality assurance study requires that aspects of health care in a given setting be surveyed to identify areas where recognized or suspected shortcomings exist and where health, economic, or intangible (for example, satisfaction, ethical) outcomes could be improved. In selecting topics for study, the time, resources, and personnel required to achieve such improvements must be taken into consideration and weighed against the benefits expected.

*Basic Considerations.* To determine whether a topic both warrants and is suitable for study, the following must be considered:

- The type and characteristics of the health problems involved.
- Their importance to society in terms of number of patients as well as health and economic costs.
- The efficacy and safety of available health care interventions.
- The effectiveness and efficiency of current clinical performance.
- The feasibility and cost of achieving improvement.

These concepts and their implications were reviewed in Chapters Four through Eight. They are briefly repeated here to illustrate their application in the first stage of a quality assurance study.

*Health problems* are a fundamental consideration in that they determine the types of complaints, signs, and symptoms to be studied to achieve clinical identification. They determine the expected health loss if untreated and the potential benefit to be expected if professional management is provided. The nature and type of health problems will ultimately determine probable earning losses and care costs to a given population.

*Importance to society* depends on the frequency of the health problem as well as on considerations of health loss and economic cost. Aside from societal importance, a practical quality assurance implication is whether the problem is of sufficient magnitude to warrant a study that can yield a sufficient number of subjects. For example, a study of physician management of malignant melanoma may be both impractical and of questionable relevance in a short-stay community hospital because of the relatively low prevalence of this health problem in this setting, while such cases may well be of sufficient frequency in a university medical center to warrant study. However, some low-frequency problems, such as dysfunction of a cardiac defibrillator, are of such high importance in any setting as to warrant study.

Many problems, regardless of their frequency in clinical practice, involve relatively little disability or economic cost. To determine whether the health and economic losses associated with a particular health problem warrant study, both its direct and indirect costs must be assessed, as well as the subjective costs of pain and suffering. Direct costs—the amount of time and resources used to manage a particular problem—can be derived from examining charges to patients or the volume of services. Indirect costs are harder to determine because they involve projected financial costs associated with morbidity and mortality, but they are equally important in both the long and short run (see Chapter Five).

Using these criteria, it is unlikely that management of self-limiting respiratory problems would warrant a study, although they are frequent in many settings and contribute to the indirect cost of illness if days lost from work are considered. Management of pneumonia, however, though involving a less frequent health problem, may well warrant a study because of its more serious health implications, the high direct costs associated with care, and the probable morbidity and mortality costs associated with lack of proper treatment. Likewise, problems involving unnecessary surgery are important because they involve health risks and direct and indirect costs: Surgery is expensive; most surgery has specific risks of disability or mortality; productive time is lost; and there are subjective costs of pain and suffering to the patient and family. An example of a topic involving high potential social costs is mismanagement of provider/patient relationships, which can lead to expensive, serious, and time-consuming malpractice suits and thus may be well worth a quality assurance study directly related to a variety of high-risk health problems and patients.

Acceptable evidence of *efficacy and safety of interventions* is necessary where quality assurance centers on specific problems of patient management (see Chapter Six). Although health problems may be important in terms of frequency, health loss, or economic costs, they may not be suitable quality assurance topics because they are not amenable to treatment (for example, advanced carcinoma of the lung). Likewise, when the use of drugs or operative procedures of unproven or controversial effect is examined, developing reliable standards or criteria for assessment of quality of care is difficult, if not impossible. Therefore, problems for which efficacious and safe interventions are available in the judgment of experts and peers are better topics for quality assurance than those involving interventions of uncertain benefit.

Quality assurance must address problems for which there is reason to believe that current performance might be substantially improved in terms of either *effectiveness* (that is, achieving the potential benefit of available interventions) or *efficiency* (that is, achieving this benefit with a more cost-effective use of resources). For example, emergency room diagnosis of trauma patients may be an appropriate topic for an effectiveness evaluation if there is reason to believe that serious internal injuries are being missed, whereas a study of perinatal deaths when there are no indications of inadequate performance would appear irrelevant. Similarly, the provision of barium enemas in the absence of rectosigmoid proctoscopy might be an appropriate topic for an efficiency evaluation if a large proportion without positive findings indicates unnecessary ordering of this test.

Finally, in selecting a topic for study, a team must consider its *improvement potential*—whether the desired improvement is feasible and can be accomplished with reasonable expenditures of time and resources. Although serious performance deficiencies may in fact exist, they are not appropriate topics for study if correcting them would be too difficult or costly. This is true, for instance, where defensive practice behavior would have to be changed in order to effect an improvement (Bertram and Brooks-Bertram, 1977). Problems of overutilization or inappropriate utilization may well exist, but when providers assume that they must protect themselves from legal action even if that means ordering costly tests of questionable value or performing cesarean sections of dubious indication, quality assurance and cost containment efforts may have little success. Selecting an appropriate topic, therefore, includes consideration of how likely a possible solution is to succeed and whether the results will be worth the effort and costs.

In summary, the first major step in a formal quality assurance program is to develop a list of topics, with priority given to those that meet the criteria just outlined. A topic selected for study should reflect a specific hypothesis that a serious problem in health care exists and that there is a realistic potential for achieving a solution.

*A Process for Selecting Topics and Setting Priorities.* To identify and select appropriate quality assurance topics, a series of practical questions must be addressed. Who and how many should be involved in this priority setting? How should those involved be organized? What information is needed? How can judgments about priorities be elicited? Research on decision theory and problem solving indicates that these elements are important to the validity of eventual decisions (Dalkey and others, 1972; Delbecq and Van de Ven, 1967).

1. *Recruitment, organization, and composition of the priority-setting team.* The person charged with executive responsibility for quality assurance and cost containment in a given institution must assemble a team capable of developing a list of high-priority topics. Ideally, this quality assurance coordinator is a physician whose interest and local clinical experience permit selection of a representative team, an interdisciplinary mix of personnel suited to the task by interest and background.

The exact composition of the team will differ in each institution; it must be able, however, to provide a balanced overview of institutional functions, especially in terms of effectiveness and efficiency of care currently provided. Physicians, nurses, pharmacists, and technical personnel should be represented. Their different perspectives and knowledge of specific problems, such as the level of present personnel performance, work loads, interpersonal relations, and condition of equipment and facilities, can prove as important as purely clinical knowledge in identifying areas of possible deficiency and in analyzing the probable benefits and costs of a recommended quality assurance project. At least one member of the board of trustees should be represented on such a team, in view of recent court rulings on the liability and accountability of the hospital board for the professional conduct of health care personnel within the institution. This fact alone requires board members to play an active role in identifying areas in which care provided in their institution may require improvement.

Hospital or clinic administrators, members of the financial staff, ancillary personnel (supply, laundry, and housekeeping services), and patient advocates who represent patient interests and values can also contribute much to priority setting. The quality assurance coordinator should make a special effort to include representatives of these vital functions. Their input for improving efficiency of operations can be substantial, and patient advocates, especially in long-term care settings, can provide important insights for achieving improved effectiveness of care and patient satisfaction. The Joint Commission on Accreditation of Hospitals has recently advocated a multidisciplinary approach in fulfillment of hospital accreditation requirements related to quality assurance.

The size of the priority team is also important. Experience has shown that to function successfully, the team should have seven to eleven members. Having at least seven representative members assures broad experience; having fewer than thirteen avoids unwieldy group dynamics and inefficient use of meeting time (Emlet and others, 1971; Dalkey, 1969; Delbecq, 1969). Experience has also shown that a core group of at least four knowledgeable and respected staff physicians is essential to provide both expertise on efficacy and safety of clinical interventions and personal judgment on present levels of clinical performance in their institution.

Finally, it is important that the team consist of people who can work well together; group intelligence should be equal to more, not less, than the sum of the individual contributors'.

2. *Information sources.* Most of the information required at this stage will come from the experience of individual team members and reflect their points of view. However, any additional available and relevant data will help the team establish more valid and reliable judgments on whether particular topics are suitable for study in light of the considerations addressed earlier. For the frequency of health problems, the sources discussed in Chapters Four

and Five offer much useful data. For example, the Vital and Health Statistics series of the National Center for Health Statistics provides an abundance of precisely categorized national data on the prevalence of health problems in both inpatient and office settings. Local utilization statistics (length of stay, diagnostic-specific discharge rates) and claims review data can provide background information on these as well as on cost aspects. Previous evaluations of quality of care in the institution, whether conducted formally or informally, can provide many clues to areas of potential improvement—for example, medical audits performed to meet PSRO and JCAH requirements, specific Medical Care Evaluation Studies (MCEs), and major tissue or death committee inquiries.

   *3. Eliciting team judgments.* Potential topics for quality assurance study can be identified through informal discussions or the more formal group judgment processes increasingly used in business management. There is evidence that the latter are a more efficient and valid method for singling out problems amenable to cost-effective solutions, and the health professions should seriously consider their use in relation to the decision process of institutional care. Such organizations as the Association of American Medical Colleges, the American Board of Medical Specialties, the American Nurses Association, and the National Board of Medical Examiners have set precedents in this respect. One approach that seems well suited to priority setting is the Nominal Group Technique, developed by Delbecq at the University of Wisconsin School of Industrial Engineering (Delbecq, Van de Ven, and Gustafson, 1975). A modified version of this approach for quality assurance purposes has been published (Williamson, 1978).

   *4. Final topic selection.* The final choice of topics must rest with those authorized to expend funds, hire and discharge staff, and authorize major structural changes within the organization. Depending on the institution, this group may be composed of the board of directors, medical staff, administrative leaders, or a combination of these. Their active participation in the quality assurance process is important because they alone can authorize commitment of funds and organizational changes needed to accomplish improvement when problems of care are discovered. Moreover, the judgments of this group should reflect not only responsibility for institutional policy but as well the ethical, legal, and political considerations that must be taken into account in efforts to achieve quality assurance or cost containment.

### Stage 2: Conducting an Initial Assessment

In the second stage of the quality assurance process, it is usually necessary to obtain objective evidence for the assumption that a problem does exist. To accomplish this, standards and criteria of care are adopted for use in an initial assessment of performance.

*Basic Considerations.* To conduct an initial assessment, it is necessary to consider a number of factors. What is the purpose of the assessment? Is assessment feasible? How should the study be designed? Is it applicable to the local setting? How will the results be analyzed so as to permit a decision whether to continue the study?

The *purpose* of initial assessment is to obtain tentative verification that a problem of care exists and is amenable to improvement. It is important to recognize that the purpose of this assessment of care differs from that of clinical research, which is conducted to develop new knowledge that can be generalized to populations other than those studied. Care assessment involves comparing measured performance against accepted standards. The results cannot be generalized beyond the study population. Consequently, initial assessment is usually best conducted by local peer review.

The second consideration is *feasibility.* In general, initial quality assessment in health care can be practical, feasible, and worth the effort and costs involved. (See, for example, Williamson, 1978; Baker, 1978; Egdahl, 1976.) If a simple topic is selected (as recommended for beginners) and the study is properly designed and conducted, such initial assessments can require less than ten hours of the time of each physician, particularly when a full-time or half-time quality assurance assistant is available and when the effort is multidisciplinary. (Some effort by nurses, record librarians, and perhaps the administrator may be required, depending on the problem to be studied). For feasibility, it is necessary to estimate the prevalence of the health problem. Can at least twenty-five cases be accumulated for study? Will complex diagnostic tests be needed to identify eligible patients? What proportion of the patients and providers can be expected to cooperate?

Concerning the third factor, *design,* measures of care based on accepted criteria reflecting reasonable standards of practice must be obtained or developed to obtain valid assessment results. Criteria of care require quantification of specific aspects of care. If the appropriateness of appendectomies in a given setting is at issue, criteria for surgery such as type and location of abdominal pain and severity of inflammation, white blood cell counts, and tissue pathology might be defined as measures that are applied to a sample of appendectomy patients. These measurements are then compared with standards that serve as benchmarks of appropriateness of medical practice. Such criteria (for example, those developed by the American Medical Association, 1976, or by Payne and Lyons, 1972) should take into account the limitations of current diagnostic procedures and other reasonable factors that would preclude perfect results. The particular method used to conduct the initial assessment depends on the problem being studied.

*Applicability to the local setting* is critical. Quality assessment criteria and standards of care should be approved or developed by local staff and must reflect scientific evidence of efficacy as well as encompass local values and resources. If the physicians whose performance is being assessed do not accept the criteria and standards applied, they are unlikely to accept assessment findings and change their practice behavior. Equally important, valid evidence must be obtained on the efficacy of health care interventions encompassed by assessment criteria and standards. Where adequate efficacy studies are lacking, development of acceptable standards may have to depend on the consensus of experts. However, for certain interventions controlled clinical trials can be cited to establish evidence of efficacy (see Chapter Six and Appendix B).

*Analysis of initial assessment results* will indicate whether and to what extent measured findings depart from accepted standards and whether any such difference is statistically significant. The latter requirement is necessary to preclude further investigation of findings that may be the result of chance distributions only. If assessment indicates care below standards, however, a more detailed investigation is generally required to determine what factors might be amenable to change so as to obtain improvement. It is always possible that, regardless of the statistical significance of findings, the original measurement instruments were invalid or the standards unrealistic. Only more detailed inquiry can establish which is the case in a given instance. Furthermore, if measured findings fall within standards, this does not necessarily imply excellence of care unless patient health outcomes can be assessed directly. In most cases, however, it can only be inferred that where standards are met, the probability of finding correctable deficiencies does not warrant additional assessment effort.

*Processes and Methods.* A number of methods exist for assessing the quality of clinical performance. They range from medical audits and chart review to direct observations of physician performance and outcome assessment of patients (see also Chapter Seven). Since both the theory and practice of quality assessment are in a state of development, these methods vary in their approach and emphasis and also in the reliability and validity of their results (Mushlin and Appel, 1977; Nobrega and others, 1977; Brook, 1974; Fessel and Van Brunt, 1972).

Familiarity with a variety of methods is as important to quality assessment as is an understanding of a variety of diagnostic methods in clinical practice. Some problems, such as physician diagnosis and follow-up of urinary tract infections, can be measured retrospectively from medical charts. However, missed infections may not be discernible from the chart if urine cultures were not ordered or salient questions were missed in obtaining a patient history. Similar problems are involved in assessing blood pressure control. If blood pressure readings are validly obtained and accurately recorded, few information problems are connected with chart review. This assumption may not be safe in many instances, however (Nobrega and others, 1977). Postdischarge health status assessment will almost always require specially designed questionnaires and patient follow-up by either telephone or visit.

Instead of dealing with each of these methods separately, I will outline a few processes that usually form part of the initial assessment.

1. *Sampling and data collection.* The range of patient sampling plans available for assessment studies is important for the implications of subsequent findings and the universe to which they can be generalized. Retrospective, concurrent, and prospective sampling designs can be used, the samples being identified either from such listings as medical charts, tumor registers, laboratory slips, and administrative records or from consecutive hospital admissions or walk-in patients upon first or follow-up contact with a clinic or hospital. Some studies use patient information available from existing sources; in others, direct patient follow-up provides the basis for assessment measures.

The study population should reflect the group of measurable sampling units that represent the universe from which the population at risk and the final study sample are drawn. Sampling frames for prospective sampling can include consecutive annual new enrollees or clinic admissions (initial visits) in a prepaid plan or consecutive hospital admissions, clinic visits (initial and follow-up), and clinic contacts (telephone calls and visits). Retrospective sampling frames can be derived from prepaid-plan enrollment files, medical record files, surgery or tumor registers, laboratory or radiology test files, administrative files, and financial or insurance records.

The study population is considered a subset of a theoretical total hospital or clinic population that cannot be enumerated for any practical purpose (Densen, 1972). A subsample comprising the population at risk for the health problem or intervention that is the assessment focus must therefore be defined from which the study sample can be obtained. Any single characteristic or combination of characteristics can be stipulated for identifying such a population subset, and depending on the study design, this subset can be either at the same risk as the parent group or at higher risk. The first type of subset is obtained by a random or consecutive selection, such as a brief time sample of an annual patient population (every third walk-in patient in one month) or a consecutive subsample of records (every tenth record in the file). More selective factors are used to identify a population subset at greater risk for a given health problem, such as demographic characteristics (all males over 65 for a study of prostatic hypertrophy), clinical symptoms, signs, or laboratory test results (all patients receiving a chest x ray or having "pneumonia" recorded on the radiology report in a study of pneumonia). From this population at risk, a further subset is identified as the study sample—that is, that subset of (or occasionally the total) population at risk to which final assessment measures will be applied.

2. *Standards of acceptable performance.* To determine whether measured performance has potential for improvement, assessment standards are adopted or developed as a benchmark or point of comparison. For example, a team studying missed congestive heart failure among hypertensive patients seen in the emergency room might set a standard of 5 percent as an upper limit for missing such cases. To apply this standard, a cohort of emergency room patients would have to be examined to determine whether they met criteria indicating heart failure. Falling short of such a standard (for example, missing 20 percent of cases) would imply that further study was necessary to confirm the finding and plan improvement actions.

It is generally advisable to obtain such standards before making assessment measures. First, if agreement on standards cannot be reached, the contemplated study should be questioned; second, this procedure permits standards to be obtained without bias from actual findings.

Standards indicating acceptable levels of performance can be obtained or adapted from the quality assessment literature or developed by local study teams. Where the latter course is chosen, the study team must obtain proof of or consensus on efficacy (see Chapter Six) of the interventions assessed and formulate standards in the light of available local expertise and facilities. A literature review of the subject prior to the standard-setting session will generally be required to augment the knowledge and experience of the team members, and expert opinion can provide an additional resource.

3. *Criteria of care.* Clinical care criteria are usually designed for two major classes: diagnostic (problem formulation) and therapeutic (problem resolution).

*Diagnostic performance* can be assessed by measurements to determine the occurrence of two types of errors—false negative (missed diagnoses) and false positives (misdiagnoses)—in each of three categories of clinical judgment: diagnostic screening, diagnostic labeling, and therapeutic planning. Diagnostic screening performance is assessed to measure the accuracy with which patients at risk are identified. For example, of new admissions with one or more indications of possible urinary tract infection, such as a history of chronic pyelonephritis, recent urological surgery, or a positive routine testuria laboratory test, how many patients were so identified by the clinic staff? False negatives here are those patients who were proved by independent assessment study to have had such indications but who were not identified as such, as shown by recorded staff notes, subsequent interventions, or personal inquiry of the physician. False positives are patients without indications who were erroneously identified as being at risk (for example, cystitis recorded in the medical chart when the patient actually had cervicitis).

Generic diagnostic performance is assessed by the accuracy with which patients who actually have a given health problem—as opposed to merely being suspected or at risk—are identified and labeled. Of patients having one or more indications for possible urinary tract infection (for example, recent pregnancy), how many do in fact have such a problem? Again, false negatives are patients with definitive evidence of the health problem subsequently verified by the study team but no positive diagnosis by local clinicians; false positives are those diagnosed as having the problem although the diagnosis was not warranted (for example, an invalid diagnosis of urinary tract infection due to a laboratory error in reporting urine culture results).

Therapeutic planning can be assessed in terms of the appropriateness with which patients requiring a particular therapeutic intervention or alteration of treatment are identified and managed. False negatives in this category refer to patients requiring but not receiving a given therapy and false positives to those who received but did not require it. Of those patients requiring a hysterectomy, how many have this procedure ordered? Of those patients receiving a hysterectomy, how many did not require it?

*Therapeutic performance* can be assessed by levels of health problem control measured by symptoms or specific impairments or levels of total patient health status and functional ability. Here, it is important to recognize that specific impairments do not necessarily correlate with general disability. For example, many patients with severe hemophilia lead normal, active lives. However, some patients with mild hemophilia are totally disabled and inactive, afraid of every possible physical trauma. If a clinician is totally oriented toward isolated health problems and fails to recognize and manage the complexity of factors generally considered outside the responsibility of medical care, therapeutic outcomes in his or her patients may be substandard. There is considerable potential for medical practitioners to improve the results of their performance by recognizing the need for increased competence in such skills as patient health education, facilitating patient self-care, and helping patients cope with general problems of life-style, such as diet, exercise, and stress management.

4. *Analysis.* Having identified the proportion of patients whose diagnosis or treatment failed to meet criteria of performance, the quality assurance team must apply statistical tests to determine whether departures from standards are due to change or within measurement error. The most important point to understand in an analysis of quality assurance study results is that failure to meet quantitative standards does not necessarily indicate poor health care. It is always possible that the quality assessment was invalid, the criteria for identifying deficient performance were incorrect, or the assessment standard was too high.

Consequently, at this stage the only valid conclusion that can be drawn is that more definitive investigation is warranted. In other words, further study will be needed to determine whether the discrepancy between measured findings and standards is due to deficient health care or deficient assessment.

## Stage 3: Definitive Assessment for Improvement Planning

The purpose of the third stage of the quality assurance study is to identify the probable cause of deficient care so that improvement plans can be devised. The results of this definitive assessment—assuming that the findings can in fact be validly attributed to poor care as opposed to poor assessment—will allow the study team to develop specific improvement goals that address the suspected cause of the departure from standards. The problem may have been caused by deficiencies in provider performance or in the organization of the delivery setting, by lack of patient compliance or patient understanding of the health problem, its management, and its course, or by some combination of these. Hence, it is necessary to identify not only probable causes of deficient care but also interpersonal relationships, organizational aspects, physician attitudes, and patient characteristics such as medical coping abilities and compliance. All these may have contributed to the orginal problem and can influence the final improvement strategy. Implementation of this stage of a quality assurance study, therefore, depends on the specific characteristics of the problem identified in initial assessment, and flexibility and perceptiveness are required to identify and establish factors that might be responsible for the departure from standards.

*Basic Considerations.* First, *causes and associated factors must be determined.* When initial assessment results indicate that standards are not being met, more definitive analysis is required to establish that care performance, not the assessment study itself, is deficient. In most cases, there are many possible explanations for the failure to meet standards, and it must always be kept in mind that the assessment study may be deficient rather than the health care provided. Even where deficiencies uncovered in the initial assessment stage are real, and even where measurements are verified, other considerations may invalidate the findings. Were the standards realistic? Is the postulated potential for improvement realistic? The definitive assessment stage must always include a reassessment of standards and of the assumption that improvement is possible.

Second, *improvement planning is required to correct poor performance.* An array of factors must be examined for improvement planning. Diagnostic and therapeutic performance may be insufficient for a wide range of reasons. For example, inadequate patient histories may impede proper diagnosis of urinary tract infections; insufficient patient health education may have rendered efficacious hypertension regimens ineffective; insufficiently precise indications for surgery may make it difficult to assess the necessity of operative interventions; a crowded physician schedule may render useless the results of what might well have been an effective laboratory screening program. The determinants of deficient care can thus vary widely in terms of both the feasibility and the cost of effecting improvement. Inadequate diagnostic results are often attributable to the provider—for example, the lack of adequate response to unexpected abnormalities in screening laboratory test results. Here, improvement planning would have to stress changes in provider behavior. Where both patients and physicians contribute to the problem, educational interventions to achieve improvement may be required for both. If the problem is one of patient compliance only, health education by nurses or trained health educators may be judged less costly than trying to inculcate physicians with these skills.

*Processes and Methods.* Because this stage of a quality assurance study is usually neglected in traditional audit activity, it deserves particular attention. In routine chart audits in short-stay hospitals, the analysis of discrepancies between measured findings and accepted standards is often left up to local hospital quality assurance personnel. Some PSROs will request a letter from the quality assurance team explaining why twice as many one-unit transfusions were being used as accepted standards. Some staff members might discuss the finding and send a letter back to the PSRO. The predominant response is usually one of justifying the measured finding so that no further action seems required. Other hospitals will undertake an educational program to remind their surgical staff about the dangers of, and lack of indications for, one-unit transfusions. In some circumstances such a response would seem reasonable, but for most serious problems uncovered by quality assessment, it is much more fruitful to follow up with a systematic, if brief, check of possible explanations for the measured deficiency. Only on the basis of such an inquiry is adequate improvement planning possible.

The first task is to develop a concise statement of the documented deficiencies. This should include measured findings and accepted standards. For example, one hospital found that, of forty-three consecutive "panic value" clinical laboratory reports (fasting blood sugar over 500 mg), thirty-eight had not been reported, as per required policy, to the attending physician within twenty-four hours (91 percent nonreports, compared with a standard of 5 percent). The next task is to have the study team examine all possible factors that might explain the performance deficiency, assuming that an invalid assessment has been ruled out. Generally, four major categories of determinants should be considered: patient factors, provider factors, organization factors, and health care environment factors. In this example, patient factors would not be applicable. Provider factors could range from physicians who were not accessible by phone to laboratory personnel remiss in trying to contact the physician. Organizational factors might range from insufficient training of laboratory personnel in their responsibilities to serious understaffing. Health care environment factors might include lack of adequate notification of the chief pathologist that he has a legal liability to assure that highly abnormal values are reported promptly, since they can signal mortal risk to the patient if the test result is valid.

If adequate data to establish the most likely determinant of the problem are missing, formal or informal inquiries must be made to identify evidence for, or at least leads to, the likely cause. In the above example, interviewing the laboratory personnel responsible for reporting highly abnormal results would be indicated. The problem might prove to be one of not knowing or of not doing what should have been done. Such information would be the key to designing an improvement plan. If the problem was lack of knowledge, an educational solution would probably be most cost-effective. If personnel shortages existed, this might require a more complicated solution involving the administrator, budgets, and personnel hiring authorizations, which might have to be deferred until more practical approaches were found ineffective.

Once such improvement priorities are set, the team must formulate strategies for achieving improvement and reach consensus on their potential cost effectiveness. Responsibility must be assigned for carrying out the most promising strategy, and a timetable must be recommended. Finally, practical constraints must be recognized and administrative support secured. In the above example, it might be necessary to inform the administrator of the improvement strategy as well as the medical chief of staff.

## Stage 4: Implementing Improvement Actions

At this stage, it is necessary to implement the actions planned in Stage 3 to accomplish improvement. Again, it must be stressed that the approach to change should correspond to the nature of the problem; thus, it can include education, training, restructuring of management or organizational procedures, use of sanctions, or attempts to initiate changes in the overall organization of delivery of services.

*Basic Considerations.* Implementing the improvement plan developed in Stage 3 is primarily a problem of getting the job done—in other words, achieving the changes originally considered feasible. Three tasks are involved: implementing planned actions, evaluating the adequacy of the methods used, and deciding when to undertake a final assessment of overall study impact (Stage 5).

It is often necessary to obtain feedback during the improvement stage to determine whether the improvement plan needs to be modified. Information gained from this feedback may lead to major changes in the improvement program or to a reconsideration of the basic assumptions underlying the original problem. For example, administering brief tests of knowledge to both physicians and patients involved in a program to improve control of hypertension may provide insight into the types of learning procedures necessary to make the educational program more effective.

*Processes and Methods.* As noted for Stage 3, there may be many alternative improvement strategies, and in principle it is best to start with the most cost-effective alternative, moving on to greater effort if necessary. Naturally, if the likely impact of a low-cost action is zero or close to it, that option will not be cost-effective. The questions to be addressed here are the extent to which new personnel or resources or value changes are required. If care of ostomy patients can be improved by providing health education, but present staff has neither the interest in providing nor the expertise to provide this service, hiring a qualified nurse may lead to a very successful program. This relatively expensive alternative will probably be more cost-effective than merely providing educational brochures or handouts, and approach that would not even begin to deal with the complex emotional issues and anxieties of such patients.

Evaluating or monitoring the implementation of the improvement plan requires both data collection and judgment about whether the plan is being carried out as intended and whether it needs to be changed. If a group of hypertensive patients is assessed for blood pressure control in Stages 2 and 3, and if health education is planned for Stage 4, then a small test of patient knowledge, pill counts, and perhaps feedback from the families might be useful information by which to judge the adequacy of the education effort before moving on to assessing its impact on a larger patient sample.

### Stage 5: Reassessing the Results of Quality Assurance Actions

At this stage of the process, the outcomes of the quality assurance study are examined to evaluate how well the improvement objectives have been met and to determine whether care has improved and, if so, whether that is the result of the quality assurance actions and not of extraneous circumstances. If reassessment shows that the improvement objectives have been met and that this result can be attributed to quality assurance, then a monitoring schedule should be developed to reassess the care at specified intervals to ensure that, once achieved, improvement is maintained. If the objectives have not been met, it is necessary to go back to Stage 3, repeating assessment of the nature of the problem or planning more suitable improvement actions. If, after further recycling, the objectives of quality assessment are still not met, a particular topic might be dropped either as not feasible or as requiring more effort than judged acceptable. A new topic would be selected (Stage 1) and the cycle repeated.

*Basic Considerations.* First, the team must *verify improvement.* Evidence acceptable to providers and observers of the impact of quality assurance must be obtained. In the best case, an assessment of the original measurements should be repeated to determine whether tangible improvement has been achieved or standards have been met. As a minimum, consensus among qualified observers should be obtained on whether intangible benefits have been achieved that seem worth the effort expended. In many instances, the nature of the problem or extraneous factors may make careful before-and-after measurements unfeasible. However, documentation of success or failure should be planned to the extent practical. Data will provide the most convincing evidence to observers, especially to regulatory bodies requiring quality assurance programs.

Next, *establish that improvement is attributable to quality assurance*. Even if improvement is confirmed, there must be acceptable evidence that the changes are due to quality assurance actions. Documentation of improvement modalities established in controlled trials and reported in the literature could be obtained. As a minimum, consensus of a group of qualified observers should be obtained regarding possible alternative explanations for any improvement observed. Since quality assurance studies are not research investigations, control groups are rarely practicable. This is no different from medical practice, where it is often not possible to provide controls for the application of therapeutic modalities. Quality assurance teams, like practitioners, must rely on other, less stringent types of evidence. For both clinical practice and quality assurance, however, assumptions about the efficacy of interventions used can be misleading, if not outright invalid. Therefore, at least some systematic effort must be made to question, if not test, such assumptions.

Finally, *establish cost-benefit*. The cost of the quality assurance effort must be measured (or at least estimated) and weighed against the benefit achieved. Ideally, unit costing of related direct and indirect costs by qualified accountants and analysis by an economist should be obtained. As a minimum, consensual cost estimates by a group of qualified observers should be weighed against the extent of confirmed improvement.

Early studies of quality assurance (Institute of Medicine, 1976) reported no conclusive evidence of improvement, let alone convincing cost-effectiveness ratios, for quality assurance efforts. More recent studies (Office of Research, Demonstration, and Statistics, 1980) have begun to demonstrate increased cost savings in the national Medicare program as PSROs have adopted more mature and focused approaches. Although at present, reimbursement is provided for some of the cost of reviewing the care of

Medicare and Medicaid patients, most quality assurance costs are assumed by the hospitals and clinics involved. Hence, it can only be suggested that whatever improvement is confirmed by reassessment must be weighed against the cost of the entire quality assurance project. It will then be largely a matter of values and of resource allocation to determine whether the benefits were worth the costs.

*Processes and Methods.* The steps to be followed in reassessment of a given problem after improvement actions usually involve replication of the original (Stage 2) assessment plan. The more comparable the specific processes of assessment, the more valid will be the results.

Planning reassessment involves several questions. First, who should be reassessed? Some quality assurance improvement actions involve only the study sample. In this case, a second measurement of the same patients and providers would be necessary. However, if the improvement plan covered the total population at risk, then a new sample might be drawn and its care assessed to determine the impact of the improvement program. It is often possible to reduce the sample size in Stage 5 if the previously measured variance is lower than expected.

Second, how should the reassessment be carried out? The same protocol as used in Stage 2 is mandatory if comparable results are to be achieved. It is tempting to alter the original assessment plan in the light of experience or of new ideas for improvement, and an astute judgment is required to determine whether possible gains in validity of the second measurement are worth the loss of comparability.

Third, when should the reassessment be accomplished? Here, a judgment must be made concerning the time necessary for the improvement plan to have taken effect. For most educational plans, the learning curve will likely peak within a few weeks and then drop off. Maximum impact can be established by reassessment as close to this peak as possible. Subsequent measurement will be equally valuable, in that it permits determination of the rate of falloff in improved practice of patient behavior. If old habits reappear and the problem recurs, educational reinforcement can then be planned. For administrative improvement actions, the behavioral change may be reflected in a gradually improving slope as continual reminders become effective. The response to improvement actions varies considerably, and it is a matter of experience and judgment to predict trends and time follow-up assessment.

To implement the reassessment plan and analyze its results, the tasks described in Stages 2 and 3 will have to be repeated. The same statistical tests should be used in Stage 5 to determine whether standards have been met. If standards have not been met, an additional test might be applied to determine whether the second measurement is statistically different from the first. It is possible that some improvement has been achieved even without meeting standards, and this finding may determine whether to repeat the cycle or apply a completely new improvement strategy. If standards have been met, the study can be terminated, with plans for future monitoring if improvement is maintained.

### Conclusions

Although much has been written on quality assurance and many methods for assessing the effectiveness and efficiency of care have been developed, proposed, implemented, and described (see also Chapter Seven; Ertel and Aldridge, 1977; Williams and Brook, 1978), most of this work has centered on the recognition and confirmation of problems. Less evidence is available on, and much less attention has been paid to, establishing the validity of assessment results. Nor has it been shown how, once deficiencies in the delivery of care have been verified and their causes identified, true and lasting improvement can be obtained. In short, it is easier to find fault than to correct it; both teachers and students should remain aware that at this time the diagnostic efficacy of quality assurance methods, though still far from perfect, is more soundly established than their potential for effecting lasting improvement.

The preceding discussion of the five stages required to assess care and to attempt and maintain improvement demonstrates these points. A range of modalities derived from clinical practice, health services research, and professional peer review are available for assessing and verifying deficiencies in care, but principles of adult learning, organizational and behavioral modification theory, and other educational means must be relied on for overcoming deficiencies. Few generally accepted and tested processes have been developed in this respect. Most writers stress that theoretically oriented procedures to assess quality of care have little relevance to daily practice and that research in the behavioral sciences has shown that to achieve even a commitment to change, the direct participation of practicing physicians in all stages of the assessment process is necessary (Riedel and Riedel, 1979). These conclusions are reinforced by three case histories that will be developed in Chapter Ten to demonstrate realistic quality assurance studies in a range of clinical settings.

# Illustrating the
# Five-Stage Approach:
# Case Studies

## John W. Williamson

ⱢⱢⱢⱢⱢⱢⱢⱢⱢⱢⱢⱢⱢⱢⱢⱢⱢⱢⱢⱢⱢⱢ

This chapter provides a practical illustration of the five stages of quality assurance. For each stage, I discuss the methods and results of an actual quality assurance study in an inpatient practice setting (Williamson, 1978). (A similar approach is used in the student volume.) Three additional case studies and a series of questions serve as practical exercises, in conjunction with the information on principles and processes in Chapter Nine.

**A Case Study Illustrating a Five-Stage Cyclic Approach**

*Selecting Topics and Setting Priorities for Quality Assurance*

An initial quality assurance effort in a 350-bed community hospital was conducted in collaboration with faculty members from a nearby state school of medicine. The physicians involved were nearly all board certified in

**207**

the major specialties of internal medicine, pediatrics, surgery, and obstetrics and gynecology.

The study team considered multiple facets of the hospital's operations and selected physician response to unexpected abnormal results of laboratory screening tests as the study topic. The assumption advanced by the chief of pathology and tentatively accepted by the team was that physicians were not responding adequately to laboratory reports of serious and unexpected test abnormalities. If this assumption was confirmed, the team believed, the problem could easily be solved by a program of continuing medical education.

This topic was considered of high priority for a quality assurance study on the grounds discussed in Chapters Four through Eight. Its social importance was clear from its frequency, the seriousness of possible disability if untreated, and the direct and indirect costs of diseases that might be identified by means of fasting blood sugars, hematocrits, and urinalyses. Ample evidence suggested that the sensitivity and specificity of the tests were acceptable in terms of diagnostic validity and that treatments of acceptable safety and efficacy were available for the most common related diseases. The staff agreed that present physician performance was likely to be substandard in detecting health problems early while the conditions involved were still relatively asymptomatic. Finally, if the study confirmed inadequate staff performance, continuing education could be used as an effective tool for improving patient management, and the health and economic benefits of improved care would far outweigh the costs involved in conducting this quality assurance project.

*Initial Health Care Assessment: Confirming the Problem*

The study of physician response to unexpected abnormal test results was directed by the chief of pathology, in collaboration with staff from a nearby state school of medicine. To confirm the original assumption that physicians were not adequately responding to laboratory reports of unexpected serious test abnormalities, an initial quality assessment was conducted.

1. *Methods.* Of a sample of 1000 consecutive admissions to the hospital, 387 abnormal laboratory test reports were identified and checked for unexpected results for

three routine admission screening tests: hemoglobin, fasting blood sugar, and urinalysis. The hospital quality assurance team set a 100 percent response rate as an assessment standard; in other words, it would not accept as satisfactory care any cases involving reports of seriously abnormal laboratory test results for which an adequate response by the attending physician could not be documented. For most patients, an adequate response was defined as a repeat test; mere chart entries that abnormalities had been noted were considered inadequate.

2. *Results.* Assessment of a systematic one-out-of-four sample of 387 abnormal test results yielded 46 unexpected abnormalities. Inadequate physician response was found in 89 percent of cases versus a standard of 0 percent; in 65 percent, there was no response whatsoever. In other words, two thirds of unexpected abnormal reports had elicited no chart notation, repeat test, or recorded follow-up inquiry on postdischarge office visits to the same physician despite serious abnormalities—for example, a fasting blood sugar of over 400 mg% in a patient with no previous history of diabetes or similar findings.

This initial assessment of the quality of care, the second stage of a study, is intended to verify the assumption that a problem does in fact exist and that it is of sufficient importance to warrant further study. As this case illustrates, initial assessment of the selected topic identified a potentially serious problem in patient care management. The extent of deficiency was unexpected, as the physicians providing care were highly respected, most of them board-certified specialists affiliated with the state university school of medicine. The standards set by the quality assurance team were not disputed, as they were based on consensus of the physicians involved. Because the deviation from the standard was so great, there was complete agreement on the need to investigate this problem further and to bring the findings to the attention of the hospital staff as quickly as possible.

*Definitive Assessment: The Basis for Improvement Planning*

To confirm initial assessment findings, a definitive assessment was conducted to provide the basis for improvement planning.

1. *Methods.* To obtain a more definitive analysis of study results, a staff meeting was organized (attended by

nearly all of the hospital medical staff) to examine the results of initial assessment. During the meeting all charts in which unexpected abnormal results were reported were made available to the physicians involved for examination. The assessment team confined its comment to asking the group for consensus on whether the problem was valid, of possibly serious health consequences to the patients, and worthy of concerted effort to seek a solution.

2. *Results.* The hospital staff offered several explanations for the findings—for instance, that laboratory report slips were not posted in the medical record early enough to permit appropriate response. However, after examining their own patients' records, the physicians on the staff were unanimous in concluding that lack of adequate response was a serious problem in terms of implications for patient health and that it required corrective action. Moreover, the physicians accepted personal responsibility for the deficient care provided in nearly every instance.

Definitive health care assessment must lay the foundation for improvement planning. This stage of the quality assurance process involves interpreting and supplementing data gathered in the initial assessment so as to (1) verify the problem identified and (2) identify correctable determinants as prerequisites for planning improvement action.

The entire physician staff was given an opportunity to refute or confirm the credibility of the assessment study. After examining the facts, the physicians accepted the results. Further, they considered the interest generated by the study an indication that improvement could be achieved promptly.

*Implementing and Monitoring Improvement Action*

The quality assurance team believed that the inadequate response to unexpected serious abnormalities established by hemoglobin, fasting blood sugar, and urinalysis screening tests was attributable mainly to physician inattention to screening test results. The first improvement action consisted in holding a hospital staff meeting, where it was decided that each physician would take responsibility for improving response to such tests in the future. To monitor the results of this action, a follow-up sampling of abnormal test results was conducted several months later, using a comparable assessment design. Again, inadequate response was found in 88 percent of unexpected abnormal test results, with no response whatever in 59 percent of reported abnormalities. Since these findings did not differ at a statistically significant level from the results of the initial assessment, the team concluded that further analysis and educational actions were required.

> 1. *Methods.* The data from the chart-review forms were retabulated and results correlated with several variables of interest (degree of abnormality, type of test, and age and specialty of the attending physician). From an educational point of view, it was attempted to reinforce the previous action by newsletters, brochures, and individual letters to the staff physicians, containing a self-addressed postcard asking for explicit acceptance of the study criteria.
> 2. *Results.* Correlation analysis revealed no association between inadequate response and the degree of abnormality, type of test, or physician specialty (with the possible exception of surgeons, whose responses were least adequate). There was a strong direct correlation, however, between physician age and lack of response, in that older physicians hardly ever responded to such test results. However, over 95 percent of the cards were returned, reconfirming general consensus on the study criteria and encouraging the assessment team that significant improvement might be achieved.

The fourth stage of a quality assurance project requires implementing specific actions to accomplish the improvement planned in the definitive assessment stage, as well as carefully monitoring the improvement plan. In principle, the general recognition by professional staff of a verified problem should suffice to produce corrective action. In practice, however, the identification of a problem is rarely tantamount to its solution; at the very least, the behavioral causes underlying it must be elucidated so as to provide not only a rational but a motivational response. In the present case, improvement was monitored and the assessment stage was repeated to provide a more solid basis for improvement planning.

*Reassessment: Determining the Impact of Quality Assurance*

The first improvement action did not lead to statistically significant improvement, and a more concentrated educational effort was undertaken. Subsequently, the original problem of insuffi-

cient response to unexpected abnormal test results was reassessed
to determine whether improvement had now been achieved.

> 1. *Methods.* Using the same sampling and analysis
> methods, a third sample of unexpected, serious laboratory
> test abnormalities was studied six months later.
> 2. *Results.* Physician response had increased to 62
> percent of 59 unexpected test abnormalities, a statistically
> significant improvement over previous assessment findings.
> However, examination of whether this improvement was in
> fact attributable to the educational measures taken led to
> the finding that the hospital's first full complement of in-
> terns had been obtained during the period between the two
> assessment studies and that most of the improvement was
> attributable to response rates for 29 laboratory reports on
> patients assigned to new interns. In the remaining 30 cases,
> the minimum adequate response rate was still only 43 per-
> cent, which was within the range of measurement error of
> the previous findings. In other words, there had been little
> change in the practice behavior of regular staff physicians.

Reassessment of the original problem (lack of physician response to
unexpected abnormal laboratory test results) indicated that no
change had occurred despite renewed effort and monitoring during the improvement stage. Although adult learning theory (involving the physicians in establishing standards and confirming the
assessment results) had been used to bring about change, and careful analysis had been employed to prevent erroneous attribution
of the apparent increase in physician response to the success of
the educational campaign, this failure was due to neglect of a
basic principle of improvement planning: valid formulation of the
problem.

Previous analysis had indicated a strong direct correlation
between physician age and response to unexpected test abnormalities. This clue, in conjunction with the lack of response to
educational exhortation, should have led to the realization that
physician management might have become routine with increasing
years and the burden of a large practice, a matter of habit rather
than of careful analysis of data. Instead, both the study team and
the physicians involved had relied on continuing education
methods, then considered a cure-all for improving health care in
this country. Moreover, they made little or no effort to evaluate
educational efficacy.

*Implementing a Revised Improvement Plan and Repeating Reassessment*

The study effort was continued by repeating Stage 3. Since ingrained habits are difficult to change, a new, noncognitive educational approach was attempted: exposure to a noxious stimulus to draw attention to a bad practice habit.

> 1. *Methods.* On the advice of an educational specialist, an opaque disc was fastened by a piece of red fluorescent tape to each laboratory slip reporting serious abnormalities for the three tests. In order to read the laboratory results, the physician had to remove both tape and disc. This procedure was followed for six weeks, to be discontinued before repeating reassessment. A final sample of sixty-nine unexpected laboratory abnormalities was collected, which was restricted to patients not assigned to interns.
>
> 2. *Results.* At this point, adequate response had increased to nearly 80 percent. Follow-up study six months later showed that over half the improvement had been maintained and that in all likelihood an educational effect had been achieved rather than a mere reflex reaction.

The final step in a quality assurance cycle is to reassess the results of the preceding stages with a view to determining whether, and to what extent, desired goals have been accomplished. It allows the team to evaluate the results of improvement actions, determine whether significant change has occurred, and establish whether such change is in fact related to the quality assurance actions taken and can be maintained over time—in other words, is not merely a monitoring effect. This step is frequently neglected and may be difficult to undertake, but only careful reassessment can provide a reliable basis for planning further action. If the study team in the case study presented had accepted at face value the findings indicating significant improvement after two cycles of the improvement plan, instead of tracing them to the admission of interns to the staff, practice habits would not have been changed. Evidence of attribution is as important in quality assurance studies as in clinical practice, and the need for controlled educational trials is generally overlooked.

Equally important is the recognition that a return to a previous assessment stage may be required to obtain improved results. The several monitoring and reassessment efforts in this study demonstrate the importance of establishing a valid educational diagnosis before prescribing educational therapy. This emphasizes again a major theme of this text—that it is essential to formulate quality-of-care problems accurately before planning how to solve them. In this instance, informational efforts, logical reasoning, and provider recognition of the importance of responding to unexpected clinical abnormalities had little effect. A more valid formulation of the problem, based on factual clues, led to a successful solution and to improvement that was maintained over time.

Finally, this case shows that it is essential to monitor learning achievement periodically and provide educational reinforcement. Learning curves tend to rise to a peak and then descend, and it is entirely possible that if the same problem were now reassessed in this community hospital, staff performance might well be as poor as that originally measured. Systematic and consistent quality assurance programs that provide regular and practically useful feedback may offer an alternative to traditional continuing medical education mechanisms, which may have little specific or measurable impact (Bertram and Brooks-Bertram, 1977).

### Suggested Projects

The following three case studies based on quality assurance projects conducted in a range of medical settings (Williamson, 1978) can be used as exercises that will allow students to apply the preceding information on conducting a quality assurance study. The questions at the end of each case require an ability to identify the stages of the quality assurance study, to supply a list of types of information that would be needed to conduct the study, to estimate direct and indirect costs of the problem if uncorrected, and to suggest ways the studies could have been carried out in those cases in which the full five stages were not completed.

*Case Study 1: Urinary Tract Infection Diagnosis in a*
*University Medical Clinic*

In a university department of medicine, the diagnostic management of urinary tract infections in new patients seen at the medical outpatient clinic was selected for quality assessment study. The topic and setting had been selected to test the twofold assumption that there might be an unacceptably high number of patients with such infections who were being missed (false negative diagnoses) and an unacceptably high number who were erroneously labeled as having such infections (false positive diagnoses). This problem, when it was substantiated, was considered both important and amenable to solution, resulting in improved health care rendered in the clinic and providing educational opportunities for clinic staff.

> 1. *Methods.* A special quality assurance team was to screen a consecutive sample of new clinic admissions for urinary tract infections regardless of their presenting complaints. A detailed history, physical examination, and laboratory tests (urinalysis and qualitative urine culture) related specifically to urinary tract infection were to be obtained before the patient was seen by regular clinic staff. Three months after the preadmission check, the patient's medical record would be examined to determine the diagnosis established by the clinic staff, using the results of the independent, detailed urinary tract infection work-up by the study team as a criterion of diagnostic performance. In consultation with a department of medicine faculty member who was internationally known for his research in pyelonephritis, the following standards were formulated as the basis for assessing diagnostic accuracy achieved by medical school outpatient clinic staff: maximum acceptable false negative diagnoses (missed diagnoses), 15 percent; maximum acceptable false positive diagnoses (misdiagnoses), 20 percent.

In other words, if the clinic staff missed more than 15 percent of the patients having a probable urinary tract infection, or if more than 20 percent of diagnoses were not adequately justified in the judgment of the study team, more definitive study of diagnostic performance would be indicated to confirm initial assessment results and to establish the potential for improving diagnostic performance.

> 2. *Results.* Sampling was concluded when the study team had screened and diagnosed 133 consecutive admis-

sions. Of these, 18 had confirmed bacteriuria and pyuria
with varying degrees of symptoms. Subsequent chart review
indicated that the rate of missed diagnoses (false negatives)
among this group was 56 percent—that is, in excess of the
established standards by a statistically significant margin
(using the binomial goodness-of-fit test; Conover, 1972;
Horn, 1977). Furthermore, this proportion of urinary tract
infections missed by clinic staff may not have reflected the
full extent of missed diagnoses, since the 115 patients classified as true negatives included an additional 14 having
counts of $10^4$ colonies/cc of urine who were not followed for
definitive diagnosis. No false positive diagnoses were found
in the sample.

Initial assessment established an unacceptably high proportion of
missed diagnoses of urinary tract infections among outpatients in a
university medical clinic, as confirmed by a three-month follow-up
of medical charts. Among the explanations for these findings, the
first and most obvious would be erroneous measurements, including the possibility that contaminated specimens resulted in an invalid assessment. Assuming that the initial assessment results were
valid, however, what went wrong with the care provided by the
clinic staff?

    1. *Methods.* The team went back over its data to check
out the possibility of inaccurate measurement on its part.
A resynthesis of the data for each patient, correlating history, physical examination, and laboratory findings, was
completed.
    To check the working knowledge of the clinic staff,
objective multiple-choice questions similar to those on certification examinations were administered. Staff problem-
solving skills were checked by a series of patient management problems requiring sequential inquiry for a simulated
patient described in a written text. Finally, the following
steps were taken to determine sequential performance in
the diagnostic work-up of the 133 patients:

- A list of major cues indicating possible urinary tract
  infections was compiled—for example, recent catheterization, history of nephrolithiasis, recent pregnancy.
- Patients having reported one or more of these cues
  were identified in the separate set of clinical data compiled by the quality assurance team for the total patient
  sample.

- Clinic records were checked to determine whether the medical staff had picked up and recorded the cues and had confirmed a possible urinary tract infection by follow-up laboratory tests, such as checks for bacteriuria.

- The number effectively diagnosed and treated was established for those with positive test results recorded in the clinic records.

2. *Results.* Reanalysis of the clinical work-up of the 133 patients yielded convincing evidence of the accuracy of the initial findings. The fact that an additional 14 patients were found to have had quantitative urine cultures in excess of $10^4$ colonies/cc of urine indicated that there might have been even more cases of urinary tract infection than the 18 found in initial assessment. More important, subsequent analysis of these data by the medical faculty did not seriously challenge these findings. The objective tests of clinical knowledge and patient management skills of the medical students, house staff, and faculty members involved yielded high scores, indicating more than adequate competence. It may be of interest that student and faculty scores were almost identical when compared in terms of both means and ranges.

However, analysis of sequential clinical performance of clinic staff and medical students revealed that, of 108 patients found by the quality assurance team to have had one or more major cues of possible urinary tract infection, only 68 had such findings recorded in their clinic charts at the three-month follow-up review. Of these 68, only 31 were given any screening laboratory tests to check for bacteriuria. Finally, of those checked, only eight were finally diagnosed. In general, it turned out that a finding of pyuria by the clinic staff was the major stimulus to subsequent screening for bacteriuria. Of 54 patients with a history of recently having had "their bladder drained by means of a rubber tube," not one had this fact recorded in his or her clinic chart. In fact, the histories of many of these patients had a note of "no history of catheterization." (It is possible that it a student asked the patient whether he or she had ever been catheterized, the patient might have said no, not understanding the question. Note that this is an example of a correctable determinant of inadequate diagnostic performance that may well be applicable beyond this study.)

Accordingly, it was concluded that although the clinic staff had adequate scientific knowledge and problem-solving skills, these were not being translated into actual clinical practice and that there were serious gaps in diagnostic performance.

In this case, a problem of inadequate quality of care was confirmed, and the focus for improvement was clearly identified as one of physician diagnostic performance. Patient compliance was not a major problem, in that the patients involved had returned, on the average, three times in the three-month follow-up period. Thus, there had been adequate opportunity to diagnose urinary tract problems. Practice arrangements did not seem to be a factor, since facilities in a university medical clinic must have been more than adequate for doing the relatively simple clinical tests required for the diagnosis in question. What was needed, then, was a more sensitive attitude among the clinic staff to cues of possible urinary tract infection and a greater readiness to follow such cues.

Subsequent discussion of the definitive assessment stage by the medical staff revealed a clear consensus that a real problem had been identified and that it was both unacceptably large in terms of the proportion of false negative diagnoses and important in terms of health implications for the patients involved. It was recognized that recurrent urinary tract infection is often not an isolated phenomenon but can be associated with diabetes mellitus and at later stages with hypertension; many of the patients involved had these health problems. Even though the potential for subsequent nephron loss and chronic renal failure in these patients may be debatable, most authorities would agree that symptomatic episodes resulting in acute care or hospitalization can probably be avoided by adequate treatment and that their prevention is important, especially in pregnant women (Naeye, 1979). Therefore, considerable improvement potential in terms of both costs and patient health was present and justified more specific improvement planning.

1. *Methods.* The faculty of the department of medicine was given copies of the quality assurance project report, which was subsequently discussed at a staff meeting. The design, implementation, analysis, and conclusions of the study were scrutinized and verified. It was concluded that the results were sufficiently valid to be taken seriously. A problem existed and seemed amenable to improvement, probably by some educational means.

2. *Results.* The project was published in a leading medical journal (Gonnella, 1970) and was the topic of much

lunchroom conversation. However, in the end no one assumed responsibility for corrective action in the form of educational programs.

*Exercises for Case Study 1*

1.  Indicate to students that the case does not involve all five stages of a quality assurance study as described in Chapters Nine and Ten. Ask them to identify which stages were completed, what approach the team used at each stage, and which stages were omitted.

2.  Ask students to assume the role of quality assurance coordinator in the university medical center described in the case and to outline a strategy to decrease the percentage of missed urinary tract infections. The following questions will have to be addressed:

    a.  Who would be involved in the problem and what roles would they play?

    b.  How would the selection of this topic be justified to the clinic staff in terms of frequency? Health and economic importance? Efficacy of diagnostic interventions? Improvement potential? (This requires searching the literature and using national and local data on frequency and costs.)

    c.  What specific improvement actions could be taken? (Students should recall the basic principles and processes for planning and implementing an improvement action.)

    d.  What immediate feedback, before reassessment of the problem, would help determine whether the plan was proceeding successfully?

    e.  How would reassessment be conducted?

3.  To include a consideration of costs,

    a.  Ask students to identify the stages in the quality assurance process where cost information should be examined and how this information should be used.

    b.  Ask students what kinds of costs would have to be examined to make an assessment of the cost-benefit of the quality assurance study.

c.	Have students estimate the direct costs of providing improved care (include such factors as laboratory tests, repeat visits, time spent with patients, personnel, and facilities).

d.	Have students estimate the indirect costs that would accrue if the health problem were left untreated in the following instances: pregnant women aged twenty-five to thirty-five; diabetic women aged twenty-five to thirty-five; women with hypertension aged twenty-five to thirty-five. (This will require knowledge of health loss and associated mortality and morbidity costs.)

e.	Ask students to identify the intangible costs (pain, suffering) associated with this condition if untreated.

f.	Estimate tentative health loss, financial, and intangible costs associated with failure to correct this problem and compare them with the estimated costs of the quality assurance study.

*Case Study 2: Hypertension Control in a Health Maintenance Organization*

In a prepaid multispecialty group clinic, hypertension control in adults aged thirty-five to sixty-five was selected as a quality assurance topic. Fourteen primary care physicians, mainly internists, participated in the study, undertaken to test the assumption that an unacceptably large proportion of patients with diastolic hypertension were out of control and at risk of serious complications (such as stroke or heart failure). The quality assurance team justified selection of this study topic on the grounds that improved follow-up and therapeutic management by the clinical staff could reduce the number of patients at risk.

1. *Methods.* To make an initial assessment of the extent of the suspected problem, the team studied a one-month consecutive sample of 248 walk-in patients having essential hypertension—that is, patients who had at least one previously recorded diastolic pressure reading greater than 110 mm Hg. The study team set a standard of 5 percent as the maximum acceptable noncontrol rate. In other words, if the average of the three readings was above 100

mm Hg in more than 5 percent of the sample of hypertensive patients, more definitive study of this problem would be indicated. On each visit during the study, three independent blood pressure readings were taken with the patient in a resting state. It was agreed that if these three readings averaged less than 100 mm Hg, diastolic blood pressure was under control.

2. *Results.* The study revealed that 36 percent of the patient sample was out of control. This represented a statistically significant deviation from the 5 percent noncontrol rate standard set by the team as a standard of therapeutic management.

Having found evidence of a potentially serious problem of patient management, the team undertook further study to verify these findings and to determine whether any of the factors involved was amenable to improvement. In view of the high noncontrol rate and the serious prognostic implications for this patient group, no questions were raised about whether the standards applied were overly stringent, although the feasibility of achieving blood pressure control in 95 percent of a group of nearly 250 patients, most of whom were poor or of working-class background, might well be questioned. It was postulated that the noncontrol rate in excess of the standard could be explained by one of two alternatives: (1) inadequate therapeutic management by providers or (2) lack of compliance by patients in following the antihypertensive regimens. Before any improvement action was advocated, the team decided to validate the initial findings and to determine the cause of the noncontrol rate.

1. *Methods.* To check the validity of the initial assessment findings, both study design and data were reanalyzed, and results of similar studies in other HMOs in the region were examined.

2. *Results.* Reanalysis of the original assessment data not only confirmed the high proportion of patients out of control but indicated that it was probably conservative in view of the criteria used. If 95 or 90 mm Hg diastolic pressure had been used as the indicator of control, over half these patients might have been considered "out of control." Comparisons of the study with related HMOs with similar patient populations (poor and working-class) revealed comparable findings, indicating that a widespread patient management problem in fact existed.

It had been decided that if the noncontrol rate was confirmed, tests of physician knowledge and patient compliance would be used to determine the probable cause of the problem.

1. *Methods.* An objective written test developed to establish clinical knowledge of hypertension management, particularly with regard to chemotherapy, was administered to the physicians to determine adequacy of therapeutic management and their acceptance of assessment standards. Physicians were also tested to ascertain their judgment of the degree of compliance by their patients with the prescribed regimen. These tests were administered to all fourteen primary care HMO physicians involved (mainly internists). A patient compliance test was used to determine patients' knowledge of their condition, medication schedules, side effects of drugs, and probable effects of absence of treatment. Pill counts were made to establish compliance in taking antihypertensive medication.

2. *Results.* Replies to the physican questionnaire indicated that physicians accepted the quality assessment design and the criteria used. None had inadequate pharmaceutical information on the management of patients with essential hypertension, but ten out of fourteen physicians (71 percent) seriously overestimated the extent of their patients' compliance with prescribed treatments, and eleven out of fourteen failed to mention patient health education as a component of hypertensive patient management.

Responses to 149 out of 248 patient questionnaires (a 58 percent response rate) showed that 15 percent were unaware that they were hypertensive or that their doctor was treating them for this problem; 20 percent lacked information on the drug regimen prescribed by their doctor; 81 percent could not state any side effects associated with the drug they were taking; and 93 percent did not know that there is little or no relation between symptoms and consequences of uncontrolled high blood pressure. Moreover, 26 percent were not taking the medication prescribed, and 28 percent took their pills sporadically, mainly when they had headaches, which they attributed to their high blood pressure. In the aggregate, 95 percent of responding patients were judged to have inadequate information regarding their condition, and 54 percent were taking or obtaining inadequate medication.

In view of the proportion of hypertensive patients who were out of control and of the consequences to patient health in terms of unnecessarily high risks of stroke, heart failure, and renal disease

(Smith, 1977, 1979; Veterans Administration Cooperative Study Group on Antihypertensive Agents, 1967, 1970, 1972), the quality assurance team acknowledged that further effort was warranted. The assessment findings confirmed studies (for example, Brook, 1974) that reported few differences in blood pressure control rates among treated and untreated patients because of poor patient compliance. Consequently, there was little doubt that intensive health education was called for to improve compliance and to enable physicians not only to provide more adequate information to patients but also to communicate this information in such a way that patients could understand and act on it. A controlled educational trial at Johns Hopkins (Inui, Yourtee, and Williamson, 1976) has shown that physicians can indeed be taught to provide more adequate health education and achieve better blood pressure control in their patients. The quality assurance team concluded that a range of factors had been identified that might be responsible for the high noncontrol rate measured and that these factors appeared amenable to improvement. The results of the patient and physician questionnaires provided the necessary details for designing a program of improvement.

      1. *Methods.* A quality assurance assistant was authorized to establish a regular return-visit schedule for hypertensive patients. The purpose of the return vists was to monitor blood pressure status, test patients' understanding of their disease, and provide education about possible complications and treatment, including the necessity to stay on medication and to be aware of possible toxic effects. Special emphasis was to be placed on ensuring patient understanding that the dangers faced in hypertension have little relation to overt symptoms, that transitory symptoms such as headaches can be entirely unrelated to high blood pressure, and that absence of symptoms should not affect an antihypertensive regimen.

      After surveying a range of health education materials that had been compiled, most of which the staff thought irrelevant to the specific needs of this group of patients, the quality assurance team designed some simple visual aids and questions to test patient understanding. Special encounter forms were prepared to record the medication being taken. A six-week revisit schedule was set up for patients who were out of control or indicated poor under-

standing of their problem. Patients were sent letters from
their physicians informing them that they would be contacted by HMO quality assurance staff to set up a series of
appointments. It was explained that this program was not a
research study but a systematic effort on the part of the
HMO to improve benefits of the health care provided by
the clinic.

The team designed a second education program for
the physicians, providing information on the degree of
therapeutic compliance by each physician's hypertensive
patients. For those who requested it or showed inadequate
understanding of the management of the essential hypertension patient, relevant literature (for example, on the
controlled clinical trials by the Veterans Administration,
1967, 1970, 1972) was provided.

2. *Results*. Over 50 percent of the patients responded
favorably and set up a series of appointments with the quality assurance assistant; others, preferring to remain with
their own physicians, retained their usual appointment
schedule. Patients who chose to visit the quality assurance
assistant were very cooperative in responding to the questionnaires and to questions probing for understanding of
their health problem. The visual aids proved successful
once certain modifications were made (for example, trans-
lation into Spanish) to compensate for such problems as
language barriers. Improved understanding was obtained,
as shown by the proportion achieving better than 80 percent overall on the written questionnaire after several
months of educational effort. Pill counts indicated apparent
success in maintaining the prescribed medication schedules.
Several patients who were not responding in terms of blood
pressure control were referred to their physicians for a
check and possible alteration of treatment. An unexpected
result was an improvement in patient satisfaction and in
provider/patient relationships. Many patients found it helpful to have someone listen to them about the stress of their
daily life and reported looking forward to the contacts with
the quality assurance assistant.

Physician cooperation with the program was satisfactory, although at first there had been some reluctance to
take formal knowledge tests. A major accomplishment was
that practically none of the physicians remained unaware of
compliance problems on the part of their patients. As a
result, physicians cooperated more fully with the quality
assurance assistant in writing letters to their patients urging
them to participate in the health education program and
spending more time on patient health education during
regular patient visits. At the end of a three-month period,
repeat testing found that none of the physicians lacked

understanding of or refused to accept health education as an essential therapeutic modality in the care of the hypertensive patient.

Six months later, hypertension control rates were reassessed by sampling the same group of patients. A marked change in health problem status was found; the overall rate of noncontrol had dropped from 36 to 19 percent, a statistically significant improvement, although still four times the standard of 5 percent set at the outset of the quality assurance study. The group of 148 patients who made regular appointments with the quality assurance assistant achieved twice the improvement observed for the 100 patients who had insisted on seeing only their own physicians for help in controlling this problem. (In percentage terms, improvement in the latter group was almost identical to that measured by Inui, Yourtee, and Williamson (1976) in a controlled educational trial, where patient health education regarding hypertension was offered only by the physicians providing care.)

Given acceptable evidence of improved blood pressure control, the team tried to determine whether the change in this group of patients could be attributed to the improvement actions.

1. *Methods.* An outside group supervising the study rechecked the data and data collection methods.

2. *Results.* The increase in the control rate of the group seeing only their physicians seemed reasonable in view of the data from the controlled educational trial. In other words, there was evidence that teaching physicians better skills in patient health education can have a beneficial effect in terms of specific measured health outcomes. The even greater improvement for patients also seen by a quality assurance assistant and instructed in aspects of compliance with prescribed regimens may reflect the effectiveness of this specific improvement modality, an assumption supported by controlled studies of patient compliance conducted by Sackett and Haynes (1976). What could not be determined was whether the significantly greater improvement in the group monitored by the quality assurance assistant was due entirely to the improvement program, which involved more frequent visits and possibly stress management as well. It may have been due in part to self-selection of a more compliant or less severely ill group of patients and to the specific health problem involved.

This study represents a successful example of planning and conducting an improvement program. It was expressly designed to correct the problem existing in this practice setting, however, and the reader should not conclude that focused health education is a panacea. The results of a controlled trial of patient education in improving household safety (Dershewitz and Williamson, 1977) show that however successful a particular improvement method may be in one setting for a particular problem, it may not prove effective in different circumstances.

*Exercises for Case Study 2*

1.  Ask students to identify the quality assurance stages that were completed in this study and discuss the approach used in each stage.
2.  Review the types of quality assurance information required (health problem importance, efficacy, effectiveness and efficiency, improvement potential). Ask students to give evidence from the case that the information obtained indicated that this health problem warranted assessment and improvement.
3.  Discuss the standard set by the quality assurance team. What evidence is there that this standard was appropriate? Inappropriate?
4.  Ask students to identify unforeseen factors of this study that may have contributed to the improvement in outcome among both physicians and patients. Discuss implications of these factors for future practice.
5.  Organize groups of about five students and instruct each group to identify other assessment topics that might be selected for study in a similar setting. Ask each group to reach consensus on an acceptable standard of performance and then document the validity of the standard by consulting the literature. Ask each group to identify criteria for comparing actual performance with standards.
6.  Using the same groups, discuss the health loss to be avoided and potential direct and indirect cost savings for each topic selected if a successful quality assurance effort were undertaken.

7.  Have each group, using the case on hypertension control as a guide, design an improvement plan for the topic selected by the group (*Reminder:* Information acquired in completing Question 5 must be taken into consideration.)
8.  Have each group predict the results of the improvement actions in terms of health benefits and cost savings and design a plan for reassessing the results of the quality assurance effort.

*Case Study 3: Postendarterectomy Status of Patients in a Fee-For-Service Multispecialty Group Clinic*

A large fee-for-service multispecialty group clinic and associated hospital elected to study the postsurgery status of patients who had undergone carotid endarterectomy. The surgeons involved were nearly all board certified. The purpose of the study was to assess the overall health status of the patients after surgery. The topic had been chosen to confirm whether too many of these patients might be unnecessarily disabled after surgery and whether improved clinical management might reduce disability.

1. *Methods.* To determine overall patient health status after carotid endarterectomy, a retrospective consecutive sample of approximately 100 patients who had undergone this operation within a four-year period was drawn from the hospital surgical register. Two standards were set: no more than 9 percent deceased at time of follow-up and no more than 34 percent incapable of performing major or daily life activities because of ill health. Each patient was interviewed either in person or by telephone (average follow-up point, eighteen months after surgery), using a standard questionnaire to measure overall functional levels, ranging from being able to return to "major life activities such as occupational work or retirement activities" or "to carry out daily living functions such as independent eating, dressing, and toileting" to partial or complete dependency (Williamson, 1978).

2. *Results.* Of a total sample of 112 consecutive patients having undergone carotid endarterectomy in the four-year sampling period, complete interview data were obtained for 104 (a 93 percent completion rate). The measured health status findings, at the average follow-up point of eighteen months after surgery, revealed that 62 percent were unable to perform major life activities and 26 percent

had died. Thus, both mortality and disability rates were in
excess of standards by statistically significant margins; the
death rate was three times that considered acceptable, given
patient age, other illnesses, or complicating conditions. The
number experiencing an unacceptable level of disability was
nearly twice the standard, involving two out of three patients sampled.

The results of the assessment thus confirmed the judgment of the
priority team that had selected this topic: The postsurgery
mortality and disability of carotid endarterectomy patients were far
greater than considered acceptable at eighteen-month follow-up.
Possible explanations included (1) invalid assessment due either to
inadequate measurements or to unrealistic standards, (2) inappropriate diagnostic judgment of operability, (3) deficient surgical
technique, and (4) lack of appropriate rehabilitation, taking into
consideration age and expected associated infirmities.

1. *Methods.* The quality assurance team, in checking
the accuracy of the findings, first examined the original
outcome standards and repeated the standard-setting process, giving particular attention to the specific clinical
characteristics of the group of patients sampled, as the surgical staff involved now claimed that the original standards
had been too stringent. The team also verified the sampling
method and results as well as the statistical analysis. Outside
specialists were contacted for informal consultation and
consensus on adequate diagnostic justification for this
operative procedure. Postoperative mortality was analyzed,
although assessment of surgical technique seemed too sensitive a question for examination at this point.
      Continuity of postoperative care was checked by
examining the extent of communication with the patients
about return for reexamination. Finally, the original patient
group was divided into three groups according to prognosis, the assumption being that most of the disability would
be in the older group having the greatest amount of associated preoperative disease and infirmity.
      2. *Results.* Examination of initial assessment findings
confirmed the original measurements. Reformulation of
outcome standards by prognostic group resulted in essentially the same distributions as originally developed.
Analysis of differential outcomes in the three prognostic
groups revealed a similar extent of postoperative disability,
including mortality, in all groups—that is, younger, low-

risk patients had the same proportion of deaths as older, high-risk patients. In all, at eighteen-month follow-up, fifteen had no postoperative care recorded and eight died of a stroke immediately after surgery; thirteen ultimately had symptoms of cerebral vascular accident before death, with twelve having an associated myocardial infarction. Further, the opinions of two outside experts who had been provided with the clinical details implied that an inappropriate group of patients may have been operated on.

Despite these definitive assessment results, the clinic and hospital staff involved ultimately disavowed the study and refused to allow the quality assurance team to reevaluate the staff's diagnostic criteria and indications of operability. The reason given was that they had wished only to do a research study into the extent to which this procedure would prevent strokes. Because the surgical staff denied the existence of a problem, no formal improvement program could be instituted. However, follow-up by the quality assurance coordinator revealed that the number of carotid endarterectomies had decreased after the study; it also appeared that a somewhat different group of patients was being operated on. It seemed possible, therefore, that the original quality assurance program had been indirectly effective, at least in terms of changed physician behavior. However, objective conclusions could not be drawn without the benefit of formal chart review, discussions with the surgical staff, and follow-up contact with patients.

*Exercises for Case Study 3*

1.   Conduct a discussion on the appropriateness of this topic as a quality assurance study in terms of health problem frequency, health loss and economic costs, and efficacy of the surgical intervention. Give particular attention to the effect on the quality assurance study of the absence of documented evidence of both criteria for operability and effectiveness of the procedure.

2.   Ask students to identify the stages of the quality assurance study that were completed and to critique the methods used at each stage.

3.  Ask students to identify both the stages that were omitted and the factors that may have contributed to the failure to complete the study.

4.  Indicate to students that this case may illustrate one of the major obstacles to assessing and improving care through quality assurance efforts. Ask them to identify that obstacle (namely, difficulty in influencing physician behavior) and to discuss modalities that could be used in overcoming it.

5.  Ask students to design improvement actions that would have been appropriate had the unacceptable mortality and morbidity rates been attributable to (1) surgical technique; (2) inappropriate diagnosis regarding operability; (3) lack of appropriate patient follow-up, including rehabilitation; (4) health care delivery, including organization of the clinical staff.

6.  Ask students to estimate the direct and indirect costs associated with this procedure and the unacceptable rates of morbidity and mortality. Compare these costs with estimated cost savings had the standards been met. Discuss the costs that could have accrued in carrying out the quality assurance improvement actions designed for Question 5 and compare these costs with the estimated health loss and economic costs of leaving the problem uncorrected.

# A Review of Selected Quality Assurance and Cost Containment Programs

*Mohan L. Garg*

🙐🙐🙐🙐🙐🙐🙐🙐🙐🙐🙐🙐🙐🙐🙐🙐🙐🙐🙐🙐🙐🙐🙐🙐

This chapter reviews the general state of the art of teaching quality assurance and cost containment in academic medical centers from 1971 to the present. It provides background on the strengths and weaknesses of existing programs so that readers can benefit from others' experience in planning and implementing quality assurance and cost containment curricula.

**Status of Quality Assurance and Cost Containment Teaching**

In 1973 Kane and Hogben surveyed departments of community and/or preventive medicine to assess ongoing and planned activities in quality-of-care assessment in U.S. medical schools. The survey, which had an 80 percent response rate, indicated that twelve departments offered a course in medical auditing or quality of care. Of these, only seven were exclusively or primarily devoted to auditing; the other five were survey courses in medical care delivery in which auditing constituted only a portion of the course. Eight schools offered auditing courses through other departments: three in schools of public health, two in departments of medicine, one in biometry, one in continuing education, and one in hospital administration (Kane and Hogben, 1974).

In 1974 the Joint Commission on Accreditation of Hospitals (JCAH) surveyed 118 accredited medical schools to determine to what extent undergraduate course work was being offered in health care evaluation research. Of the 107 schools responding, 83 stated that no courses were offered in this area. In the 24 schools where some course work was available, the offerings ranged from a one-hour lecture to five full courses. In only seven of the 24 schools was evaluation research a requirement rather than an elective (Carroll and Becker, 1975).

To create additional support for curriculum development efforts, the Association of American Medical Colleges (AAMC) organized a symposium in Washington, D.C., in June 1975. The participants, a limited number of medical school faculty members plus representatives of the Department of Health and Human Services (then DHEW), were invited to explore ways in which quality assurance, specifically peer review, could be effectively introduced at the undergraduate and graduate levels of medical education. Four of the medical schools (University of California, San Francisco; University of Utah; University of Illinois Rockford School of Medicine; Medical College of Ohio, Toledo) presented an overview of their programs, which are discussed briefly in this chapter. The symposium recommended that peer review and chart audit be introduced as an important ingredient of undergraduate medical education; that quality evaluation be taught throughout the continuum of undergraduate and graduate medical education; and that this teaching not be restricted to any particular academic department or division.

Subsequently, AAMC conducted two workshops, one in

1977 and another in 1978, as a practical step to promote the development of quality assurance programs at academic medical centers. The workshops, funded by the National Fund for Medical Education, were to assist medical schools in developing quality assurance and cost containment programs.

Stimulated partly by these activities and partly by escalating public concern about quality and cost of care, several other academic medical centers initiated some curricular activities at various points in their educational cycle. In July 1978, AAMC again surveyed all 118 accredited medical schools to reassess progress in teaching program development. The survey, which had a 100 percent response rate, indicated that 41 schools had identifiable programs in quality assurance and cost containment, of which 21 were operational and 20 in the planning phase. A follow-up survey of these 41 schools was conducted to obtain more specific information on program goals, objectives, methods of approach, and early evaluation results.

The following section briefly describes selected quality assurance teaching programs conducted in five medical schools and affiliated teaching hospitals in the early 1970s. The next section discusses in greater detail four programs instituted after 1975 that focus specifically on quality assurance and cost containment. Finally, the last section summarizes several new approaches to quality assurance and cost containment teaching initiated since 1978, with a view to presenting the most recent developments in the field at the time of this writing.

### Early Teaching Programs

By 1973 five academic medical centers—Medical College of Ohio, Toledo (MCOT); University of Utah; University of Illinois, Rockford School of Medicine; University of California, San Francisco (UCSF); and Michigan State University—had initiated modest teaching programs in quality assurance and cost containment. Each of these medical centers had its own goals and objectives as well as its own methods and level of involvement. Student responses to these programs differed greatly. As a result, some were discontinued, and the others were modified in accordance with student demands or emerging societal concerns.

Although each of these programs developed rather independently, they shared the following characteristics:

- In each program the educational experience was built around management of individual patients and emphasized assessment of care provided to individual patients.
- Chart audit was the predominant method used, with standards and criteria developed by peer groups (that is, students and residents). In two instances (Rockford and MCOT), the programs used peer review in the strict sense (students reviewed each other's charts), whereas in other settings students conducted audits by reviewing charts of staff physicians and faculty members as well as of students and residents.
- In each program students developed their own criteria based on local practice even though nationally derived criteria for inpatient chart audit were available (for example, AMA guidelines). Faculty members considered the process of developing criteria an excellent learning experience.
- Each program was evaluated, although the precise method of evaluation differed across sites.
- None of the programs continued as originally designed; three were discontinued and two were significantly modified.

In the programs at MCOT, Utah, and UCSF, quality assurance teaching centered on the use of the problem-oriented medical record. In addition, a major objective of two of the programs (MCOT, UCSF) was to familiarize students with PSRO activities and requirements: utilization review, peer review through chart audit, medical care evaluation studies, and profiling.

The major strengths of these early programs lay in the commitment and competence of the faculty, in that program developers were knowledgeable about quality-of-care assessment and highly motivated to integrate it into student training and educational experience. Moreover, most faculty members felt that the involvement of students and residents in setting criteria and standards for quality-of-care evaluation had improved patient management skills.

However, a number of weaknesses detracted from the effectiveness of these early programs. Most were elective and had to compete with other learning experiences that responded more immediately to the students' general orientation to biomedical science and clinical proficiency. As a result, programs were not popular among students and house staff, and evaluation showed little positive educational benefit. Methods for assessing care were limited to utilization review, peer review, chart audit, and physician profiling (that is, PSRO activities). Cost and resource utilization were not formally considered except in hospital utilization review activity. Health care assessment using aggregated data for larger populations was neglected in analyzing practice patterns for quality and cost management.

Table 11.1 summarizes the goals, objectives, student level, learning activities, and evaluation results of these early programs.

## A Second Generation of Programs

On the basis of an evaluation of their early programs, the Medical College of Ohio at Toledo and the University of Illinois Rockford School of Medicine instituted modified and improved quality assurance curricula. New teaching programs were developed at the University of Missouri, Kansas City, the University of Wisconsin, and the University of Pennsylvania. A brief description of these programs follows.

*Curriculum Changes and Modifications*

*Medical College of Ohio, Toledo.* Guided by the evaluation results of its previous four years of teaching peer review and medical audit, the faculty at MCOT restructured and broadened its teaching programs in 1975. The new goal was to teach a wider range of methods to evaluate the quality and cost of care, emphasizing the importance of self-assessment and peer review for the practicing

**Table 11.1. Early Quality Assurance Teaching Programs.**

| | | | Institution | | |
|---|---|---|---|---|---|
| | *Medical College of Ohio, Toledo* | *University of Utah* | *University of Illinois, Rockford* | *University of California, San Francisco* | *Michigan State University* |
| Program goal(s) | To prepare students for participation in PSROs | To teach medical care auditing | To develop positive attitudes toward peer review and quality assurance | To teach medical record-keeping skills and peer audit | To teach peer review processes early in professional training |
| Student objectives | To become familiar with PSROs<br>To learn patient and practice profiling<br>To learn medical audit methods<br>To participate in student peer review | To be aware of various forms of medical care evaluation<br>To maintain and audit a problem-oriented record<br>To develop audit criteria<br>To evaluate quality from chart | To become comfortable with peer review<br>To develop and apply patient care criteria | To understand need to assess care efficiency and professional accountability<br>To understand areas of professional and institutional liability | To learn goals and objectives of peer review<br>To develop criteria of care<br>To participate in peer review |
| Program length | One month | 24 hours | Continuous over six-month period | 24 hours | During twelve-week clerkship |
| Student level | Senior clerkship in ambulatory care | Open to all medical students and family practice residents | Second-and third-year medical students in community health centers | Third-and fourth-year medical students, residents, pharmacy and nursing students | Second-year medical students |

**Table 11.1. Early Quality Assurance Teaching Programs, Cont'd.**

| | (Mandatory) | (Elective) | (Mandatory) | (Elective) | (Elective) |
|---|---|---|---|---|---|
| Program activities | Introductory two-hour seminar on general issues<br>Student development of diagnostic and management criteria<br>Student design of a quality assurance study<br>Student sampling of charts and records<br>Student utilization of POMR and other record systems | Eight two-hour didactic sessions on principles of auditing<br>Two three-hour field sessions with students conducting medical audits in community settings | Student development of care criteria for individual patients<br>Chart review by student peers<br>Student review of individual audited charts<br>Student review of faculty-generated criteria | Eight two-hour lectures and lab sessions on POMR and medical audit for students<br>Four two-hour lectures on data systems, outcome measurement impact on local community, utilization review for students<br>Student participation in "mock audit" committee<br>Lectures on UR, criteria development, and auditing for residents<br>House-staff development of criteria for utilization and quality | 12 two-hour sessions of lectures and practical exercises (planned)<br>Orientation to peer review (completed)<br>Student generation of minimal criteria at initial stage (completed)<br>Student refinement of consensus criteria (planned)<br>Student review of peers (planned) |

Table 11.1. Early Quality Assurance Teaching Programs, Cont'd.

| | | | | | |
|---|---|---|---|---|---|
| Evaluation results | Students had improved attitudes toward PSRO and peer review | Students found course relevant, suggested that it be made mandatory, gained in skills but retained negative attitudes toward peer review | Students showed little improvement in objective measures of diagnosis and therapy and retained negative attitudes toward audit and peer review | Students improved record-keeping skills through use of POMR but remained indifferent to utilization review  Residents' skills in and knowledge of UR varied despite uniform program content in three different sites | Program was discontinued at midpoint because students felt inadequate to develop criteria and uncomfortable with peer review |
| References | Mulligan and others (1976) | Kane (1973a, 1973b) | Barr and others (1976) | Barbaccia (1976) | Greenbaum and Hoban (1976) |

physician (Mulligan and others, 1976). PSRO activities and their effect on physician practice continued to be emphasized, but new objectives were developed as well. Students were to examine other methods of assessing care, develop implicit and explicit criteria, expand chart audits to cover both inpatient and outpatient care, explore the issue of inflation in health care cost, and understand the role of the physician in generating costs (Garg, Kleinberg, and Gliebe, 1978). Quality assurance and cost containment teaching was expanded beyond the original senior clerkship ambulatory care and integrated into every phase of the medical student's education.

Some of these changes became part of the ongoing curriculum in quality assurance and cost containment. For example, a ninety-minute lecture given as part of the course "Introduction to Clinical Medicine" is used to present quality assurance legislation (the Social Security Act of 1965 and the 1972 amendments) and to discuss the implications of peer review for medical practice. Quality assurance and cost management issues are also discussed at revised clinicopathological conferences (CPCs) conducted as part of the body system curricula. During each CPC, students review subjective and objective findings of patient work-up and the treatment plan, noting discrepancies between findings and treatment as well as examining the utility of each diagnostic test ordered in light of its charges and appropriateness. Students are supplied with a listing of all diagnostic procedures performed in the hospital and associated charges.

During the one-month clerkship in ambulatory care and community medicine, three weekly seminars center on quality assurance and cost-effective clinical decision making. At the first seminar, different methods of quality assessment and their appropriateness are discussed (for example, the tracer condition method and disease staging). Alternative methods for improving quality of care are also examined (for example, JCAH standards, mandatory continuing medical education, and specialty recertification). During the second seminar, the focus is on cost control and health care cost inflation, with attention given to the role of the PSRO, the federal government, and third-party payers in controlling costs. Students also perform one or more chart audits for patients with selected problems during this month; reports of these audits, which are conducted by using implicit and explicit criteria, are discussed during the third seminar.

The major aim of the program is to involve students in evaluating the total patient care process in terms of both quality and costs (Garg, Gliebe, and Elkhatib, 1978a, 1978b; Garg, Gliebe, and Kleinberg, 1977; Garg, Kleinberg, and Gliebe, 1978a; Garg and others, 1975, 1978; Kleinberg, Garg, and Gliebe, 1979; Mulligan and others, 1976).

*University of Illinois Rockford School of Medicine.* In response to student evaluations of its 1973-1975 program, the faculty invited students to plan, implement, and evaluate the quality assurance program. The faculty acted as advisers, and a student steering committee controlled policy and procedures. Because in the preceding years students had felt that the purpose of chart auditing was primarily educational and that its principal value lay in developing, as opposed to applying, criteria (Barr and others, 1976), the goal was changed from making students comfortable with peer review and quality-of-care assessment to educating them in common ambulatory care problems. On the basis of their frequency as visit diagnoses and their educational potential, four topics were selected for the program; oral contraception, depression, assessment of coronary risk factors, and low back pain. After reviewing the literature on these problems, students prepared a bibliography and developed criteria, which were discussed with experts during grand rounds. The students ran the criteria development sessions; the goal was to achieve consensus on a list of minimum performance criteria that would integrate the scientific basis for criteria, the opinions of experts, and documented student experiences.

To evaluate this student-run program, the faculty surveyed attitudes toward the quality assurance curriculum among enrolled students. These surveys, in which 85 percent of the students participated, indicated substantially improved attitudes toward quality-of-care assessment after participation in the program. For a description of the program during 1976-1977, see Dennis and others (1977).

In 1977-1978, the independent criteria development by students and peer review systems, as well as a sophisticated weighting scheme for evaluating student behavior, were abandoned. A greater variety of auditing methods were introduced, with implicit chart audit considered the most beneficial. Two other changes were development of an outcome audit on obesity and inclusion of audit on a portion of the routine physical examination. The latter differed from other approaches in that it dealt with the diagnostic process used by the students in their examination of patients rather than with specific health problems (Barr, Wollstadt, and Campobello, 1978).

An overview evaluation of these years showed that the goal of educating students in quality assurance had been achieved. The faculty is proposing to continue the Ambulatory Care Audit program and to bring emphasis on cost containment to the same level as that on quality of care.

*University of Missouri, Kansas City, School of Medicine.* A quality assurance and cost containment curriculum was introduced in 1976 by means of three pilot studies to determine the feasibility of incorporating education in quality-of-care evaluation and cost awareness into a required inpatient rotation. The goal of the pilot studies was to make teaching and learning of patient care evaluation relevant to both faculty and students by associating it with patient care responsibility and clinical problem solving. Thirty-eight students from the last four years of the six-year curriculum and three faculty physicians participated in the pilot studies, conducted during three successive rotations over a seven-month period. Assessment methods included medical record audit; questionnaires on hospital charges for drugs, laboratory tests, radiology, and hospital services; and audits of clinical methods for history taking, physical examination, and patient management. The topics examined were pneumonia, decreased hemoglobin, and congestive heart failure (in that order).

Evaluation of these pilot studies showed that the majority of participants considered education in patient care evaluation appropriate to their needs; most found disease-specific auditing helpful in gaining clinical knowledge about the audit topics; half indicated willingness to participate on a medical audit committee. The evaluations also found an increased knowledge of costs generated by physicians, improvement in clinical performance in management of decreased hemoglobin, and high compliance with pneumonia audit criteria (Mulligan, 1979).

Faculty members on all departmental teams agreed to continue these activities during inpatient rotations with some modifications (for example, discussion time was reduced to allow more time for assessment of patient care). Criteria have been developed or revised for nineteen clinical problems and diseases; sessions on topic selection and criteria formulation have been used as means of setting and learning clinical practice standards for diagnostic and therapeutic outcomes of care.

In addition to participating in this program, students also serve as members of interdisciplinary patient care evaluation committees in the department of medicine. The curriculum has been expanded to include additional pilot studies; more explicit use of cost and efficacy considerations in the evaluations of the interdisciplinary patient care committees is serving as a means of integrating quality and cost instruction with clinical practice. The objective of these continuing efforts is to bring quality assurance and cost containment issues and methods to the management of individual patient care and to incorporate knowledge about costs of care into teaching about quality. A 1979 pilot project in the Department of Medicine teaches students standards of quality of care for the diagnosis and treatment of such problems as severe chest pain and informs them of patient charges for related diagnostic tests and therapy.

The students involved appeared to have favorable attitudes toward the educational benefits gained from developing and applying audit criteria in patient care, an approach that is favored over learning about quality assurance in isolation.

*University of Wisconsin Medical School.* Since 1974, the Department of Family Medicine and Practice has offered an elective in Quality Assessment and Assurance and Medical Records to fourth-year medical students. The objective is to impart understanding of the need for, and appropriate use of, the medical record, including the problem-oriented record, and to provide techniques to assess the quality of care. The students are introduced to various peer review methods, to the role of third parties in utilization review and medical audit, and to the practical role of the physician in influencing the quality and cost of patient care in different medical settings (Renner and others, 1979). Seminars are conducted by local and regional experts on quality assurance and cost containment. Students participate in practical workshops to gain an understanding of the concepts and state of the art of assessment and quality assurance for short-term inpatient care, ambulatory care, and long-term care and are directly exposed to PSROs and similar agencies. Students also develop the skills necessary to design and write process and outcome criteria, audit medical records, and analyze audit data. This is accomplished through "mock" audit sessions and through active participation in two ongoing audit projects.

Evaluation results of this course are not available at this time. Faculty members at Wisconsin hope that quality assurance can be introduced across departments and that a better integration of the hospital quality assurance activities and the teaching of this issue can be achieved.

*University of Pennsylvania.* A cost containment program for house staff at the Hospital of the University of Pennsylvania (HUP), designed as a research evaluation project, had as its major goal to educate physicians about the appropriate use of ancillary services. The program was designed in four phases. In the first phase, baseline data were collected to obtain information on physician overutilization of ancillary services. In the second, or didactic, phase, the history and economics of increases in health care expenditures were reviewed during grand rounds; a videotaped patient simulation dealing with diagnosis and treatment was shown during a medical management conference; and newsletters containing information about the diagnostic value and limitations of particular procedures relative to fees charged were distributed monthly to faculty and house staff. The third phase, a program to provide feedback to house staff, consisted in notifying physicians of instances of ordering unnecessary tests. The final, or participatory, phase involved conferences with residents to discuss the design and purpose of the program. The program was directed to medical residents at HUP; surgical residents at HUP as well as medical residents at Thomas Jefferson University Hospital served as controls. Results of this effort are currently being evaluated (Eisenberg, Williams, and Pascale, 1979).

A companion learning unit for medical students was also developed and integrated into a four-week medical clerkship. This program consisted of lectures, readings, seminars, and case discussions on cost containment. Each group of students was shown the videotaped patient simulation used in the house-staff program, received copies of patient bills, and participated in cost-utility discussions related to care of current patients. Residents who had been sensitized to cost containment issues acted as role models to provide reinforcement to participating medical students. Evaluation consisted of before-and-after tests that included an attitude scale, a knowledge questionnaire, and patient management problems. Control groups were set up among students in medical clerkships at affiliated hospitals as well as among students at HUP who did not receive didactic instruction on cost containment but were in contact with residents participating in the house-staff cost containment program.

*Changes in Emphasis: Common Trends Despite Greater Diversity*

The five programs just described were able to draw on the experience of an earlier group of independently developed programs. This second generation of programs is characterized by far more diversity and complexity than the first. Two programs (Medical College of Ohio and University of Wisconsin) have offered a thorough and comprehensive review of quality assurance techniques; one program (Medical College of Ohio) makes frequent use of the clinical pathological conference (CPC) for detailed discussion of cost management; and one program (Rockford School of Medicine) has evolved as an almost entirely student-run program. Nonetheless, they share a number of characteristics that may indicate a common trend in the evolution of quality assurance teaching programs (see Table 11.2). Among these are:

- Less emphasis on any one prescribed group of activities (for example, PSRO, JCAH) but continued emphasis on developing appropriate skills and knowledge related to quality assurance and cost containment methodologies.
- More emphasis on strategies to make students and residents conscious of the costs of care.

**Table 11.2. Second-Generation Programs, 1976–1979.**

|  | Institution | | | | |
|---|---|---|---|---|---|
|  | *Medical College of Ohio, Toledo* | *University of Illinois, Rockford* | *University of Missouri, Kansas City* | *University of Wisconsin* | *University of Pennsylvania* |
| Program goal(s) | To teach quality assurance and cost containment methods emphasizing peer review | To educate students in common ambulatory care programs | To make teaching and learning of care evaluation relevant to faculty and students | To impart understanding of appropriate use of record  To provide quality assessment techniques | To encourage voluntary cost containment among physicians-in-training |
| Program objectives | To understand effect of PSRO on physician practice  To examine other assessment methods  To explore issues in health care cost inflation  To develop implicit and explicit criteria | To develop criteria for common ambulatory care problems with educational potential  To gain familiarity with a variety of auditing methods | To associate clinical care evaluation with patient care responsibility and clinical problem solving | To develop skills in formulating process and outcome criteria  To understand UR and MCEs  To understand physician role in controlling quality and costs | To gain information necessary for appropriate decision making in use of diagnostic services  To understand financial consequences of medical decisions  To understand personal cost-generating behavior |

Table 11.2. Second-Generation Programs, 1976–1979, Cont'd.

| | | | | |
|---|---|---|---|---|
| **Student level** | All undergraduate years<br>Integrated into "Introduction to Clinical Medicine," CPCs, "Ambulatory Care Clerkship"<br>(Mandatory) | Throughout ambulatory experience in community clinics<br>Third-year students<br>(Mandatory) | Continuous during clinical rotations in last four years of six-year curriculum<br>(Mandatory) | Six weeks<br>Fourth-year students in department of family medicine and practice<br>(Elective) | Throughout residency<br>Four weeks for medical students during medicine curriculum<br>(Mandatory/Elective) |
| **Program activities** | Introductory lecture on general issues in "Introduction to Clinical Medicine"<br>Regularly scheduled CPCs on cost and quality<br>Quality assurance and cost-effective clinical decision-making topics discussed during ambulatory and inpatient clerkships<br>Seminars during clinical clerkships | Students plan, implement, and evaluate program<br>Students prepare bibliography on care management and then develop criteria for assessing quality of care on certain specific diseases/problems | Seminars are offered on criteria development and care evaluation<br>Students participate in medical record audit, development of criteria<br>Students complete questionnaire on hospital charges for services and ancillary services<br>Students serve as members of interdisciplinary evaluation committee | Seminars on basic quality assurance/cost containment concepts<br>Students participate in "mock" audit sessions<br>Students participate in ongoing audit procedures within department of family medicine and practice<br>Students participate in workshops on existing quality assurance approaches | Discussion of history and economics of increase in health care expenditures during grand rounds<br>Monthly medical management conferences using videotaped patient simulations to discuss use of diagnostic procedures<br>Distribution of monthly newsletter to educate physicians on value and limitations of specific |

| | | | | |
|---|---|---|---|---|
| | | | | diagnostic procedures<br>Dissemination of charges for most frequently used diagnostic tests through news-letter<br>Use of computer-based system to identify excessive users of certain procedures<br>Didactic sessions for students |
| Evaluation results | Improved understanding of quality and cost considerations in evaluating patient care process | Improved knowledge of costs generated by physicians<br>Improved clinical performance<br>Favorable attitude toward educational benefits of developing criteria | Markedly improved student attitudes toward quality assurance | In process |
| References | Garg and others (1975); Mulligan and others (1976) | Mulligan (1979) | Barr, Wollstadt, and Campobello (1978) | Renner and others (1979) | Eisenberg, Williams, and Pascale (1979) |

- More emphasis on self-review and self-assessment as an essential element in the self-correcting activities of professional providers.
- Continuous evolution of each program and changes in its goals and objectives in response to internal evaluation studies.

Although the second generation of quality assurance teaching programs have a common scope, there is now greater diversity in the educational experiences offered to students and exposure to a variety of quality assurance methodologies. Health care cost management is emphasized as a part of quality assurance, and students' involvement in self-assessment is increasingly stressed so as to prepare them for similar efforts in future practice. Of particular importance is the trend toward continuing program evaluation, with modifications made on the basis of evaluation results.

A major weakness of these programs is that they continue to place emphasis on individual care management and give scant attention to aggregated population data and the use of such data in analyzing entire practice profiles.

### New Points of Departure

Consistent with current national concerns, programs developed since 1978 have tended to emphasize teaching students about health care cost management. Several approaches have been introduced. Instead of listing all new programs, I have selected a few for detailed discussion because they reflect present trends in integrating cost containment and ethical principles into the teaching of quality assurance. Where appropriate, programs similar in content and goals are cited in the text; general characteristics of the selected programs are summarized in Table 11.3.

*Focus on Cost and Ethics*

*Jefferson Medical College.* Second-year students at Jefferson had previously participated in an interdisciplinary program, Medicine and Society, which included lectures on cost containment, utilization review, quality assurance, and PSROs. When this approach proved inadequate for changing attitudes and behavior, an experimental program more directly related to clinical problem solving was designed to maximize student involvement in problems of cost containment. Current objectives of the program, entitled Student Model Utilization Review Committee Project, are to increase awareness of actual health service charges, define the functions of personnel responsible for peer review, recognize how coding and data collection techniques are currently used in utilization review, identify potential areas where physicians can contribute to the reduction of costs, and gain understanding of different mechanisms of and approaches to health care cost control (Zeleznik and Gonnella, 1979).

As part of the junior six-week clinical clerkship rotation at the Thomas Jefferson University Hospital, students participate as members of a mock hospital utilization review committee. In ninety-minute weekly meetings, the following techniques are used to familiarize students with economic and quality issues that may arise in their own future practices: collection of preexperimental and postexperimental data; discussion of admission of a patient; review of cases presented both by representatives of the university hospital quality assurance committee and, for purposes of comparison, by the quality assurance representative from another hospital; and presentation of cases by representatives of PSRO, Blue Shield, and other agencies concerned with costs.

*University of Oregon School of Medicine.* At the University of Oregon, an attempt is being made to integrate the teaching of quality assurance, cost containment, and medical ethics into already existing curricula. The overall goal is to establish a flexible program that will give medical students a reasonably accurate awareness of issues of health care costs and quality. Specifically, students are expected to acquire cost information at several levels, including a working knowledge of costs of common medical procedures used in providing diagnostic, therapeutic, and rehabilitative services, as well as an overview of systems of health care financing and reimbursement, current methods and concepts of quality assurance, and individual and professional responsibility for allocating medical resources. Cost and allocation information is examined in light of socioethical principles (Garland and others, 1979).

**Table 11.3. Programs Developed Since 1978 (Selected Listing).**

| | Institution | | | |
|---|---|---|---|---|
| | *Jefferson Medical College* | *University of Oregon* | *SUNY-Buffalo* | *Medical College of Georgia* |
| Program goal | To maximize student involvement in problems of cost containment | To provide students with awareness of health care costs within the context of ethical decision making | To integrate quality assurance and cost containment into four years of curriculum and to promote cost-effective decision making | To educate students and residents to greater awareness of health care costs |
| Student objectives | To develop awareness of health services charges<br>To define functions of peer review personnel<br>To become familiar with coding and data collection<br>To understand different approaches to health care cost control | To become familiar with health care financing and reimbursement<br>To understand current concepts and methods of quality assurance<br>To be aware of ethical dimensions of cost, quality, and allocation decisions | To understand various quality assurance methodologies<br>To be able to analyze and measure quality of care<br>To identify and describe methods of determining cost effectiveness<br>To recognize physician's role and responsibility in cost containment | To know charges of common hospital and laboratory procedures<br>To become aware of personal patterns of overutilization |
| Program length and student level | Nine hours<br>Third-year medical students<br>(Elective) | Integrated throughout curriculum<br>All four years<br>(Mandatory plus electives) | Integrated throughout curriculum of school of medicine; all four years<br>(Mandatory plus electives)<br>Second-year students in | Integrated into four medical services at Talmadge Hospital<br>Second-, third-, and fourth-year students |

| | | | "Social and Preventive Medicine" (Mandatory) | Internal Medicine and Family Practice residents (Mandatory) |
|---|---|---|---|---|
| Program activities | 1½-hour weekly meetings Seminar discussions and lectures Student collection of preexperimental data Student participation in model utilization review committee Student review of cases presented by hospital quality assurance committee Guest lecturers from PSRO and quality assurance programs | Lectures, case study presentations, and discussions throughout four years First year: "Public Health and Epidemiology"—broad overview of cost data, quality measurement ethics Second year: "Patient Evaluation"—discussion of costs and ethics as part of case presentations on patient treatment Third, fourth years: Clerkships—discussion of cost and quality Elective—open to all students: "Ethics and Health Care" | Competency-based learning modules in cost-effectiveness strategies included in: First year: "Biometry" Second year: "Epidemiology," "Organization and Delivery of Health Care," "Social and Legal Aspects of Medicine" Third year: Clerkships in medicine and pediatrics Fourth year: Four-week elective in quality assurance and cost containment | Student work-up of simulated patients via Computer Assisted Patient Simulation (CAPS) with cost of hospitalization and procedures tabulated as feedback Biweekly cost containment conferences in department of medicine Development and provision of daily cumulative bills posted on each patient's chart Laboratory reports containing results and charges of tests |
| References | Zeleznik and Gonnella (1979) | Garland and others (1979) | Matthews (1979) | Lewis (1979) |

This examination of issues of cost, quality, and ethics is integrated into the four years of undergraduate medical education. In a required first-year course ("Public Health and Epidemiology"), students receive a broad overview of cost data, quality measurement, and social and professional ethics. In the second-year course on patient evaluation, which also is required, seven case discussions of initial patient evaluation and subsequent treatment plans are scheduled, including discussions of costs and ethics. An elective course ("Ethics and Health Care"), open to medical, nursing, dental, and graduate students, also uses the case study approach and relates cost information to social and individual ethics. During the required third- and fourth-year clerkships, substantial cost-of-care information is being disseminated, and additional discussions pertaining to the acquisition of cost information will be included in routine student evaluations of individual clerkships. An experimental three-week clerkship designed as a PSRO rotation is in the planning stage.

Two other programs are similar to that at Oregon in their examination of health care costs from a societal and ethical perspective.

The *Eastern Virginia Medical School* conducts a mandatory program for third-year students during a six-week Family Practice Clerkship. The program consists primarily of seminar discussions of health care economics, the health care system, PSRO responsibilities and functions, and techniques for measuring quality of care. Students are assigned readings and prepare class presentations on specific topics.

The *University of Southern Illinois* includes discussions of quality assurance and cost containment in its required curriculum on Medical Education, Society, and the Humanities. Students rotate through this curriculum three times during their clinical year, for a total of six weeks. The objectives related to quality assurance and cost containment include familiarizing students with the effects of limited resources on the delivery of health care, reimbursement mechanisms, and federal, voluntary, and consumer-generated cost containment measures; introducing students to the economic consequences of physician decisions; promoting understanding of various health care cost components and current proposals for curbing costs; and preparing students to conduct cost-benefit analyses, particularly for extended life support and extensive diagnostic workups (Davis, Begley, and Jarrett, 1978). Learning experiences for these topics vary from seminars and discussions to field observations.

*State University of New York, Buffalo, School of Medicine.* A quality assurance and cost effectiveness component was introduced into the second-year curriculum in the department of social and preventive medicine in 1979. Students are expected to analyze and apply methods of evaluating and assuring the quality of care and to become familiar with the state of the art of quality assessment studies and methods. They are instructed on the responsibility and the role of the individual practitioner for quality assurance and cost containment activities, and they gain an understanding of the intent and requirements of PSROs. Specifically, they are taught to differentiate between cost-effective and cost-escalating decisions and are expected to identify and describe two methods of determining the cost effectiveness of clinical decisions (Matthews, 1979).

The School of Medicine of the State University at Buffalo has also initiated a project to develop a cross-curricular sequence of competency-based learning modules in cost-effective intervention strategies for use throughout the four years of undergraduate medical education. The underlying argument for this interdisciplinary approach is that quality assurance and cost containment are interrelated and that distributive learning providing broad exposure will have a significant impact on both cost-effective decision making and student values. The learning modules will be incorporated into a first-year course in biometry, second-year offerings in epidemiology, organization and delivery of health care, social and legal aspects of medicine, and the family practice sequence; third-year medicine and pediatric clinical rotations; and a four-week concentrated program in cost containment and quality assurance offered twice during the senior year (Matthews, 1979).

*Medical College of Georgia.* This quality assurance and cost containment program had its beginnings as a residency program for educating house officers on various issues related to cost containment in health care. The program is now supported by a two-year grant from Blue Shield and conducted through the department of medicine (Lewis, 1979). Its major objective is to bring medical students and house officers to a greater awareness of the cost of common laboratory and hospital procedures and to encourage them to minimize patient expenditures. Program activities include use of the computer-assisted patient simulation system to allow students to work up simulated patients on a computer terminal, with the cost of hospitalization and procedures tabulated as feedback; use of a laboratory reporting system for four major clinical services at Talmadge Hospital; and daily generation of the cumulative hospital bill on each patient. Cost containment conferences within the department of medicine for house staff and students are held biweekly.

The program is being designed so as to allow for a prospective evaluation of its impact on the medical services at Talmadge Hospital. Two medical services will serve as study groups, two others as control groups.

The University of Arkansas, the University of North Dakota, and the University of California at Davis have programs similar to that of the Medical College of Georgia in that they emphasize awareness of charges for particular procedures. Arkansas and North Dakota are directed primarily toward residents. An interesting difference is that one of these programs centers on outpatient care provided in hospital clinics.

At the *University of Arkansas College of Medicine,* a computer-based ambulatory care information system developed as a pilot program for patient management education is being used to provide information on costs of care generated by residents. This program was recently instituted for all residents in medicine. It not only provides resident utilization profiles (that is, diagnostic-specific calculations of costs to the average patient receiving the prescribed care) but also permits peer review and comparison with national cost data for similar medical problems. In addition, the information system allows residents to determine the frequency of health problems seen in their practice, evaluate resource utilization, and select cases for medical audit (Monson, 1979).

At all family practice residency sites of the *University of North Dakota School of Medicine,* residents are required to learn the charges for all procedures and analyze randomly selected cases with regard to management, follow-up, consultation, and referral for both quality and appropriateness of care. Quality and cost containment are interrelated in this process (Dunnigan, 1978). Residents are required to justify each hospital admission on the basis of appropriateness, timeliness, and cost/quality benefit. Additionally, a seminar program discussing a variety of issues related to cost containment has been developed in collaboration with the National Association of Blue Shield plans and will be available to all residency programs throughout the state through a special communications system developed by the University of North Dakota.

At the *University of California, Davis, Medical Center,* the experimental program in cost containment for medical students also emphasizes knowledge of charges. The purpose of the program is to enable students to gain an understanding of the multiple factors affecting health care costs and of the role physicians can play in helping contain those costs. Students are asked to complete a standardized worksheet for at least one patient during clinical rotations. A sample price file of charges for clinical services, supplies, pharmaceuticals, laboratory, radiology, nuclear medicine, cardiology, and professional fees is supplied. Students record daily the major charges generated and analyze their medical appropriateness in view of treatment patterns and specificity and sensitivity for the diagnosis in question. A similar worksheet is prepared for outpatient cases.

*Characteristics of Third-Generation Programs*

Most recently developed programs reflect a change from quality assurance to cost containment as a principal focus. Despite their diversity of objectives, teaching methods, and type of educational experiences offered at different levels in the medical curriculum, there is a common emphasis on educating residents in principles of quality assurance and cost containment. A wider span of programs now exists throughout the undergraduate curriculum, with involvement of medical students in the programs designed for residents during clinical clerkships.

The principal strengths of these new programs thus appear to lie in their multidisciplinary approaches, which seem to have replaced emphasis on specific quality assurance methods, and in their reinforcement of principles throughout the medical curriculum. Discrete evaluative components have been built into most of these programs, although program effectiveness in attaining these goals cannot be measured until evaluation results are available for analysis. Even now, however, it is clear that because of the diversity of objectives and educational methods, a uniform comparative evaluation of these programs will be difficult.

### Conclusions

In 1970–1973, a handful of institutions had developed formal programs to educate medical students and house officers in quality assurance and, to a lesser extent, cost containment methods. Some of these programs were later discontinued; others were developed into more complex programs. During the mid seventies, new programs began to emerge, many of which utilized experiences gained through earlier programs. The last three years have been marked by a proliferation of numerous programs featuring greater diversity, joint involvement of house staff and medical students, a tendency to present a general overview of all methods of quality assurance (not just those currently required by PSRO, JCAH, and such agencies) and above all, increased emphasis on cost containment.

Although no single program can justly be described as a model for future curriculum development, particularly since evaluation results are not yet available, certain attributes are worth noting. It seems appropriate, for example, to include a general discussion of national issues in quality assurance and cost containment in seminar or lecture courses during the first two years of the medical curriculum. It must be realized, however, that this material will appear more remote to students at this stage than during the clinical clerkship years, when cost management and quality assessment can be incorporated into clinical problem-solving exercises. In addition, because this is a rapidly developing field, it would appear more appropriate to provide students and house officers with an overview of various methods in quality assurance and cost management than to concentrate on chart audit and peer review.

Learning will take place more effectively when the learner is involved in experiences directly related to future practice. For example, clinical problem-solving exercises for students in clinical clerkships will seem to have a direct relation to perceived activities during residency years, whereas for residents, involvement in quality assurance and cost management programs for aggregates of patients in the hospital and clinic setting will be perceived as relevant to future activities as practicing clinicians and staff/faculty members. Wherever possible, students should be exposed to practical experiences involving quality assurance activities and cost management procedures as they relate to aggregate groups of patients rather than to individual patients. Programs that stimulate and reinforce the idea that a practicing physician must be a lifelong learner and a self-assessing and self-correcting clinician will undoubtedly have the greatest eventual impact.

꙰꙰꙰꙰꙰꙰꙰꙰꙰꙰꙰꙰꙰꙰꙰꙰꙰꙰꙰꙰꙰꙰ 12

# Future Trends
# and Needs

*John W. Williamson*
*James I. Hudson*
*Jay Noren*

꙰꙰꙰꙰꙰꙰꙰꙰꙰꙰꙰꙰꙰꙰꙰꙰꙰꙰꙰꙰꙰꙰꙰꙰

Achieving and maintaining health care quality and efficient allocation of health care resources will remain an urgent issue throughout the coming decade. Systematic efforts to measure quality of
care have documented numerous deficiencies in the provision of
the most basic health care services (Williamson, 1978; Brook and
Lohr, 1979; Ballantine, 1980). Recent investigations (Couch and
others, 1981; Steel and others, 1981) again show the magnitude
of surgical mishaps and iatrogenic illnesses even in institutions
known for their high standards of care. Moreover, the rate of increase in health care expenditures is a major concern of both the
public and private sectors. Despite government regulations and
programs designed to curb rising health care costs, Freeland, Calat,
and Schendler (1980) have predicted that expenditures will continue to escalate during the 1980s.

Faculties of medical and other health professional schools can expect increased pressure to include quality assurance and cost containment education in their curricula. Whether these educational efforts succeed in improving quality and containing costs may depend, in large measure, on factors beyond the control of individual faculty members. However, faculty members might have substantial influence on future success by recognizing a few critical issues concerning both the *content* and *methods* of quality assurance education. This chapter will examine these issues and formulate implications that might facilitate the planning of relevant educational strategies in the coming years.

## Future Content of Quality Assurance Education

The goals of quality assurance education are to enhance the capacity of future clinicians in making wise decisions about effective and efficient care for individual patients, in reviewing and self-correcting their practice patterns for groups of patients, in acting prudently on behalf of their patients and society at large in terms of health resources allocation, and in assuring that the system for which they are responsible maintains a standard of quality for all.

A number of disciplines include the knowledge or content base for attaining these goals. Biostatistics, epidemiology, economics of health care, organization development, systems analysis, information theory, decision theory, learning and behavioral theory, sociology, anthropology, and some fundamentals of clinical practice can be called the "basic sciences" of quality assurance/cost containment. Those proficient in these areas might be considered exquisitely equipped to teach or conduct research in quality assurance, technology assessment, decision analysis, health science information management, and the host of other activities related to an institution's risk management, quality control, and cost management. However, few faculty members claim high proficiency in all these content areas. Most programs at academic institutions are conducted by an interdisciplinary group consisting of persons with varying degrees of knowledge and experience who maintain regular communication with the major groups responsible for quality monitoring (for example, JCAH and PSRO) and remain informed on current literature related to quality assurance.

Undoubtedly, the group as a whole should be familiar with the literature base suggested in this text. In addition, the growing body of information on health status measurement, health scales, patient satisfaction, health indexes, and health risk estimation needs to be incorporated into quality assurance education. A working familiarity with the "basic sciences" enumerated above would appear to characterize the effective teacher-model in this field. Quality assurance and cost management research in the coming decade undoubtedly will be based on those content areas. However, two major issues require special emphasis in planning future educational content in quality assurance: (1) proposed strategies for controlling health care costs and (2) structured methods for solving problems, making rational decisions, and managing health science information. The following sections will review these issues and discuss their implications for quality assurance education.

*The Problem of Rising Health Care Costs: Proposed Solutions.* Despite some modest successes in curbing the rise of health care expenditures—successes attributed to PSRO program implementation (Office of Research, Demonstration and Statistics, 1980) and to the activities of state ratesetting agencies (Solomon and Cohen, 1978; Biles, Schramm, and Atkinson, 1980), the rate of increase in these expenditures has exceeded the rate of inflation for the past fifteen years. Much of this increase in aggregate expenditure on health services might have been expected as the result of widespread application of more advanced, technology-oriented interventions to a larger population covered by public and private insurance mechanisms. However, this reason is not sufficient to account for the rapid and steady rise of health care costs. Some current explanations have attributed the problem to external factors that increase the demand for services; others have argued serious inefficiencies within the health care system. Even though wide regional and institutional variations in hospital occupancy rates, lengths of stay, costs per hospitalization, and rates of surgery could be explained by differences in case mix or access to services (Rafferty and Hornbrook, 1979), it is difficult to dismiss out of hand the view that a large amount of redundant medicine has been, is being, and will continue to be practiced unless vigorous steps are taken to curb this trend (Enthoven, 1978a). In the current, predominantly fee-for-service, reimbursement system, almost no incentives exist for physicians to behave differently in ordering tests and procedures—or for patients to question the necessity of certain practices.

Feldstein and Taylor (1977) and Feldstein (1979) maintain that the rise in hospital costs, a major contributor to rising health care expenditures, is not a form of price inflation, but rather reflects an increase in the quantity of services that are packed into a day of care. Greenspan and Vogel (1980) convincingly link multiple tax subsidies to the increase in demand for health insurance, which in turn causes a greater demand for services. They further maintain that increases in reimbursement rates in the private sector exert pressure on federally financed program prices, and vice versa.

Factors contributing to the present situation are numerous, complex, and interrelated, affecting all dimensions of the supply-demand equation. For example, demographic factors—such as the aging of Americans that will continue to increase demand for services—cannot be controlled by changes in policy or reorganization of services. Other influences originate on the supply side, such as medicine's preoccupation with curative measures at the expense of prevention (Hiatt, 1975; Somers and Somers, 1977), the growing power of corporate laboratories (Bailey, 1979), and a predicted oversupply of physicians (Fordham, 1979).

The range of proposed solutions is equally diverse. For example, Moloney and Rogers (1979) propose that physicians find ways to cut back appropriately on the thousands of technology-related actions they perform daily, and Relman (1980) suggests that restraint in use of marginal procedures and services and elimination of obsolete ones would result in a single, sustained 5 percent reduction in present expenditures. Others maintain that more radical reforms of the current health care system are needed to achieve reductions in expenditures. Among the proposed strategies are (1) enhancing competition and/or adopting new approaches to regulation, (2) changing reimbursement procedures and insurance payer incentives, (3) altering the basic organization of health care providers, (4) scrutinizing particular diagnostic and therapeutic procedures, and (5) changing provider behavior through the educational process.

Each of these strategies has implications for future quality assurance activities and education. Therefore, each will be described and its implications discussed.

*The Competition Approach.* Several plans call for restructuring the system and reorganizing health care financing so as to provide incentives for physicians and patients to act prudently in using health care resources. Enthoven (1978b) has proposed a "competition approach" in his Consumer Choice Health Plan (CCHP) that would reduce the tax subsidy for health insurance, provide for consumer choice among competing plans while offering incentives to purchasers to select the less expensive options, and use copayments to discourage overuse by consumers at the point of seeking care.

Feldstein (1979) suggests reducing tax subsidies and increasing copayments as an alternative to hospital cost-containment legislation. In fact, several procompetition bills were introduced in Congress during 1979 and 1980, including the Health Care Cost Restraint Act of 1979 (H.R. 5740), the Health Incentive Reform Act of 1979 (S. 1968), the National Health Care Reform Act (H.R. 7527), the Comprehensive Health Care Reform Act (S. 1590), and the Consumer Health Expense Control Act (H.R. 7528).

Although these proposals have evoked interest in a number of quarters, including organized medicine and segments of the practicing community (Ackerman, 1980), many urge caution about implementing them. Fein (1980), for instance, argues that existing inequities in access must be attacked before problems of inefficiency can be solved. Ginzberg (1980) agrees and questions the popularity of an arbitrary "tax" among workers and the plan's eventual appeal to physicians and consumers. Foreseeing problems in reconciling teaching and research support with the provision of services, academic medical centers have also expressed their concerns (Association of American Medical Colleges, 1980).

Some view the competition approach as a desirable alternative to regulation, although McNerney (1980) called for a proper balance between competition and regulation. Predictably, the debate over competition versus regulation has become quite politicized (Enthoven, 1981). Some of the proposed actions would affect quality assurance activities as well. For example, certain parts of the competition package, such as a ceiling on nontaxable health insurance benefits, could be passed by Congress as part of tax reform legislation. The national PSRO program could eventually be dismantled as a result of the perception that the savings in use of health resources attributed to the program have not been sufficient to warrant continuing to support the program's operational costs on a national scale.

Passage of procompetition legislation and/or reduction in federal programs to regulate costs does not mean that quality assurance and cost containment activities would be abandoned, however. Formal hospital-based quality assurance activities, as recently organized (Affelt, 1980), will undoubtedly continue. Moreover, it is likely that the recent state-initiated efforts to control hospital costs, such as those currently underway in Massachusetts, New Jersey, Maryland, New York, and Washington, will be adopted by others. In addition, industry has shown some interest in contracting with individual PSROs to conduct utilization review. These types of quality assurance and cost containment activities are sufficient to warrant continued quality assurance education in medical and health professional schools.

*Changes in Reimbursement Through Health Insurance Initiatives.* As mentioned before, the present reimbursement system has also been cited as the source of the ills in rising health care expenditures. Moloney and Rogers (1979), for example, claim that the system encourages physicians to use technology as a way of making the most economical use of their time. An analysis based on the California Relative Value Scale (RVS) by Hsiao and Stason (1979) supports this view, demonstrating the dramatic discrepancies between existing reimbursement levels and resource-cost values for office visits compared with surgical procedures. Similar variations were noted by Delbanco, Meyers, and Segal (1979), who suggest, as a first step in reform, redistribution in Blue Shield panels, removal of secrecy from fee-payment protocols, and elimination of physician majorities on Blue Shield boards.

However, it is difficult to document great enthusiasm for attempting major changes in the reimbursement system. The American Academy of Pediatrics has repeatedly argued that across-the-board reductions are unequal for the various forms of practice and discourage primary care physicians from delivering quality care (Blim, 1974). Showstack and others (1979) see little likelihood of broad changes that would limit physician autonomy. Despite these objections, Moloney and Rogers (1979) maintain that real savings would come not from leveling of physicians' fees but from a decrease in the use of technology, which, in turn, would reduce the accompanying costs of personnel to apply and service the technologies and of follow-up of false positive tests. Despite the belief that changes in the reimbursement system are necessary and would improve the present situation, the exact mechanism for producing these changes remains unclear. Egdahl and Walsh (1979) have proposed that the insurance industry continue to develop strong utilization review in a variety of prepaid plans, including those with fee-for-service arrangements with physicians. Others have suggested that premium structures be altered to offer financial incentives for health promotion activities (Brailey, 1980) or that wider coverage of preventive services be considered (Institute of Medicine, 1976).

Representatives of the insurance industry as well as of management and labor are skeptical about the cost savings that could be achieved by health promotion. They believe that major changes are unlikely until undisputed cost benefits from prevention and screening can be demonstrated—a difficult undertaking.

Although no specific program has been adopted from the proposed initiatives, the health insurance industry has undertaken one activity that appears to be bearing fruit in reducing utilization. It has formed an alliance with employers and labor groups and with PSROs to carry out utilization review and quality assessment in the private sector. This effort has demonstrated savings in areas where it has been rigidly applied.

*Changes in Organization of Health Care Providers.* Over the past few decades, providers have shown increased interest in alternative forms of organizing the delivery of health services. These alternatives also have potential for cutting health care costs. For example, health maintenance organizations (HMOs) have demonstrated consistently lower hospitalization rates (Luft, 1978), and the reduction in health care expenditures in regions saturated by HMOs has been impressive (Christianson and McClure, 1979; Christianson, 1980). However, HMOs have not grown sufficiently in other regions to demonstrate similar effects on health care costs. In fact, the HMO movement must overcome considerable resistance from physicians and consumers before it can grow to the point of having a significant impact on health care expenditures during the coming decade.

Multispecialty group practices have expanded over the past thirty years, however, and many believe that the projected increase in the number of physicians will enhance this growth. These groups, essentially competing with one another, are likely to feature built-in incentives for reducing unnecessary expenditures.

These new forms of organizing services will also need to show that quality care is being provided. This should stimulate interest in refining quality assurance methodologies, especially those that can be applied to ambulatory care in both fee-for-service and large prepaid group practices.

*Other Proposed Strategies.* Among other proposed strategies for curbing the rise in health care costs are regionalization of certain surgical interventions (Luft, Bunker, and Enthoven, 1979) and second-opinion surgery programs, which have demonstrated some results in reducing unnecessary surgery (McCarthy and Finkel, 1979, 1980). Longmire and Mellinkoff (1979), while supporting the concept of regionalization, point out that there may be problems in selecting institutions for regional assignment. In addition, there are controversies over the definition of unnecessary surgery and marginal or outdated procedures and services. Here technology assessment, appropriately applied, could play a major role. Enthoven (1978a), Hiatt (1975), and Relman (1979) have offered convincing arguments for a bold, national program of technology assessment that would involve support and participation of both the academic and practicing communities. Relman (1980) has also stated that "assessment techniques and clinical decision making should be taught and practiced in academic centers, and careers in this field should be encouraged by appropriate faculty recognition."

*Decision Methods Most Relevant to Quality Assurance.* The more we recognize that few health care decisions—and quality assessment decisions as well—are based on hard data, the more we become interested in the decision process itself. Health professionals are beginning to recognize the multiple biases inherent in current decision methods; hence the increased interest in problem solving, decision theory, and information management. The following sections provide a brief discussion of structured group judgment, decision analysis, and cost/benefit and cost-effectiveness analyses. These methods, when applied to problems in health care, hold the potential for providing informed estimates—where no definitive data are available—for medical problem solving and decision making.

*Structured group judgment* methods can be divided into two major types, those in which panel members meet together (nominal group technique) and those in which they remain apart and anonymous (Delphi technique). Both have a body of supportive research literature indicating their strengths and limitations (Delbecq, Van de Ven, and Gustafson 1975; Dalkey, 1969; Piper, 1974; Lindstone and Turoff, 1975).

In the future it can be expected that the results of carefully implemented structured group processes will be recognized as clearly more reliable and valid than haphazard judgments of individuals or open-interaction panels (see also Chapter Ten), and the bias of open-interaction group judgments will be considered as unacceptable as bias introduced by an inappropriate statistical test or low response rates.

Structured group judgment techniques will be most effective and successful if certain guidelines are applied. For example:

• The type of group effort to use will be dictated by the importance of the problem to be solved: Critical problems will be subjected to large-group judgment, such as the Delphi technique, whereas most issues can be effectively and efficiently managed by small-group processes, such as the nominal group technique.
• Criteria for the relevance of the information should be explicit.

Systematic protocols should be applied to assure the validity of the data provided. Search strategies should be designed carefully, with networking or telephone pyramid methods used when applicable to ensure the relevance and validity of the documents submitted.

- Group judgments should be elicited by structured methods requiring the contribution of each panel member. To the extent possible, implicit assumptions of team members should be made explicit for the purpose of group analysis and as the basis for subsequent judgments.

- Mathematical consensus techniques, in contrast to forced consensus, should be used to aggregate the individual judgments. Documenting dissent is as important as establishing consensus. Input from differing points of view derived from different professional experiences is an asset and contributes to the improved validity of the group median discussion point.

*Decision analysis* applies probability analysis to alternative decision paths as a means of improving decision making. Until recently, methods of quality (effectiveness-efficiency) evaluation have concentrated on retrospective review of provider performance as recorded in some form of health care record or on concurrent analysis as viewed by a silent observer. These methods examine primarily the provider's knowledge (of various examination and surgical procedures) and some skills (data acquisition through patient interview, follow-up of abnormal laboratory results). Evaluation of the provider's analytical thought processes, clinical judgment, or decision making is beyond the scope of these methods, even though the decision process or clinical judgment critically influences the quality of health care. Much research is being conducted at present to improve decision processes. Bunker, Barnes, and Mosteller (1977) summarized several studies on this topic as they relate to surgery, and Weinstein and others (1980) recently produced an excellent comprehensive text on this subject.

Decision analysis techniques are now being applied experimentally to health care problems and have considerable potential for application to quality assurance. The present interest in decision analysis stems from the fact that physicians are faced with an increasing volume of medical information, yet must make diagnostic and treatment decisions under conditions of considerable uncertainty. Providing additional information does not solve this uncertainty problem. Rather, the physician needs methods that will enable him or her to interpret the information more rationally and to apply it more readily. The degree of uncertainty ranges along a continuum that begins with simple decision problems for which common sense provides an answer and progresses through problems of increasing complexity for which intuition is inadequate to reach rational decisions but for which mathematical guides are helpful. Decision analysis provides a set of guides to enhance clinical decision making, and its value increases with the complexity of the clinical decision problem.

The following example of the major decisions and uncertainties underlying an appendectomy problem was taken from Pliskin and Taylor (1977). Figure 12.1 illustrates the various levels of decision making involved in this case. The first decision point is to operate or wait and see how the patient progresses. If the decision is to operate, the surgeon may find a perforated, an inflamed, or a normal appendix. If the decision is made to wait and see, the patient may get worse, stay the same, or improve. Each of these possibilities has its own subsequent decision possibilities regarding surgery, and surgery's subsequent results. Figure 12.2 also supplies measured data, or "informed guesses" of the possibilities. By mathematically combining probability values along various branches, one can compute the decision branches for any given patient in terms of probability of the final outcome.

Although such methods seem unnecessary for simple decisions, applying these principles systematically to more complex decisions, such as those involved in open-heart surgery, provides a powerful resource for clinical decision making. The major difficulty with this approach does not involve its theory so much as the present lack of precise probability values for each branch of complex decision trees. This problem can be partly resolved by the use of a "sensitivity analysis" (Pauker and Kassirer, 1975). Here the largest and smallest values consistent with each key probability and patient preference/utility are entered into the formal analysis, and

Level 1      Level 2      Level 3      Level 4

Patient's
Symptoms
if No Surgery
Initial Act      at Level 1      Act      Surgical Findings

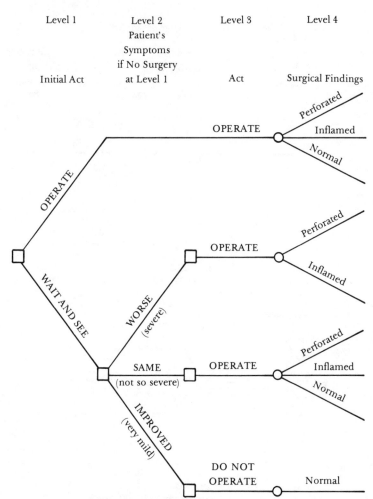

**Figure 12.1. Appendectomy Decision Tree for Patients Under Suspicion
for Appendicitis.**

*Source:* Pliskin, N., and Taylor, A. "General Principles: Cost-Benefit and
Decision Analysis." In J. Bunker, B. Barnes, and F. Mosteller (Eds.), *Costs,
Risks and Benefits of Surgery.* New York: Oxford University Press, 1977.

their effect on the final outcome is determined. Often, such an
analysis indicates that the degree of uncertainty does not alter the
original conclusion.

    Structured group data estimates may provide a means for
managing the probability-value problem more sucessfully than by

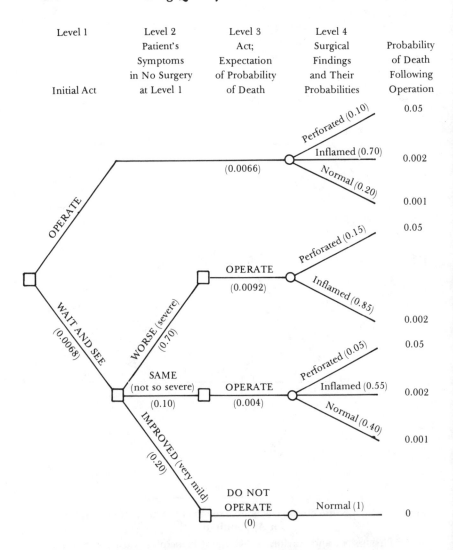

| Level 1 | Level 2<br>Patient's<br>Symptoms<br>in No Surgery | Level 3<br>Act;<br>Expectation<br>of Probability | Level 4<br>Surgical<br>Findings<br>and Their | Probability<br>of Death<br>Following |
|---|---|---|---|---|
| Initial Act | at Level 1 | of Death | Probabilities | Operation |

**Figure 12.2. Appendectomy Decision Tree for Patients Under Suspicion for Appendicitis, with Mortality Data.**

The numbers along the tree are judgmental estimates of Benjamin A. Barnes, M.D. The analysis based on these numbers shows a slight preference for operating on this type of patient as the risk of death, .0066 is less than the .0068 associated with "wait and see." *Source:* Pliskin and Taylor: 1977, p. 14.

using a single individual's informed guesses. Consequently, for areas in which acceptable data or data estimates are available, decision analysis will likely prove extremely useful. For the remaining areas, further refinement in the technology must await the development of more precise probability values, which may come from (1) more experience, (2) structured consensus development, or (3) controlled clinical trials.

*Cost/benefit and cost-effectiveness analyses* have been extolled, along with decision analysis, as being among the most important means for improving clinical judgment in the future (Donabedian, 1978a). In Donabedian's opinion, the very essence of quality resides in choosing the most appropriate strategy for the management of any given situation. Donabedian also believes that the necessary tools—namely, decision analysis and analysis of cost effectiveness and cost benefits—now exist for specifying and testing such strategies, which means that the mysteries of clinical judgment are amenable to yielding of their darkest secrets.

Health care cost/benefit analysis is a method for determining the costs associated with a particular health care program and the resulting relative benefits. To carry out the analysis, one must decide what costs and benefits should be included and what values should be attached to them. All possible advantages and disadvantages of the program analyzed must be weighted, both individuals and society must be considered, and costs and benefits must be valued in common units (Pliskin and Taylor, 1977).

Cost-effectiveness analysis partly avoids the difficult task of assigning dollar values to benefits by specifying a program or intervention objective without assigning a fiscal value to it. For example, the objective might be to increase average survival for a defined population of cancer patients by six months. The analytical task then is to compare costs of several alternative interventions or programs that achieve this objective so that the least costly, most cost-effective program or intervention can be chosen. Cost/benefit analysis can be applied across the entire health care delivery system for resource allocation among programs with different objectives. Cost-effectiveness analysis is limited to allocation decisions associated with one specified objective.

Several current characteristics of the health care system inhibit the impact of this kind of analysis, however (Office of Technology Assessment, 1980a). First, there is a tendency for every institution to adopt the best and latest health care technology. This tendency is based on the traditional medical practice of doing the most for every individual patient and is fueled by current methods of third-party reimbursement for services. Second, data showing links between health care intervention input and outcome are often inadequate. We must accept the fact that wherever there is contention over the purely moral aspects of one action over another, it is almost certain that the outcome of the attendant cost/benefit study will vary according to which of the opposing value systems is adopted (Muir Gray, 1979).

For all the problems and constraints of application of cost/benefit and cost-effectiveness analyses—and these have been very well reviewed in a recently published report of the Office of Technology Assessment (1980b)—the advantage in these methods lies in their formal, objective, empirical, logical, open, and explicit approach (Enthoven, 1978b; Starr and Whipple, 1980; Fuchs, 1980). If some constraints in health services utilization are inevitable, then we agree with Fuchs that the principles of cost/benefit and cost-effectiveness analyses offer the most rational basis for this aspect of cost control. Deciding to whom resources should be allocated is extremely difficult, requiring complex value judgments. Decision-analytic techniques aid in that decision process. They provide a medium through which the views of society as a whole can be more fairly reflected. Clearly, health care providers can and should provide valuable input to this process, but consumers, epidemiologists, economists, politicians, and others have equally important contributions to make (Mooney, 1980; Parsons and Lock, 1980).

As clinicians become more comfortable with structured group judgment, decision analysis, and cost/benefit and cost-effectiveness analyses, undoubtedly they will begin to discover more opportunities for the appropriate application of these decision aids. All of us—health consumers, providers, and the public at large—become the benefactors. That is, after all, the ultimate goal of quality assurance.

## Future Educational Methods in Quality Assurance

The preceding sections of this chapter reviewed expected economic and decision-making developments in health care that will have immediate implications in planning the *content* of quality assurance education. Equally important are the critical issues related to the incentives, motivation, and commitment to quality assurance that have immediate implications for planning *methods* of quality assurance education. These goals involve the "affective domain of learning"—the domain that encompasses educational objectives related to developing personal interests, achieving satisfaction, clarifying values, and making commitments. This section emphasizes these affective learning goals as they relate to career development and attitudes that affect the continued competence and excellence of health professionals, particularly in what is termed the "art" of caring. For the health professional, this means caring not only about one's patients as human beings, but equally about one's performance in terms of effectiveness and efficiency, and about the likely outcomes of one's professional activities in terms of health and economic benefits achieved.

A large component of the quality of care is the interpersonal relationship between the health professional and the patient, or what Donabedian (1980) and Brook and others (1976, 1979) call the art of care. This art relates to the provision of services in a manner appropriate to the values, expectations, and aspirations of individual patients; to the "caring" functions; and to the way patients are treated personally. Methods for assessing quality of care have barely begun to address this aspect of health care delivery even though it may be an area in which the most grievous breaches of quality occur. Because our instruments for measuring the art of caring are still rudimentary (Ware, Davies-Avery, and Stewart, 1978), it is difficult to assess the true scope of deficiencies in this realm. Nevertheless, a number of outcome-oriented studies conducted over the past decade (Williamson, 1978; Brook, 1979; Brook and others, 1977) offer ample evidence to support the view that as much total benefit, or more, could be expected to accrue from improving this element of care as through continuously increasing efforts to study rare underlying causes of disease or adopting increasingly technology-intensive diagnostic and therapeutic procedures.

It is difficult to predict how much improvement in the art of caring could be achieved by reorienting the educational process for future health professionals. Earlier works by Becker and others (1961), Meyer (1960), and Eron (1955) described the deleterious effect of our education system to the idealism and altruism of medical and nursing students. More recent investigations have documented that medical students and residents feel or perceive that they lack control in their personal lives (Edwards and Zimet, 1976; Frey and others, 1975; Frey, Demick, and Bilbar, 1981; Boufford, 1977), suffer a loss of autonomy and of self-determination (Rosenberg, 1971), are dealt with in a less than responsible and human manner (Keniston, 1967), eventually come to a passive acceptance of the "system" (Huebner, Royner, and Moore, 1981), and learn to "play the game" (Rosenberg, 1971). It is easy to understand the subsequent effect of these self-perceptions on idealism, altruism, and caring for others, particularly in situations of stress.

When one adds conventional emphasis on technology and technological competence in the student's learning experience, one can begin to understand the decrease in the student's will or ability to make *human* contact with patients, a phenomenon cited by a number of observers (Reiser, 1973; Burra and Bryans, 1979; Meyer, 1960; Rosenberg, 1971; Lesserman, 1980). The lessening of this sense of caring for the welfare of the patient, we suggest, can result in serious, unfavorable consequences in quality of medical care.

Learning to care about the continued excellence of one's professional performance is also an important part of one's professional education. Quality, particularly as defined in this book, means providing *both* effective and efficient care—that is, achieving an optimal health result for individual patients and in so doing avoiding unnecessary expenditure of resources. Ultimately, caring must encompass concern for outcome. In medical practice, caring requires the physician to act so as to improve the ultimate outcome with respect to disease or disability while taking into consideration the values of the patient and his or her family. In this sense, caring is benefit-oriented and not a preoccupation with the technical process alone. It demands a continual objective appraisal of outcomes so as to seek and achieve the highest benefit consistent with the patient's needs within constraints set by society and current health care technology. This continual reassessment of the outcomes of one's performance (that is, quality assurance) is an indispensable and integral part of providing care. Many health care practitioners maintain that they are too busy providing care to devote time to systematic quality assurance endeavors. This is equivalent to a pilot's being too busy flying the plane to have time to check his compass bearings to see where he is in relation to where he wants to be.

The essence of quality assurance education is to revitalize that concern for where we are going (the outcomes of care) and to identify the most effective and efficient means of getting there. One of the major objectives of quality assurance education is to motivate students to want to understand and conduct systematic appraisals of the level of benefits presently achieved so as to improve the care they are providing. These educational objectives are both affective and cognitive. The major portion of this book has been concerned with the cognitive aspects of education that can be transmitted by didactic lectures and readings. It is equally important to use methods such as case studies, role playing, field trips, and actual participation in quality assurance programs to achieve the goal of influencing students' attitudes and values.

There are relatively few educational texts in the health field that are specifically designed to facilitate achieving educational goals in the affective domain. Krathwohl and others (1964) provide one of the most insightful resources for this purpose. This work outlines a complete taxonomy of educational objectives that range from effecting simple feeling responses to influencing complex value and philosophic systems. Illustrative examples are provided at each taxonomic level for planning effective learning experiences and evaluating learning accomplishments. This topic is also addressed in works concerning adult learning and continuing education. One of the more definitive reviews in the medical field is "Continuing Education of Health Professionals: Proposal for a Definition of Quality" (Suter and others, 1981). This resource was developed as a joint project of the Veterans Administration and the Association of American Medical Colleges. The reader is urged to refer to such resources in planning more effective pedagogic methods in future quality assurance education programs.

## Conclusions

Changes in health services organizations and financing will undoubtedly affect quality assurance activities and education. In addition, they will influence quality assurance research. Donabedian (1978b, 1980, 1981) has identified several topics for future research, including further investigations of the relation between quality and costs; studies of particular components of care that affect quality, such as the client/practitioner relationship, continuity and coordination of care, and physician behavior; and refinement of decision analysis, criteria mapping, and information management as tools for quality assessment. Brook and others (1977, 1979) suggest other research issues for the 1980s, such as continued refinement of short-term, disease-specific outcome measures and improvement in methods of measuring the art of care. To these topics, we would add: further refinement of methods of assessing and ensuring the quality of long-term care, expanded review of the quality of ambulatory care, improvement in technologies for concurrent review (Sheber, 1980), development of practical and equitable methods to assess physician competence (Senior, 1977), and application of quality assurance findings to learner-oriented continuing education (Rubenstein and others, 1979; Osborne, 1980).

Undoubtedly there are other areas of investigation that will require urgent attention. The knowledge base and content for quality assurance activity and education have expanded rapidly and will continue to broaden as we develop a clearer picture of the complexity of the health care cost problem and make more sophisticated attempts to solve it. The number of researchers and educators concerned with quality assurance has likewise increased. This increase in activity and research is bound to have its effect on quality assurance education. Future health care professionals will need knowledge and skills to enable them to meet the demand for quality and cost control in providing health services under different systems for organizing and financing care. It is our hope that the content and processes described in this book will assist faculties of medical and other health professional schools to develop the types of educational programs in quality assurance and cost containment that can prepare future health care providers to meet these needs.

# Appendix A

## A Historical Perspective on Quality Assurance and Cost Containment
*Elizabeth Fee*

ЖЖЖЖЖЖЖЖЖЖЖЖЖЖЖЖЖЖЖЖЖЖЖЖЖЖ

Quality assurance can be described on two levels: It is, in its strictest sense, a set of techniques for assuring the maintenance and improvement of standards and of the effectiveness and efficiency of medical care. More broadly, it is an effort to regulate and control medical practice. As such, it involves a set of relationships between the medical profession and the public and between the medical profession and the government.

Like other professionals, physicians have traditionally

278

insisted on complete professional control over their own work process, including their fees; they have resisted pressures toward public accountability, on the argument that it is within the nature of a profession to set and enforce its own standard of services. The fact that their ministrations have as their goal the relief of pain and suffering and the restoration of health sets them apart from other, more mundane providers of services. Thus, theirs has been one of the few occupations to maintain the independent status once associated with all skilled crafts, although licensure and safeguards against excessive fees have often, if not consistently, been mandated by government.

As long as the medical profession was organized on an individual practitioner basis, it was indeed possible, by means of self-regulation and internal control, to avoid public interference in strictly medical affairs. Today, however, medicine is highly organized and institutionalized: It involves a complex social organization and is practiced by means of sophisticated technology. The view of medical practice as a private transaction between the physician as healer and the patient as a mere recipient of services no longer holds. The relationship between physician and patient is now mediated on many levels by third-party payers, insurance companies, and government. It is in this context that demands for public accountability in the process of medical care are being heard. These demands are fueled by many concerns with the present conditions of medical care, among them anxiety over the vast and rapid inflation of its cost.

If we are to understand how this situation has come about and how to reconcile legitimate professional and public concerns, we will need to review the history of medical professionalization and medical organization, paying attention to the social context of medical practice and also to the question of medical fees and costs in the United States.

### Growth of the Medical Profession in the United States

The history of medical care in the thirteen British colonies in North America from the seventeenth to the eighteenth centuries reveals not one type of medical practice but many competing forms. Until well into the latter half of the nineteenth century, there was no one uniform standard of medical care, no single type of practitioner. The elite of the profession were highly educated—either in European medical schools or, later, in the best of the American colleges. They had medical degrees, were of high social status, considered themselves scientific practitioners, and charged correspondingly high fees. These were, however, the minority; they were physicians to the well off. The majority of practitioners were of lower social status and had little formal education. Most were trained by apprenticeship; they had few pretensions to "book learning" but were practical men who had learned their craft through practice and experience. Generally their fees were considerably lower than those of the elite; they provided medical care to a population that could not afford the services of the college-educated men. Fees for service were usually set on a sliding scale, depending on patients' ability to pay. Set fees also were influenced by the number of practitioners in a given geographical area, and complaints about fee cutting were common, as were early attempts to hold down fees considered excessive—for example, in the colony of Virginia in 1645.

*Remuneration of Physicians and Costs of Medical Care.* Physicians obviously preferred to treat the well off, since their incomes depended largely on the incomes of their patients. The most successful made small fortunes from medical practice; others barely made enough to support themselves and combined medical practice with other occupations, such as farming or the manufacture of drugs. (In drug manufacture also, a few became rich from sales of successful patent medicines, some simply conducted a small business enterprise on the side, and others undoubtedly failed entirely.)

In some areas, physicians undertook contract practice, a form of prepayment. They would attend individuals, families, or organized groups at a set price per year. Indeed, even when physicians were paid on a fee-for-service basis, they were often paid on the "credit system"—bills were paid annually and sometimes in kind; at times they were not paid at all. Once medical societies were organized in the eighteenth century (the first in New Jersey in 1766), they attempted to formalize these methods of payment. The medical societies came to oppose contract practice and the credit system. As a group in Cincinnati suggested, "Regular patrons should have their bills presented as soon as the treatment of a case is completed. The service is then fresh, and gratitude for attention at its height" (*Cincinnati Medical Observer*, 1857).

Fee bills were established in many states by cooperation between physicians who agreed to a minimum regular charge for their services and avoided competitive pricing. Physicians' fees varied considerably throughout the country; they were much higher in cities than in rural areas, and charges for all specialized services were high. Special charges were made for the use of medical instruments such as the stethoscope, the forceps, and the vaginal speculum. Even in its infancy, medical technology carried special status and correspondingly high costs.

However, it was part of physicians' professional ethics not to refuse services to those unable to pay; then, as now, provision was made for treating those unable to pay a fee for services rendered. Most fee bills allowed the poor to be treated gratis; the standard fees were for those able to pay (Rosen, 1946). During the colonial period, medical care of those on poor relief was assumed as a charge on the local town or county government. Churches, the traditional dispensers of services to the poor in Europe, also undertook responsibility for medical care to the sick poor in America and paid a physician on an individual case basis. By the late seventeenth century, there were salaried "town physicians" to care for the sick poor (Roemer, 1945). As the population in the colonies increased in the early eighteenth century, large towns built almshouses and engaged salaried physicians. For those needing treatment but not shelter, free consultation and treatment was provided in dispensaries. Attending physicians and apothecaries were paid an annual salary by a board of governors, the money being raised by charitable subscription. All these forms of medical care were patterned after the English poor relief system and provided a minimal level of service. Recipients were the carefully screened "deserving poor" who were expected to be suitably grateful for any assistance; this system was organized by the prominent local citizens and combined Christian charity with social control. Access to care was firmly regulated, as were the hours, salaries, and conduct of the physicians involved.

Several other forms of "free" medical care coexisted with this fee-for-service system. In the antebellum South, for example, slave owners provided some medical care for their slaves, if only to protect their investment. In 1798, the United States Congress established an early form of compulsory health insurance for merchant seamen, deducting a small sum from each sailor's wages to operate marine hospitals (Terris, 1944). These wage deductions failed to cover hospital costs, and the Congress was forced to make up the deficit, thus providing the first federally organized health service. State governments assumed responsibility for the mentally ill on the same basis as they provided jails—more to protect the social order than for the benefit of the inmates. For both physicians and patients, the various forms of public or privately funded medical care represented resorts for the desperate—a minimum level of professional care, at minimal cost, in the uncomfortable context of charitable institutions organized by respectable citizens for their social inferiors.

In contrast to the fee-for-service system based on the individual's ability to pay and the charitable free care to the poor or mentally ill, each of which left control of access and quality in the hands of the physicians or the funding source rather than within the power of the patients, certain forms of contract practice based on the concept of health insurance began to develop. The contract practice of fraternal societies and mutual benefit associations was based on organizations of working men to provide sickness insurance in the form of cash benefits. Fraternal societies were often ethnic group associations; one of the first, founded in 1787, was the Free African Society in Philadelphia, followed by La Société Française de Bienfaisance Mutuelle and the German Benevolent Society (Schwartz, 1965). The latter two organizations also operated their own hospitals. Fraternal orders became most active in offering medical benefits in the last decades of the nineteenth century; by World War I, they provided an estimated half to three quarters of all health insurance in the United States, the remainder being provided by trade unions and commercial insurance companies (Sydenstricker, 1917). Today they still constitute a large sector of Latin American systems of health care—for example, in Argentina.

"Lodge practice," or medical prepayment, plans were popular forms of contract practice, although these were bitterly opposed by the American Medical Association and termed the layman's method of exploiting physicians (*Journal of the American Medical Association*, 1906, 1907, 1911). Many physicians, however, were glad to have the financial security afforded by contract practice and were willing to work for fraternal societies and trade unions, just as they were willing to staff the urban dispensaries and hospital outpatient clinics that provided services to those unable to pay the fees of private physicians.

*Quality of Care.* Examination of the quality of medical care in terms of therapeutic efficacy, safety, and effectiveness, measured by the current norms of scientific medicine, forces one to conclude that, until the middle of the nineteenth century, the efficacy of available therapies and the effectiveness of their use were largely unproved. This judgment is equally valid whether we consider the practice of the medical elite or that of the ordinary rural practitioners.

Physicians used remedies that were believed effective by virtue of custom or authority or by virtue of successful experience. Even when a physician had no firm convictions about the usefulness of a particular drug, he might be likely to prescribe it for the patient, for lack of anything better; in the physician/patient relationship a prescription could help convince both parties that some concrete effort was being made to alleviate distress and disease.

Even then, the main criticisms of medical practice were that physicians used too many drugs, that the drugs prescribed often did more harm than good, and that physicians were overly fond of surgical interventions, such as bleeding and lancing their patients. In contemporary terms, the problem as seen by critics of medicine was "overutilization."

In the American colonies as elsewhere, the only methods of regulating the quality of medical practice were those imposed by a competitive market. Each physician had to convince his patients or potential patients of the value of his services and had to build his own reputation as a practitioner. This reputation depended in part on salesmanship; in part on personal qualities; in part on knowledge, erudition, and wisdom; and to a large degree on the testimony of customers satisfied with the outcomes of their treatment. In available accounts of medical practice, largely confined to diaries and letters, we find happy patients who were "cured" by the most improbable remedies. New medical sects were often formed when an unorthodox treatment cured a patient who had previously been given up as lost; new medical theories were developed on the basis of a small number of successful cases. Quality control, to the extent that it existed, was administered directly by patient satisfaction. One sign of the quack medicine man was the speed of his travels; he did not stay in one area long enough to be accountable for the success of his remedies, and he therefore depended on his abilities for instant persuasion.

The question of the quality of medical care, however, was argued vigorously by physicians. The elite of the profession, both in Europe and in the Americas, attempted to raise standards and to introduce into their art the principles of scientific inquiry that had been developed in the natural sciences. Examples are the treatises by Stahl (1698) and Miller (1814) and Bartlett's *Inquiry into Certainty in Medicine* (1848). At the same time, these academically oriented physicians defended their own superiority to the mass of uneducated practitioners and were concerned with elevating the general status of the profession. These early attempts at ensuring the standards of the medical profession, or "quality assurance," led to concerted efforts to control through licensing laws the numbers and qualifications of persons seeking to practice.

*Medical Education and Licensure.* The first local societies for physicians, formed in colonial towns in the mid eighteenth century, admitted physicians with medical degrees and others whom they considered reputable but excluded the lowest ranks of the profession. There were no state licensure requirements until 1760, when New York established licensure of practicing physicians; in 1763 the Connecticut legislature vigorously opposed an attempt by physicians to control their own licensure. After the Revolution, however, between 1780 and 1830, state medical societies energetically advocated the licensing of medical practitioners, and several state governments responded by establishing examining boards or by giving the medical societies the power to test and license new applicants (Shryock, 1960). After the first American medical schools were established in the late eighteenth century (for example, the College of Philadelphia in 1765), several state legislatures adopted the rule that graduation from a chartered medical school constituted licensure to practice. Licensing regulations were formalized by 1830.

This development toward regulated access to the profession was turned back in the Jackson era, when egalitarian philosophy led to the repeal of government-controlled physician licensure in almost every state between 1830 and 1840; the market was to regulate the quality of medical care. During the next half century, many proprietary, or private, medical schools were established by physicians and operated primarily for profit; students paid their fees, obtained a more or less cursory medical education, and gained their licenses. In addition to the competition among these regular medical schools was the competition among a growing number of medical sects, each with its own theory, its own practice, and its own appeals to patients. Botanics, homeopaths, osteopaths, chiropractors, Grahamites, Thomsonians, eclectics, and many others challenged orthodox, or allopathic, medicine with claims to a safer and more effective form of medical practice. Allopathic physicians who protested against sectarian medicine faced a largely unsympathetic public; they were accused of seeking a medical monopoly in their own interest. The republican ideology, antagonistic to their efforts to regulate medical practice, stressed instead the freedom of each citizen to choose his or her own physician. In 1847 these allopathic physicians formed the American Medical Association to defend their interests. The national association represented only the "regular" medical societies; it hoped to reestablish licensing standards and to promote educational reforms, thereby improving the quality of medical practice.

During the latter half of the nineteenth century, the elite of the medical profession again included many who had obtained their medical education at European schools, particularly the German universities. On returning to America, they emphasized the importance of scientific training and research as a basis for medical practice. They wanted to reform medical education along European lines, to take licensing power away from the hundreds of small proprietary medical schools, and to remake the medical profession in the continental European pattern.

Efforts to reform medical education had, however, a built-in obstacle. The majority of the regular physicians were graduates of existing proprietary medical schools and had thus obtained their licenses to practice; they were not enthusiastic about advocates of reform. Some, indeed, had a financial interest in the existing schools.

In 1876 reform-minded physicians on the faculties of medical schools founded the Association of American Medical Colleges. The organization folded in 1883 and revived again in 1890 when the struggle for higher licensing requirements gained intensity. In 1901 the AMA was reorganized, producing a reform leadership willing to push for the overhaul of medical education.

In this struggle, the medical elite gained some new and very powerful allies, the great corporate foundations interested in medical education and research, such as the Rockefeller and Carnegie foundations. Although older charitable institutions had traditionally provided local support of medical services for the poor, and wealthy persons had endowed private hospitals or established free clinics, the new philanthropy was on a much larger scale, with more ambitious aims. Private fortunes were dedicated to the reorganization and reform of American institutions on a national and international level; the reform of medical education, the endowment of medical research, and the reconstitution of the medical profession were appropriately large tasks. The AMA Council, in turn, knew that to institute the kind of medical education it desired required a new financing structure; these schools could not be run as profit-making ventures but would have to be supported by public or private funds. They turned to the foundations. In 1905 Andrew Carnegie established the Foundation for the Advancement of Teaching, and in 1909 this body undertook a national survey of medical schools. The director of the survey, Abraham Flexner, published his famous study, the Flexner Report, in 1910, condemning the standards of proprietary colleges. Foundation grants were given to colleges meeting the standards laid down in the Flexner Report; state legislatures and licensing boards helped bring pressure to bear on those schools declared inferior. As the new standards were instituted, many of the existing schools closed. Following the closing of medical schools, the ratio of physicians to population declined from 1:600 in 1910 to 1:763 in 1938 (Shryock, 1960).

The American Medical Association, aided by powerful foundations and state legislatures, had achieved its aims: a higher standard of medical training and control of access to the profession. Medicine was now oriented toward the basic medical sciences and toward medical research; the association among medical schools, universities, and hospitals had been consolidated. Specialization was developed by hospital residencies between 1880 and 1920, and later organizations of specialists set up their own processes of certification.

During the Flexnerian reforms, all emphasis had been on medical education and licensure, not on medical practice. Medical practice, however, was transformed in the process. The lower ranks of physicians were eliminated; most of the schools that had provided access to medical education for women, minorities, and working-class people were abolished. The status and income of medical practitioners rose rapidly, as did the overall costs of medical care. Emphasis on scientific and laboratory medicine tied newly trained physicians to urban centers and hospital practice; following European traditions, specialty knowledge and academic status came to be more highly valued than the skills of the general practitioner. The family doctor was to become a romantic figure, representing values that had been lost in the new scientific enthusiasm.

At the turn of the century, many of the older practitioners complained that the new passion for medical research did little to enrich medical practice. The medical reformers assumed that a new medical science would produce, in turn, a more effective practice—but the theory came first. Most historians of medicine and commentators on medical care, at least until very recently, have accepted the claims of scientific medicine quite uncritically, and some have regarded all medical history before the Flexner Report as a dark age of error and confusion. Ertel (1977), for example, states that "as long as medicine simply presided in sympathetic ceremonies to the inevitable, that is, officiated over the course of the disease about which it could do little or nothing, it was virtually irrelevant to inquire whether physicians in general were doing a good job. It really did not matter. Now it does." His graph depicting the hypothetical evolution of therapeutic effectiveness shows medical care suddenly and dramatically becoming effective in the twentieth century. This perception is very widely shared. Others have argued that the fall in mortality rates associated with the decline of infectious disease predated any effective medical therapies and must be attributed to broader social causes, such as better diet, housing, and sanitary conditions, and other public health measures (Dubos and Dubos), 1953; Powles, 1973). In any case, scientific medicine, until recently, has maintained an unquestioned reputation for therapeutic efficacy, and control over quality was the prerogative of its practitioners.

### Society and the Profession: The Limits of Growth

*Access to Medical Care.* At the turn of the century, in valuing theory and scientific advances over everyday practice, medicine had now lost its much-prized independence. Medical schools could no longer be operated without the financial assistance of either corporate or state funds, and the orientation to scientific medicine could not be maintained without the research institutes, laboratories, and expensive equipment of the academic centers. Increasingly, medical men concentrated in the cities, and their geographical distribution exacerbated the effects of their reduced numbers. Increasing costs of care, and the recognition that medical services should be available to the growing population incapable of making large out-of-pocket payments for care, led to societal concern and to government involvement in mechanisms for ensuring the availability of services.

Around the turn of the century, Germany and other European countries established compulsory health insurance systems in response to working-class pressures (Dawson, n.d.). In 1911 the British Parliament passed a National Insurance Act, providing national health insurance for industrial workers. It was the British act that generated most interest in the United States; reformers saw health insurance as one means of mitigating increasingly evident social disparities of wealth and of thus achieving a balance between "the known evils of laissez faire and the anticipated evils of socialism" (Fine, 1956). In 1904 the American Socialist Party had called for sickness insurance; in 1912 Theodore Roosevelt's Progressive Party adopted a similar platform. Also in 1912, the American Association for Labor Legislation created a Committee on

Social Insurance to prepare a model bill for introduction to state legislatures (Numbers, 1978). This bill provided income protection and complete medical care for manual laborers earning less than $100 a month, with premiums to be divided among workers, employers, and the state. Initially, the organized medical profession supported the legislation; many physicians felt that some form of social health insurance was inevitable and that it was politic to cooperate rather than to fight such moves. Indeed, general practitioners might benefit from a more secure method of financing medical costs.

Commercial insurance companies, however, violently opposed national health insurance and waged a vigorous campaign to convince physicians and legislators that a national health system would be a disaster for the medical profession, would lower incomes, and would again produce an inferior form of medical care. Organized labor was divided on the issue; in many states, labor actively campaigned for compulsory health insurance, but Samuel Gompers, president of the American Federation of Labor, argued that the solution to the problem of medical care was not compulsory insurance but higher wages (Commission to Study Social Insurance, 1916). The medical profession was eventually persuaded to adopt a strong stand against any form of compulsory health insurance, and by 1920 the prospect of any such legislation was dead.

What survived, however, were fragmented efforts by government and public agencies to provide care for those in need. In 1921, for example, the Sheppard-Towner Bill provided federal funds to the states for establishing prenatal care centers, conducting child health conferences, supporting visiting nurse programs, and distributing informational literature. The Great Depression of 1929 brought a crisis in medicine, as in all areas of the economy; hospital income from endowments and patient fees declined precipitously, while the patient load increased dramatically. Hospitals were forced to find new methods of financing patient care and began to experiment with insurance schemes to cover hospital costs (Williams, 1932). These became the Blue Cross plans, promoted by the American Hospital Association in competition with commercial insurance companies.

Prepaid hospital insurance provided an immediate solution to the problem of hospital financing, but political pressures for broader social security legislation intensified. Reflecting the emphasis on government intervention where private initiative was insufficient, the original draft of Franklin D. Roosevelt's Social Security Bill of 1934 included compulsory health insurance. However, the traditional insistence of the medical profession on control over practice as well as fees prevailed, and this provision was deleted from the Social Security Act of 1935. Instead, some federal funds were given to the states to support local public health programs. The boundaries of subsequent legislation had been set: Congress provided funds for specific programs, preventive health measures, and education but did not question the basic organization of the system of medical care. In 1937, establishment of the National Cancer Institute provided research grants to search for solutions to some pressing health problems. Authority to provide research grants on a broader basis to institutions and individuals was extended to the National Institutes of Health in 1944.

During World War II, the questions of medical care organization, facilities, and financing reappeared. The Wagner-Murray-Dingle Bill of 1943 again called for federally financed health insurance through extension of the Social Security program. Again this legislation was defeated. Unions then began organizing for group health insurance to meet rapidly rising medical costs, thus bringing the financing of health care into collective bargaining agreements. This strategy of unions, then the most powerful political force favoring national health insurance, redirected attention toward voluntary, or commercial, insurance, which was endorsed by the American Medical Association.

The continuously increasing costs of providing modern hospital care, however, inescapably led to a growing provision of federal funds and, as inescapably but not necessarily effectively, of federal control and regulation. Funding for construction and modernization of hospital facilities was provided through the Hill-Burton program, the Hospital Survey and Construction Act of 1946. This legislation represented the first federal attempt at health planning; states were required to survey their needs for health care facilities and to plan hospital construction (Taft and

Levine, 1976). The actual planning done, however, was little more than a formality, and later federal analysis showed that the geographical location of new health facilities built under the Hill-Burton program bore little consistent relation to areas where health needs were greatest (Levin, 1972).

Health manpower legislation also attempted to include a rational planning component and was also conspicuously unsuccessful in this goal. Funds were given to educational institutions, with virtually no local or state control over expenditures. The federal government was reluctant to reinforce a verbal commitment to planning with any form of strict accountability; there was little political resistance to the provision of funds but much resistance to any attempted control of expenditures. Planners warned that this type of unrestricted funding would inflate medical costs without accomplishing the desired objectives, but the dimensions of the problem were not apparent until after the Social Security Amendments of 1965 instituted the Medicare and Medicaid programs (Taft and Levine, 1976).

Despite the numerous bills passed to improve access to availability of health care resources, and the growth of health insurance plans, there still remained a sizable portion of the American population for whom the costs of care were prohibitive and who were ineligible for health insurance: the elderly and the poor. To remedy this situation, Congress passed the Social Security Amendments of 1965 (PL 89-97) to provide hospital and medical protection to these two groups. Through Medicare (Title XVIII), the federal government was to provide hospital and medical protection to those sixty-five years of age and older, to those under sixty-five receiving cash benefits from the Social Security program or from the railroad retirement program because of disability, and to certain patients with chronic kidney disease. Under Medicaid (Title XIX) the federal government was to provide joint funding with state governments for medical care to the needy.

To restrain costs and to ensure quality of care provided to those served under the new legislation, PL 89-97 included requirements that hospitals institute utilization review committees as a condition for receiving funds to review the appropriate use of medical services. (This requirement was extended to Medicaid programs by the 1967 Social Security Amendments, PL 90-248.) In addition, the law established standards and requirements for hospitals involved in the Medicare program and certification of individual providers. These standards were intended to ensure a minimum level of acceptable medical care. Agencies of state governments were responsible for assessing compliance with the utilization review and physician certification requirements. However, survey teams did not have the expertise to determine whether the utilization review had been conducted in an effective manner. No hospital was ever barred from the program for failure to meet requirements, even though in most cases compliance was *pro forma* (Goran, Roberts, and Rodak, 1976).

With the enactment of the Social Security Amendments, the federal government became one of the largest third-party payers for medical services. Nearly 25 million people became eligible for coverage under the law, increasing demand for health services throughout the country. It soon became apparent that national expenditures for health care were increasing at a level that caused serious concern (see Department of Health, Education, and Welfare, 1972). These costs escalations prompted further legislative action. In 1969 Senator Wallace Bennett introduced a bill to establish Professional Standards Review Organizations as an amendment (No. 851) to the Social Security Amendments of 1969 (H.R. 17550). In 1972 this bill was reintroduced, with some modifications, as Amendment No. 823 to the Social Security Amendments of 1971 (H.R. 1). It was in discussion of these bills that the interrelationship between cost control and quality assurance was first expressed (Gosfield, 1975). In the same year, Professional Standards Review Organizations were established as part of the Social Security Amendments of 1972 (PL 92-603). Under this legislation responsibility for review of medical services to patients receiving care under Medicare and Medicaid programs was given to local organizations of practicing physicians. These PSROs were to assure that services were medically necessary and provided in accordance with professional standards. Gosfield (1975), in summarizing the provisions of the PSRO legislation, cites the methodology for PSRO review prescribed in the law as follows: "Each PSRO shall apply professionally developed norms of care, diagnosis, and treatment based upon typical patterns of practice in its regions (including typical lengths of stay for institutional care by age and diagnosis) as principal points of evaluation and review." The approach and methodologies developed by PSROs to carry out this mandate are discussed in Chapter Seven of this text.

PSROs are not the only form of systematic quality assurance and cost containment programs. A number of other programs and approaches to cost and quality control are being proposed, including Peer Review Organizations, sponsored by the American Medical Association; the Health Outcomes Commission, sponsored by InterStudy; and the Commission on the Quality of Care, a section of the "Health Security Act," Senator Kennedy's national health insurance bill supported, at least initially, by organized labor (Gosfield, 1975). In addition, the Health Maintenance Organization Act of 1973 requires that federally qualified HMOs have an ongoing internal quality assurance program, and several of the national health insurance proposals include requirements for quality and cost review.

Moreover, a number of quality assurance programs have been developed or are being proposed in the private sector. More recently, as private industry has grown increasingly concerned with the rising costs of health care and its effects on the costs of the benefit packages to employees, many large companies have become interested in the work of the medical care foundations in the area of utilization review. In 1977 the American Association of Professional Standards Review Organizations joined with the American Association of Foundations of Medical Care to form a nonprofit organization, Peer Review Network, Inc. (PRN). Recently PRN has negotiated with large companies and labor groups and with their numerous health insurance carriers to provide organized utilization and peer review of all services offered employees through the various health insurance plans. Industry's interest in controlling health resource expenditures and its willingness to participate in programs to review utilization of these resources indicate that quality assurance activities may well extend more fully into the private sector.

It is clear from this brief overview of the history of quality assurance and cost containment that the recent trends in both the private and public sector betoken a commitment to establishing systematic procedures for assessing the cost and quality of health care. Although there are many difficulties yet to be resolved (for example, clarifying the relation between quality assurance and cost containment as well as selecting appropriate and cost-effective methods for assessing and improving care), quality assurance and cost containment have become an integral part of contemporary medical practice.

## References

Bartlett, E. *An Inquiry into the Degree of Certainty in Medicine; and into the Nature and Extent of its Power over Disease.* Philadelphia: Lea and Blanchard, 1848. Abridged version reprinted in G. H. Brieger, *Medical America in the Nineteenth Century: Readings from the Literature.* Baltimore and London: Johns Hopkins University Press, 1972.

*Cincinnati Medical Observer.* II, 1857, p. 79. Cited by G. Rosen, "Fees and Fee Bills: Some Economic Aspects of Medical Practice in Nineteenth Century America." *Bulletin of the History of Medicine,* 1946, *6* (Supplements), 35.

Commission to Study Social Insurance and Unemployment. *Hearings Before the Committee on Labor, House of Representatives, 64th Congress, April 6 and 11, 1916.* Washington, D.C.: U.S. Government Printing Office, 1918.

Dawson, W. H. *Social Insurance in Germany, 1883–1911.* New York: Scribner's, n.d.

Dubos, R., and Dubos, J. *The White Plague–Tuberculosis, Man, and Society.* Boston: Little, Brown, 1953.

Ellwood, P. M., Jr. "Models for Organizing Health Services and Implications of Legislative Proposals." *Milbank Memorial Fund Quarterly,* 1972, *50,* 73–101.

Ertel, P. Y. "Perspectives of Medicine and Society: Evolution and Role of Peer Review in Medical Practice." In P. Y. Ertel and M. G. Anderson (Eds.), *Medical Peer Review: Theory and Practice.* St. Louis: Mosby, 1977.

Fine, S. *Laissez-Faire and the General Welfare State: A Study of Conflict in American Thought, 1865–1901.* Ann Arbor, Mich.: University of Michigan Press, 1956.

Fuchs, V. R. *Who Shall Live? Health, Economics, and Social Change.* New York: Basic Books, 1974.

Goran, M. J., Roberts, J. S., and Rodak, J., Jr. "Regulating the Quality of Hospital Care—An Analysis of the Issues Pertinent to National Health Insurance." In R. H. Egdane and P. P. Gertman (Eds.), *Quality Assurance in Health Care.* Germantown, Md.: Aspen, 1976.

Gosfield, A. *PSROs: The Law and the Health Consumer.* Cambridge, Mass.: Ballinger, 1975.

Hirschfeld, D. *The Lost Reform.* Cambridge, Mass.: Harvard University Press, 1970.

*Journal of the American Medical Association.* 1906, *47,* 1923. 1907, *49,* 2028–2029. 1911, *57,* 145.

Levin, A. L. "Health Planning and the Federal Government." *International Journal of Health Services,* 1972, *2,* 367–376.

Numbers, R. L. *Almost Persuaded: American Physicians and Compulsory Health Insurance, 1912–1920.* Baltimore and London: Johns Hopkins University Press, 1978.

Powles, J. "On the Limitations of Modern Medicine." *Science, Medicine and Man,* 1973, *1,* 1–30.

Roemer, M. I. "Government's Role in American Medicine—A Brief Historical Survey." *Bulletin of the History of Medicine,* 1945, *18,* 146–168.

Rosen, G. "Fees and Fee Bills: Some Economic Aspects of Medical Practice in Nineteenth Century America." *Bulletin of the History of Medicine,* 1946, *6* (Supplements), 35.

Schwartz, J. L. "Early History of Prepaid Medical Care Plans." *Bulletin of the History of Medicine,* 1965, *39,* 450–475.

Shryock, R. H. *Medical Licensing in America, 1650–1965.* Baltimore: Johns Hopkins University Press, 1960.

Stevens, R., and Stevens, R. *Welfare Medicine in America: A Case Study of Medicaid.* New York: Free Press, 1974.

Sydenstricker, E. "Existing Agencies for Health Insurance in the United States. Proceedings, Conference on Social Insurance, 1916." *Bulletin of the U.S. Bureau of Labor Statistics,* 1917, no. 212.

Taft, C., and Levine, S. "Problems of Federal Policies and Strategies to Influence the Quality of Health Care." In R. H. Egdahl and P. M. Gertman (Eds.), *Quality Assurance in Health Care*. Germantown, Md.: Aspen, 1976.

Terris, M. "An Early System of Compulsory Health Insurance in the United States, 1798–1884." *Bulletin of the History of Medicine,* 1944, *15,* 433–444.

U.S. Department of Health, Education, and Welfare. *Program Analysis: Delivery of Health Services for the Poor.* Washington, D.C.: U.S. Government Printing Office, 1967.

U.S. Department of Health, Education, and Welfare. *Legislative History of Professional Standards Review Organization of the Social Security Act Amendments.* Washington, D.C.: U.S. Government Printiing Office, 1972.

Welch, C. E. "Professional Standards Review Organizations— Problems and Prospects." *New England Journal of Medicine,* 1973, *289,* 291–295.

Williams, P. *The Purchase of Medical Care Through Fixed Periodic Payment.* New York: National Bureau of Economic Research, 1932.

# Appendix B

## Efficacy of Selected Common Interventions for Coronary Artery Disease

*Daniel M. Barr*

ㅊㅊㅊㅊㅊㅊㅊㅊㅊㅊㅊㅊㅊㅊㅊㅊㅊㅊㅊㅊㅊㅊㅊㅊ

This appendix reviews the efficacy of some common and controversial interventions for coronary artery disease. From evidence of this type one can propose criteria of care for quality assurance (Avery and others, 1976) and estimate the potential benefit of an intervention in relation to costs for groups (Weinstein and Stason, 1977) and individuals (Pauker, 1976). The evidence reviewed illustrates both the concept of efficacy and the scarcity and complexity of efficacy studies for important interventions. It can be used in conjunction with the student volume to indicate the range of factors to be considered in an efficacy search as well as to demonstrate selection of relevant literature.

The efficacy review tried to establish whether there is documented evidence that (1) the interventions of primary prevention of coronary artery disease alter the screened person's outcome by reducing the risk of developing disease; (2) stress electrocardiograms are useful in further diagnosing symptomatic patients with angina and possible angina as presumptive diagnoses; (3) coronary arteriography is diagnostic of coronary artery disease; (4) surgery or medical treatment is the treatment of choice for newly detected patients with angina; (5) the coronary care unit is the best place for an otherwise healthy patient with acute myocardial infarction; (6) timely postcoronary exercise improves immediate and long-term symptoms and survival.

Each question can be formulated as a matrix diagram with cells showing how well the intervention works in relation to a "more valid" test of patient symptoms and survival, as shown in Figures B.2 and B.3. For comparability, this is done here as if the study were performed on 100 patients, unless otherwise noted. How these diagrams are prepared should reflect the nature and context of the study or the quality assurance and cost containment effort in which the reader is involved. For example, five-year survival rates are not useful (unless actuarially corrected) for a one-year study of patients with newly detected angina. However, in constructing the charts, the reader should also consider the state of the literature.

## Prevention

Three major risk-factors—hypertension, cigarette smoking, and hypercholesterolemia—have been shown to be consistently associated with increased risk of coronary artery disease (Wright and Fredrickson, 1973). Persons with one or more risk factors, as a group, develop initial major coronary events (largely acute myocardial infarction and sudden death) four times as often as persons with no risk factors (Wright and Fredrickson, 1973). These three risk factors plus glucose intolerance and left ventricular hypertrophy have been validated in relation to coronary angiography in terms of both the presence and the extent of coronary artery disease (Salel and others, 1977). Recently, the low-density lipoprotein fraction of cholesterol has been placed in the villain's role, whereas a high-density fraction may be protective (Kannel, Castelli, and Gordon, 1979).

Risk factors with sparser evidence include a sedentary lifestyle without regular exercise (Morris and Crawford, 1958; Paffenburger and Hale, 1975) and a Type A behavior pattern (Frank and others, 1978; Jenkins, Rosenman, and Zyzansk, 1974; Jenkins, 1976). Other risk factors studied recently include coffee, alcohol, and exogenous estrogen ingestion, corneal arcus, diagonal earlobe crease, and the weather. Though not a "risk factor" in the sense of being subject to alteration, family history is a clinically important predictor of increased risk.

Of the coronary risk factor interventions, only antihypertensives have been shown to be clearly efficacious. Cigarette smoking cessation programs and similar interventions have been of uniformly low efficacy (80 percent or more have continued smoking in long-term follow-up studies). Cholesterol manipulation by either diet or drugs has not been shown in controlled trials to be an efficacious intervention (Mann, 1977; Glueck, Mattson, and Bierman, 1978; Blackburn, 1975; Oliver, 1978).

Balancing this grim view is the declining cardiovascular mortality rate since 1964. By 1975 this decline exceeded the overall decrease in the death rate by 60 percent (Walker, 1977). Two thirds of the 32 percent reduction in the age-adjusted cardiovascular death rate over the past thirty years has occurred in the past ten years (Levy, 1979). The start of this decline, in 1964, followed the first warning on smoking by the Surgeon General of the Public Health Service and the American Heart Association's public recommendation to limit dietary intake of saturated fats and cholesterol. Other events during this period have included a national blood pressure program, alteration in dietary fat intake, reduction in per capita cigarette consumption and in toxicity of cigarette contents, coronary care units, rescue teams, improved cardiovascular surgical interventions, increased exercise, and the introduction of beta blocks. Consequently, the cause of the decline is uncertain.

The cells of Figure B.1 will therefore remain blank until the efficacy of the interventions for primary prevention is better established.

## Detection

The search for better methods of detecting coronary artery disease is intense. Some methods, such as myocardial lactate production in response to atrial pacing, left ventriculography, stress ventriculography, and ST-mapping are more useful in defining the degree of disease or myocardial damage. Others, such as radioisotopic imaging, apexcardiology and systolic time intervals, and echocardiography, may have a role in early detection of myocardial ischemia (Waters and Forrester, 1978). Combinations of methods have been advocated (Cohn and others, 1972). That better methods are needed is obvious from the observation that 40 percent of myocardial infarctions remain unrecognized (the range in other studies is 20 to 60 percent). Half of these were asymptomatic; symptoms in the other half were atypical (Medalie and Goldbourt, 1976).

The two most widely used detection methods are stress electrocardiography and coronary angiography. The efficacy of stress electrocardiography is usually evaluated using coronary angiography as the "true test." The test is usually regarded as positive if there is one millimeter or more of ST-segment depression. The median reported sensitivity of stress electrocardiography is 55 percent, and the range is 33 to 80 percent (Hartley, 1975). Sensitivity increases with increasing severity of coronary artery disease. Although a sensitive indicator of severe and symptomatic coronary artery disease, this test is not consistently sensitive to mild degrees of stenosis. The predictive value of a test is more useful clinically than its specificity. The median reported predictive value of exercise electrocardiography is 92 percent; the range is 87 to 97 percent. Consequently, a positive test is usually diagnostic (Hartley, 1975). Various proposed methods to increase the sensitivity of stress electrocardiography include Bayesian analysis of the extent

Patients develop any major events
of coronary artery disease?*

Yes                    No

Intervention programs
eliminate major risks

Yes

No

*Events refers to myocardial infarction and sudden death due or presumed due to coronary artery disease.

**Figure B.1. Existing Data on Efficacy of Preventive Interventions for Coronary Artery Disease.**

of ST-depression (Rifkin and Hood, 1977), evaluation of the slope of the ST-segment (Goldschlager, Selzer, and Cohn, 1976), incorporation of change in heart rate and mean arterial blood pressure in an exercise index (Balnave and others, 1978), and twenty-four-hour ambulatory electrocardiographic monitoring (O'Rourke and Ross, 1974; Ryan, Lown, and Horn, 1975). Because angiographically rarely detectable myocardial infarction can result from coronary spasm alone or spasm preceding thrombosis (Braunwald, 1978; Maseri and others, 1978), coronary angiography is not a completely valid measure of the diagnostic efficacy of stress electrocardiography. However, the efficacy of stress electrocardiography is established, though subject to modification in the future (Figure B.2). It is an "insensitive if negative, yet very predictive if positive" test for coronary artery disease.

The efficacy of coronary angiography is usually evaluated using post-mortem examination, including arteriograms, as the "true" test. Disagreement about the degree of stenosis of 25 percent or more and disagreement about a substantial reduction in arterial lumen have been used as criteria for diagnostic disagreement. (Reduction of 50 percent in arterial lumen diameter is equivalent to 75 percent reduction in lumen area. These represent the definition of *substantial*.) The most recently reported sensitivity of

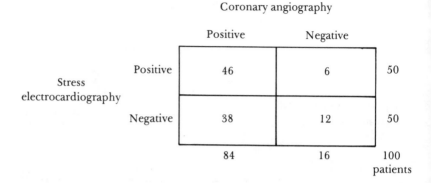

Figure B.2. Diagnostic Efficacy of Stress Electrocardiography Compared with Coronary Angiography (Adapted from Hartley, 1975).

coronary angiography is 65 percent (Galbraith, Murphy, and de Soyza, 1978), with a range in the three most recent studies of 50 to 75 percent (Galbraith, Murphy, and de Soyza, 1978; Hutchins and others, 1977; Schwartz and others, 1975). The most recently reported predictive value is 56 percent, with a range in these three studies of 56 to 88 percent. In other words, in at best 80 percent of instances coronary angiograms are in agreement with post-mortem studies. These studies related pathological examination of arterial sections to coronary angiograms. No study has been reported in terms of patients diagnosed falsely positive or falsely negative. Moreover, because the authors of these articles do not present their results in the manner suggested in Chapter Six and exemplified in the figures in this appendix, the results of two of the studies could have been misinterpreted here owing to inability to determine the number or percentage of true positive, as distinct from true negative, results. A review by an authoritative source in this area is needed.

Agreement between angiograms and autopsies has been said to be greater when the prevalence of lesions is lower (Galbraith, Murphy, and de Soyza, 1978). However, for diagnostic tests generally, decreased prevalence has been found to be associated with decreased predictive value (Galen and Gambino, 1975). Studies are not consistent on the issue of whether there are more false positive or false negative angiograms, although generally more false negatives have been reported. Missed lesions in one study (Hutchins and others, 1977) occurred at the ostia of the diagonal branches of the left anterior descending coronary artery, perhaps because of overlapping radiographic images of two vessels near the branch point. Overestimated lesions were few and were due to coronary spasm. Angiogram interpretive accuracy will probably be increased in the future by radioisotope scans and other means. At this point angiography represents the "gold standard" (Hutchins and others, 1977) and is fairly sensitive and fairly specific (Figure B.3).

Two additional points should be made regarding these diagnostic methods. First, both sensitivity and predictive value are increased by increasing disease prevalence. Most of the subjects of most efficacy studies are diseased. Consequently, as new tests are introduced and evaluated in university hospital populations (with presumed higher disease prevalence), their reported sensitivities and predictive values may be greater than when evaluations are performed on populations with lower disease prevalence (as for coronary artery disease in primary care practice). Second, all diagnostic methods involve observer variability, whose extent in stress electrocardiography is uncertain. One study on coronary arteriography reported complete interobserver agreement in 37 percent of readings and disagreement in stenosis estimates of 20 percent or more in about 40 percent (Bjork, Spindola-Franco, and Van Houten, 1975). Another study reported that majority opinions of cardiologists were accurate in 50 percent of false positive or false negative interpretations in relation to the pathologic lesions. "This suggests that even with group opinion or consensus opinion, an incorrect interpretation is likely to be accepted by the majority rule at least half the time" (Galbraith, Murphy, and de Soyza, 1978). It also suggests the extent of caution needed in interpreting the results of a relatively accurate diagnostic procedure.

## Management

Once a patient is diagnosed as having coronary artery disease or succumbs to an acute myocardial infarction, many therapeutic and management decisions are made. Two of these,

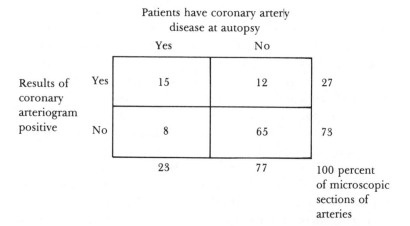

Figure B.3. Diagnostic Efficacy of Coronary Angiography for Coronary
Artery Disease Compared with Autopsy (Including
Postmortem Coronary Angiograms). (Adapted from Galbraith,
Murphy, and de Soyza, 1978.)

whether to use a principally surgical or medical approach for angina and whether to admit a patient with an acute myocardial infarction to a coronary care unit, are considered here.

Resources expended on myocardial revascularization for angina approach 1 percent of the health care budget in the United States. Patient survival and symptomatic or functional status are the accepted end points for determining the efficacy of this surgical procedure. Patients with 50 percent or more reduction in the arterial diameter of the left main coronary artery represent from 2 to 15 percent of patients studied for ischemic heart disease. The principal study of this form of coronary artery disease found that 71 percent of medically treated and 93 percent of surgically treated patients survived an average of twenty-four months follow-up. The proportion with morbid events and symptoms was lower in the surgical group (Takaro and others, 1975). In contrast, in one study of patients with unstable angina or coronary insufficiency, virtually all patients in both groups survived four months. In the surgical group 90 percent were functional Class I or II, compared with 36.8 percent of medically treated patients (Selden and others, 1975). In the most recently reported study of stable angina, 90 percent of medically treated and 92 percent of surgically treated patients survived an average of three years, whereas 50 percent of medically treated patients were in functional Classes I and II, compared with 71 percent of surgical patients (Kloster and others, 1979). These data suggest that myocardial revascularization is better palliation for these forms of coronary artery disease than medical treatment and that surgery increases patient survival for significant left main-stem lesions over medical approaches. Whether the palliative effects of myocardial revascularization persist is uncertain (McIntosh and Garcia, 1978). Thus, the efficacy of myocardial revascularization is established. It is palliative and increases longevity for left main-stem lesions. It is only palliative for other lesions (Figure B.4).

The coronary care unit serves many functions. Its principal function (indication) is to provide care for patients with suspected or proven myocardial infarctions. Since first proposed by Day (1963), such units have increased use of services without necessarily increasing survival (Martin and others, 1974). The most definitive study (a randomized, controlled clinical trial, as described in Chapter Six) compared home and hospital care, the latter initially in an intensive care unit. There was no difference in mortality between the two groups (Mather and others, 1976). Although it has been said that in-hospital myocardial infarction survival has increased from 67 to 85 percent as a result of this special unit, the basis for these figures is not as carefully derived as in Mather's study (Edwards and Jones, 1979). Clearly, control of arrhythmias in the first few hours is best accomplished there. Yet some seriously argue that the psychic trauma of the ambulance, monitoring, and special care in fact contributes to anxiety and production of arrhythmias (Colling, Carson, and Hampton, 1979). Early discharge from the hospital has been found safe also (Ross, 1978). Thus, the efficacy of the coronary care unit is not established (Figure B.5). Existing evidence, which is sparse and conflicting, shows little survival benefit.

### Rehabilitation

The effects of exercise training on mortality and symptoms following myocardial infarction have not been the object of large,

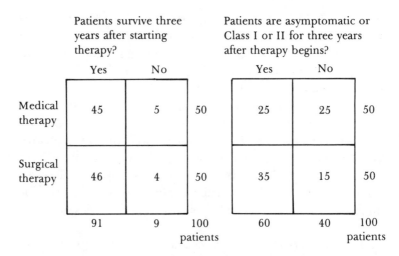

Figure B.4. Efficacy of Medical and Surgical Approaches to Stable Angina (Modified from Kloster and others, 1979).

randomized studies with follow-up over five years (Kellerman and Denolin, 1977). Three studies are underway. Available data from the Goteborg study indicate no significant survival advantage for patients involved in long-term exercise training programs, although symptoms and quality of life may be improved (Sanne, 1977). Thus, the efficacy of cardiac rehabilitation is uncertain (Figure B.6). Evidence is sparse.

## References

Avery, A. D., Lelah, J., Solomon, N. E., Harris, J., Brook, R. H., Greenfield, S., Ware, J. E., and Avery, C. H. *Quality of Medical Care Assessment Using Outcome Measure.* Vol. 2: *Eight Disease-Specific Applications.* Santa Monica, Calif.: Rand Corporation, 1976.

Balnave, K., Scott, M. E., Morton, P., and Murtagh, J. G. "Reliable Prediction of Coronary Disease Using Treadmill Exercise Testing." *British Medical Journal,* 1978, *i,* 958–959.

Bjork, L., Spindola-Franco, H., and Van Houten, F. X. "Comparison of Observer Performance with 16 mm Cinefluorography and 17 mm Camera Fluorography in Coronary Arteriography." *American Journal of Cardiology,* 1975, *36,* 474–478.

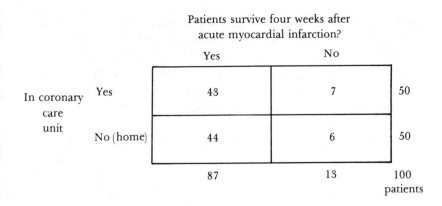

**Figure B.5. Efficacy of the Coronary Care Unit as Measured by Patient Survival (Modified from Mather and others, 1976).**

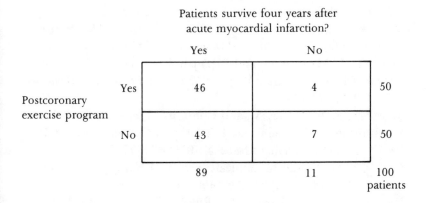

**Figure B.6. Efficacy of Postcoronary Exercise as Measured by Patient Survival (Modified from Sanne, 1977).**

Blackburn, H. "Contrasting Professional Views on Atherosclerosis and Coronary Disease." *New England Journal of Medicine,* 1975, *292,* 105–107.

Braunwald, E. "Coronary Spasm and Acute Myocardial Infarction—New Possibility for Treatment and Prevention." *New England Journal of Medicine,* 1978, *299,* 1301–1303.

Cohn, P. F., Gorlin, R., Vokonas, P. S., Williams, R. A., and Herman, M. V. "A Quantitative Clinical Index for the Diagnosis of Symptomatic Coronary Artery Disease." *New England Journal of Medicine,* 1972, *286,* 901–907.

Colling, A., Carson, P., and Hampton, J. "Home or Hospital Care for Coronary Thrombosis?" *British Medical Journal,* 1979, *i,* 1254–1259.

Day, H. H. "An Intensive Coronary Care Area." *Dis Chest,* 1963, *44,* 423–427.

Edwards, S. R., and Jones, R. J. "The Decline in Coronary Heart Disease Mortality and the Coronary Care Unit." *Journal of the American Medical Association,* 1979, *241,* 403.

Frank, K. A., Heller, S. S., Kornfeld, D. S., and others. "Type A Behavior Pattern and Coronary Angiographic Findings." *Journal of the American Medical Association,* 1978, *240,* 761–763.

Galbraith, J. E., Murphy, M. L., and de Soyza, N. "Coronary Angiogram Interpretation: Interobserver Variability." *Journal of American Medical Association,* 1978, *240,* 2053–2056.

Galen, R. S., and Gambino, S. R. *Beyond Normality. The Predictive Value and Efficiency of Medical Diagnoses.* New York: Wiley, 1975.

Glueck, C. J., Mattson, F., and Bierman, E. L. "Diet and Coronary Heart Disease: Another View." *New England Journal of Medicine,* 1978, *298,* 1471–1474.

Goldschlager, N., Selzer, A., and Cohn, K. "Treadmill Stress Tests as Indicators of Presence and Severity of Coronary Artery Disease." *Annals of Internal Medicine,* 1976, *85,* 277–286.

Hartley, L. H. "Value of Clinical Exercise Testing." *New England Journal of Medicine,* 1975, *293,* 400–401.

Hutchins, G. M., Bulkley, B. H., Ridolfi, R. L., Griffith, L. S. C., Lohr, F. T., and Piasio, M. A. "Correlation of Coronary Angiograms and Left Ventriculograms with Postmortem Studies." *Circulation,* 1977, *56,* 32–37.

Jenkins, C. D. "Recent Evidence Supporting Psychologic and Social

Risk Factors for Coronary Disease." *New England Journal of Medicine,* 1976, *294,* 987–994.

Jenkins, C. D., Rosenman, R. H., and Zyzansk, S. J. "Prediction of Clinical Coronary Heart Disease by a Test for the Coronary-Prone Behavior Pattern." *New England Journal of Medicine,* 1974, *290,* 1271–1275.

Kannel, W. B., Castelli, W. P., and Gordon, J. "Cholesterol in the Prediction of Atherosclerotic Disease: New Perspectives Based on the Framingham Study." *Annals of Internal Medicine,* 1979, *90,* 85–91.

Kellerman, J. J., and Denolin, H. (Eds.). *Critical Evaluation of Cardiac Rehabilitation.* Basel: Karger, 1977.

Kloster, F. E., Kremkau, L., Ritzmann, L. W., Rahimtoola, S. H., Rosch, J., and Kanarek, P. H. "Coronary Bypass for Stable Angina: A Prospective Randomized Study." *New England Journal of Medicine,* 1979, *300,* 149–157.

Levy, R. "Stroke Decline: Implications and Prospects." *New England Journal of Medicine,* 1979, *300,* 490–491.

McIntosh, H. D., and Garcia, J. A. "The First Decade of Aortocoronary Bypass Grafting, 1967–1977: A Review." *Circulation,* 1978, *57,* 405–431.

Mann, G. V. "Diet-Heart: End of an Era." *New England Journal of Medicine,* 1977, *297,* 644–650.

Martin, S. P., Donaldson, M. C., London, C. D., Peterson, O. L., and Colton, T. "Inputs into Coronary Care during 30 years: A Cost Effectiveness Study." *Annals of Internal Medicine,* 1974, *81,* 289–293.

Maseri, A., L'Abbate, A., Baroldi, G., Chierchia, A., Marzilli, M., Ballesura, A. M., Severi, S., Parodi, O., Biagini, A., Distante, A., and Pesola, A. "Coronary Vasospasm as a Possible Cause of Myocardial Infarction: A Conclusion Derived from the Study of 'Preinfarction' Angina." *New England Journal of Medicine,* 1978, *299,* 1271–1277.

Mather, H. G., Morgan, D. C., Pearson, N. G., Read, K. L. Q., Shaw, D. B., Steed, G. R., Thorne, M. G., Lawrence, C. J., and Riley, I. S. "Myocardial Infarction: A Comparison Between Home and Hospital Care for Patients." *British Medical Journal,* 1976, *i,* 925–929.

Medalie, J. H., and Goldbourt, U. "Unrecognized Myocardial Infarction: Five Year Incidence, Mortality, and Risk Factors." *Annals of Internal Medicine,* 1976, *84,* 526–531.

Morris, J. N., and Crawford, M. D. "Coronary Heart Disease and Physical Activity of Work: Evidence of a National Necropsy Study." *British Medical Journal,* 1958, *ii,* 1485–1496.

Oliver, M. F. "Cholesterol, Coronaries, Clofibrate, and Death." *New England Journal of Medicine,* 1978, *199,* 1360–1362.

O'Rourke, R. A., and Ross, J. "Ambulatory Electrocardiographic Monitoring to Detect Ischemic Heart Disease." *Annals of Internal Medicine,* 1974, *81,* 695–696.

Paffenburger, R. S., and Hale, W. E. "Work Activity and Coronary Heart Mortality." *New England Journal of Medicine,* 1975, *292,* 545–550.

Pauker, S. G. "Coronary Artery Surgery: The Use of Decision Analysis." *Annals of Internal Medicine,* 1976, *85,* 8–18.

Rifkin, R. D., and Hood, W. B. "Bayesian Analysis of Electrocardiographic Exercise Stress Testing." *New England Journal of Medicine,* 1977, *197,* 681–686.

Ross, R. S. "Early Discharge After Heart Attacks and the Efficient Use of Hospitals." *New England Journal of Medicine,* 1978, *198,* 275–276.

Ryan, M., Lown, B., and Horn, H. "Comparison of Ventricular Ectopic Activity during 24-Hour Monitoring and Exercise Testing in Patients with Coronary Artery Disease." *New England Journal of Medicine,* 1975, *292,* 224–229.

Salel, A. F., Fong, A., Zelis, R., Miller, R. R., Borhani, N. O., and Mason, D. T. "Accuracy of Numerical Coronary Profile." *New England Journal of Medicine,* 1977, *296,* 1447–1450.

Sanne, H. "Physical Training after Myocardial Infarction." In J. J. Kellerman and H. Denolin (Eds.), *Critical Evaluation of Cardiac Rehabilitation.* Basel: Karger, 1977.

Schwartz, J. N., Kong, Y., Hackel, D. B., and Bartel, A. G. "Comparison of Angiographic and Postmortem Findings in Patients with Coronary Artery Disease." *American Journal of Cardiology,* 1975, *36,* 174–178.

Selden, R., Neill, W. A., Ritzmann, L. W., Okies, J. E., and Anderson, R. P. "Medical Versus Surgical Therapy for Acute Coronary Insufficiency: A Randomized Study." *New England Journal of Medicine,* 1975, *293.*

Takaro, T., Hultgren, H. N., Lipton, M. J., and Detre, K. M. "The Veterans Administration Cooperative Randomized Study of Surgery for Coronary Arterial Occlusive Disease: II. Subgroup with Significant Left Main Lesions." *Circulation,* 1975, *54* (Supplement III), 107–117.

Walker, W. "Changing United States Life-Style and Declining Vascular Mortality: Cause or Coincidence?" *New England Journal of Medicine,* 1977, *197,* 163–165.

Waters, D. D., and Forrester, J. S. "Myocardial Ischemia: Detection and Quantitation." *Annals of Internal Medicine,* 1978, *88,* 239–250.

Weinstein, M. C., and Stason, W. B. "Foundations of Cost-Effectiveness Analysis for Health and Medical Practices." *New England Journal of Medicine,* 1977, *196,* 716–721.

Wright, I. S., and Fredrickson, D. T. (Eds.). *Cardiovascular Diseases: Guidelines for Prevention and Care.* Pub. No. 1727–0035. New York: Intersociety Commission for Heart Disease Resources; Washington, D.C.: U.S. Government Printing Office, 1973.

# References

Abt, C. C. "The Social Costs of Cancer." *Social Indicators Research,* 1975, *2,* 175–190.

Ackerman, F. "Competition and Regulation: The Consumer Choice Health Plan Alternative." *Medical Group Management,* 1980, *27,* 58–64.

Acton, J. P. *Evaluating Public Programs to Save Lives: The Case of Heart Attacks.* Santa Monica, Calif.: Rand Corporation, 1973.

Acton, J. P. *Measuring the Social Impact of Heart and Circulatory Disease Programs: Preliminary Framework and Estimates.* Santa Monica, Calif.: Rand Corporation, 1975.

Acton, J. P. *Measuring the Monetary Value of Lifesaving Programs.* Santa Monica, Calif.: Rand Corporation, 1976.

312

Affelt, J. "New Quality Assurance Standard of the JCAH." *Western Journal of Medicine*, 1980, *132*, 166–170.

American Hospital Association. *International Classification of Health Problems in Primary Care. World Organization of National Colleges, Academies, and Academic Associations of General Practitioners/Family Physicians.* Chicago: American Hospital Association, 1975.

American Medical Association. *Sample Criteria for Short-Stay Hospital Review: Screening Criteria to Assist PSROs in Quality Assurance.* Chicago: American Medical Association, 1976.

American Psychiatric Association, Committee on Nomenclature and Statistics. *Diagnostic and Statistical Manual on Mental Disorders.* (3rd ed.) Washington, D.C.: American Psychiatric Association, 1980.

Association of American Medical Colleges. "Testimony on S.1968, the Health Incentives Reform Act." Submitted to the Subcommittee on Health, Committee on Finance, U.S. Senate, March 18, 1980.

Bailey, R. *Clinical Laboratories and the Practice of Medicine: An Economic Perspective.* Berkeley, Calif.: McCutchan, 1979.

Bain, S. T., and Spaulding, W. B. "The Importance of Coding Presenting Symptoms." *Canadian Medical Association Journal,* 1967, *97,* 953–959.

Baker, H. T. *Quality of Medical Care: Research in Methods of Assessment and Assurance.* Kaiser Permanente Medical Care Program, Southern California Region, 1978.

Ballantine, H. "Peer Evaluation." In E. Carels, D. Neuhauser, and W. Stason (Eds.), *The Physician and Cost Control.* Cambridge, Mass.: Oelgeschlager, Gunn, and Hain, 1980.

Banta, H. D., and Thacker, S. B. *Costs and Benefits of Electronic Fetal Monitoring: A Review of the Literature.* National Center for Health Services Research, Research Report Series. DHEW Pub. No. (PHS) 79-3245. Washington, D.C.: U.S. Government Printing Office, 1979.

Barbaccia, J. "Introducing Quality Assurance and Medical Audit into the UCSF Medical Center Curriculum." *Journal of Medical Education,* 1976, *51,* 386–391.

Barr, D. M., Wollstadt, L. J., and Campobello, P. L. *Annual Report*

*1977–1978: Ambulatory Care Audit Program of the Primary Care Experience.* Rockford: Rockford School of Medicine, University of Illinois College of Medicine, 1978.

Barr, D. M., Wollstadt, L. J., Goodrich, L. L., Pittman, J. G., Booher, C. E., and Evans, R. L. "The Rockford School of Medicine Undergraduate Quality Assurance Program." *Journal of Medical Education,* 1976, *51,* 370–377.

Barr, D. M., Wollstadt, L. J., and Kinast-Porter, S. "Will Physicians Learn to Like Quality Assurance? The Effect of a Curriculum on Medical Student Attitudes." *Journal of Medical Education,* 1979, *54,* 649–650.

Becker, H., Geer, B., Hughes, E., and Strauss, A. *Boys in White: Student Culture in Medical School.* Chicago: University of Chicago Press, 1961.

Becker, M. H., Drachman, R. H., and Kirscht, J. P. "A New Approach to Explaining Sick Role Behavior in Low-Income Populations." *American Journal of Public Health,* 1974, *64,* 205–216.

Becker, M. H., and Maiman, L. A. "Sociobehavioral Determinants of Compliance with Health and Medical Care Recommendations." *Medical Care,* 1975, *13,* 10–24.

Beckhard, R. *Organizational Development: Strategies and Models.* Reading, Mass.: Addison-Wesley, 1969.

Bennis, W. G. *Organizational Development: Its Nature, Origins, and Prospects.* Reading, Mass.: Addison-Wesley, 1969.

Bentley, J. D., and Butler, P. W. *Describing and Paying Hospitals— Developments in Patient Case Mix.* Washington, D. C.: Association of American Medical Colleges, 1980.

Berk, A. *Costs of Illness and Disease, 1900.* Public Services Laboratory of Georgetown University, Report No. B5. Springfield, Va.: U.S. Department of Commerce, National Technical Information Service, Report No. PB-280-300, 1977a.

Berk, A. *Costs of Illness and Disease, Fiscal Year 1930.* Public Services Laboratory of Georgetown University, Report No. B2. Springfield, Va.: U.S. Department of Commerce, National Technical Information Service, Report No. PB-280-299, 1977b.

Berk, A., Paringer, L., and Mushkin, S. J. "The Economic Cost of Illness, Fiscal 1975." *Medical Care,* 1978, *16,* 785–790.

Berry, C. J., Brewster, A., Held, P. J., Kehrer, B. H., Manheim, L. G., and Reinhardt, U. *A Study of the Responses of Canadian Physicians to the Introduction of Universal Medical Care Insurance: The First Five Years in Quebec. Final Report.* Princeton, N.J.: Mathematica Policy Research, 1978.

Bertram, D. A., and Brooks-Bertram, P. A. "The Evaluation of Continuing Medical Education: A Literature Review." *Health Education Monographs,* 1977, *5,* 330–362.

Biles, B., Schramm, C., and Atkinson, J. "Hospital Cost Inflation Under State Rate-Setting Programs." *New England Journal of Medicine,* 1980, *303,* 664–668.

Birnbaum, H., Schwartz, M., Wilson, D., Naierman, N., and Weinstein, R. *A National Profile of Catastrophic Illness.* Cambridge, Mass.: Abt Associates, 1977.

Blim, R. "The American Academy of Pediatrics Involvement in Health Care Financing." *Pediatrics,* 1974, 54(1), 98–105.

Bloom, B. S. (Ed.). *Taxonomy of Educational Objectives.* Handbook I: *The Cognitive Domain.* New York: McKay, 1956.

Bouchard, R. E., and Tufo, H. M. "Problem-Oriented Approach to Practice, II: Development of the System Through Audit and Implication." *Journal of the American Medical Association,* 1977, *236,* 502–505.

Boufford, J. "Primary Care Residency Training: The First Five Years." *Annals of Internal Medicine,* 1977, *82,* 359–368.

Brailey, A. "The Promotion of Health Through Health Insurance." *New England Journal of Medicine,* 1980, *302,* 51–52.

Breslow, L., and Somers, A. R. "The Lifetime Health-Monitoring Program: A Practical Approach to Preventive Medicine." *New England Journal of Medicine,* 1977, *196,* 1–8.

Brook, R. "Studies of Process-Outcome Correlations in Medical Care Evaluation." *Medical Care,* 1979, *17,* 868–873.

Brook, R., Davies-Avery, A., Greenfield, S., Harris, J., Lelah, J., Solomon, N., and Ware, J. "Assessing the Quality of Medical Care Using Outcome Measures: An Overview of the Method." *Medical Care* (Supplement), 1977, *15.*

Brook, R., and Lohr, K. "Quality Assurance in Medical Care: Lessons from the U.S. Experience." In *Proceedings of the Bosch*

*Conference on Quality Assessment of Medical Care.* Stuttgart, West Germany, Autumn 1979.

Brook, R., Ross Davies, A., and Kamberg, C. *Selected Reflections on Quality of Medical Care Evaluation in the 1980's.* Santa Monica, Calif.: Rand Corporation, 1979.

Brook, R. H. *Quality of Care Assessment: A Comparison of Five Methods of Peer Review.* DHEW Pub. No. (HRS)74-3100. Rockville, Md.: Department of Health, Education and Welfare, 1974.

Brook, R. H., Williams, K. N., and Avery, A.D. "Quality Assurance Today and Tomorrow: Forecast for the Future." *Annals of Internal Medicine,* 1976, *85,* 809–817.

Brown, C. R., Jr. "Assessing Quality of Patient Care: The Bi-Cycle Concept." In E. Scheye (Ed.), *The Hospital's Role in Assessing the Quality of Medical Care—Proceedings of the Fifteenth Annual Symposium on Hospital Affairs, May 1973.* Chicago: University of Chicago, 1973.

Brown, C. R., Jr., and Fleisher, D. S. "The Bi-Cycle Concept: Relating Continuing Education Directly to Patient Care." *New England Journal of Medicine,* 1971, *284* (Supplement), 88–97.

Brown, C. R., Jr., and Uhl, H. S. M. "Mandatory Continuing Education: Sense or Nonsense?" *Journal of the American Medical Association,* 1970, *213,* 1660–1668.

Bunker, J. P., Barnes, B. A., and Mosteller, F. *Costs, Risks, and Benefits of Surgery.* New York: Oxford University Press, 1977.

Burra, P., and Bryans, A. "The Helping Professions Group: Interpersonal Dimensions in Health Sciences Education." *Journal of Medical Education,* 1979, *54,* 35–41.

California Medical Association/California Hospital Association. *Educational Patient Care Audit Manual.* San Francisco: California Medical Association/California Hospital Association, 1975.

Carden, T. S. "Tonsillectomy—Trials and Tribulations." *Journal of the American Medical Association,* 1978, *240,* 1961–1962; and 1979, *240,* 2005–2006.

Carroll, J., and Becker, S. "The Paucity of Coursework in Medical Care Evaluation." *Journal of Medical Education,* 1975, *50,* 31–37.

Christianson, J. "The Impact of HMO's: Evidence and Research Issues." *Journal of Health Politics, Policy and Law,* 1980, *5,* 354–367.

Christianson, J., and McClure, W. "Competition in the Delivery of Health Care." *New England Journal of Medicine,* 1979, *301,* 812–818.

Cochrane, A. *Effectiveness and Efficiency: Random Reflections on Health Services.* London: Nuffield Provincial Hospitals Trust, 1972.

Codman, E. A. *A Study in Hospital Efficiency.* Boston: Thomas Todd, 1916.

Commission on Professional and Hospital Activities. *Hospital Adaptation of the ICDA; H-ICDA.* (2nd ed.) 2 vols. Ann Arbor, Mich.: Commission on Professional and Hospital Activities, 1973.

Conover, W. J. "A Kolmogorov Goodness-of-Fit Test for Discontinuous Distributions." *Journal of the American Statistical Association,* 1972, *67,* 591–596.

Cooper, B. S., and Rice, D. P. "The Economic Cost of Illness Revisited." DHEW Pub. No. (SSA) 76-11703. *Social Security Bulletin,* February 1976.

Cooper, J. "Medical Education and the Quality of Care." *Journal of Medical Education,* 1976, *51,* 363–364.

Couch, N., Tilney, N., Raynoer, A., and Moore, F. "The High Cost of Low-Frequency Events: The Anatomy and Economics of Surgical Mishaps." *New England Journal of Medicine,* 1981, *304,* 634–637.

Dalkey, N. C. *The Delphi Method: An Experimental Study of Group Opinion.* Memorandum RM-5888-PR. Santa Monica, Calif.: Rand Corporation, 1969.

Dalkey, N. C. (Ed.), Rourke, D. L., Lewis, R., and Snyder, S. *Studies in the Quality of Life: Delphi and Decision Making.* Lexington, Mass.: Lexington Books/Heath, 1972.

Davis, P., Begley, C. E., and Jarrett, I. *Program Descriptions.* Springfield: Southern Illinois University School of Medicine, 1978.

Delbanco, T., Meyers, K., and Segal, E. "Paying the Physician's Fee: Blue Shield and the Reasonable Charge." *New England Journal of Medicine,* 1979, *301,* 1314.

Delbecq, A. L. "The World Within the 'Span of Control': Managerial Behavior in Groups of Varied Size." *Business Horizons,* 1969, *10*(4), 47–56.

Delbecq, A. L., and Van de Ven, A. H. *Nominal Group Techniques for*

318                                                      References

*Involving Clients and Resource Experts in Program Planning.*
*Academy of Management Proceedings.* Seattle: Graduate School of
Business Administration, University of Washington, 1967.

Delbecq, A. L., Van de Ven, A. H., and Gustafson, D. H. *Group
Techniques for Program Planning.* Glenview, Ill.: Scott, Foresman,
1975.

Dennis, J. E., Dust, E. P., Kaplan, C. B., Pechman, K. J., Rohlfing,
M. B., Styczynski, R. M., Barr, D. M., Wollstadt, L. J., and
Pechman, I. *Ambulatory Care Audit Program of the Primary Care
Experience: Annual Report 1976–77.* Rockford: Rockford School
of Medicine, University of Illinois College of Medicine, 1977.

Densen, P. M. *Guidelines for Producing Uniform Data for Health Care
Plans.* Pub. No. (HSM)73-3005. Rockville, Md.: Department of
Health, Education, and Welfare, 1972.

Dershewitz, R. A., and Williamson, J. W. "Prevention of Childhood
Household Injuries: A Controlled Clinical Trial." *American Journal of Public Health,* 1977, *67,* 1148–1153.

Dewey, J. *Experience and Education.* New York: Macmillan, 1935.

Dobson, H., Greer, J. G., Carlson, R. H., Davis, F. A., Kucken,
L. E., Steinhardt, B. J., Ferry, T. P., and Adler, G. S. "PSROs:
Their Current Status and Their Impact to Date." *Inquiry,* 1978,
*15,* 113–128.

Donabedian, A. "The Quality of Medical Care: Methods for Assessing and Monitoring the Quality of Care for Research and for
Quality Assurance Programs." *Science,* 1978a, *200,* 856–864.

Donabedian, A. "Needed Research in the Assessment and Monitoring of the Quality of Medical Care." NCHSR Research Report
Series, DHEW Pub. No. (PHS) 78-3219, 1978b.

Donabedian, A. "The Definition of Quality and Approaches to Its
Assessment." In *Explorations in Quality Assessment and Monitoring.*
Vol. 1. Ann Arbor: Health Administration Press, University of
Michigan, 1980.

Donabedian, A. "The Criteria and Standards of Quality." In *Explorations in Quality Assessment and Monitoring.* Vol. 2. Ann Arbor:
Health Administration Press, University of Michigan, 1981.

Dresnick, S. J., Roth, W. I., Linn, B. S., Pratt, J. C., and Blum, A.
"The Physician's Role in the Cost-Containment Problem." *Journal of the American Medical Association,* 1979, *241,* 1606–1609.

Drexler, A., Yenney, S. L., and Hohman, J. "OD: Coping with

Change." *Hospitals, Journal of the American Hospital Association,* 1977a, *51,* 58–60.

Drexler, A., Yenney, S. L., and Hohman, J. "OD Team Building: What It's All About." *Hospitals, Journal of the American Hospital Association,* 1977b, *5,* 99–104.

Dunnigan, R. J. Personal communication, 1978.

Edwards, M., and Zimet, C. "Problems and Concerns Among Medical Students—1975." *Journal of Medical Education,* 1976, *51,* 619–625.

Egdahl, R. H. *Quality Assurance in Health Care.* Gaithersburg, Md.: Aspen, 1976.

Egdahl, R. H., and Walsh, D. "Private Cost Containment: The Art of the Possible?" *New England Journal of Medicine,* 1979, *300,* 1330–1332.

Eisenberg, J. M., Williams, S. V., and Pascale, L. A. "An Education Program for Reducing the Overutilization of Diagnostic Procedures." *Proceedings of the 8th Annual Conference on Research in Medical Education,* 1979, 403–405.

Emlet, H. E., Williamson, J. W., Casey, L., and Davis, J. L. *Alternative Methods for Estimating Health Care Benefits and Required Resources.* Vol. 1: *Summary.* Falls Church, Va.: Analytic Services, 1971.

Enthoven, A. "Shattuck Lecture—Cutting Cost Without Cutting the Quality of Care." *New England Journal of Medicine,* 1978a, *298,* 1229–1238.

Enthoven, A. "Consumer Choice Health Plan." *New England Journal of Medicine,* 1978b, *298,* 650–658; 709–720.

Enthoven, A. "The Competition Strategy: Status and Prospects." *New England Journal of Medicine,* 1981, *302,* 109–112.

Eron, L. "The Effect of Medical Education on Medical Students' Attitudes." *Journal of Medical Education,* 1955, *30,* 559–566.

Ertel, P. Y., and Aldridge, M. G. (Eds.). *Medical Peer Review: Theory and Practice.* St. Louis: Mosby, 1977.

Evans, R., Pittman, J., and Peters, R. "The Community-Based Medical School: Reactions at the Interface Between Medical Education and Medical Care." *New England Journal of Medicine,* 1973, *288,* 713–719.

Fein, R. "Social and Economic Attitudes Shaping American Health Policy." *Milbank Memorial Fund Quarterly,* 1980, *158,* 349–385.

Feldstein, M. *Economic Analysis for Health Service Efficiency.* Amsterdam: North Holland, 1967.

Feldstein, M. "Limiting the Rise in Hospital Costs Without Regulations." Testimony before the Senate Health Committee, March 1979.

Feldstein, M., and Taylor, A. *The Rapid Rise of Hospital Costs. Report to the Executive Office of the President.* Washington, D.C.: Council on Wage and Price Stability, 1977.

Fessel, W. J., and Van Brunt, E. E. "Assessing Quality of Care from the Medical Record." *New England Journal of Medicine,* 1972, *286,* 134–138.

Festinger, L. *A Theory of Cognitive Dissonance.* Evanston, Ill.: Row, Peterson, 1957.

Fetter, R. B., Mills, R. E., Riedel, D. C., and Thompson, J. D. "The Application of Diagnostic Specific Cost Profiles to Cost and Reimbursement Control in Hospitals." *Journal of Medical Systems,* 1977, *1,* 137–149.

Fetter, R. B., Shin, Y., Freeman, J. L., Averill, R. F., and Thompson, J. D. "Case Mix Definition of Diagnosis-Related Groups." *Medical Care,* 1980, *18* (Supplement).

Fetter, R. B., Thompson, J. D., and Mills, R. E. "A System for Cost and Reimbursement Control in Hospitals." *Yale Biology Journal,* 1976, *49,* 123–126.

Fink, A., and Kosecoff, J. *An Evaluation Primer.* Washington, D.C.: Capitol Publications, 1978.

Fink, R., Shapiro, S., and Lewison, J. "The Reluctant Participant in Breast Cancer Screening Programs." *Public Health Report,* 1968, *83,* 479–490.

Flach, E. *Participation in Case Finding Programs for Cervical Cancer. Administration Report, Cancer Control Program.* Washington, D.C.: U.S. Government Printing Office, 1960.

Fletcher, R. H., and Fletcher, S. W. "Clinical Research in General Medical Journals." *New England Journal of Medicine,* 1979, *301,* 180–183.

Fordham, C. "Cost Implications of Current Health Manpower Policy." Paper presented at annual meeting of Association for Academic Medical Centers, Phoenix, Arizona, 1979.

Freeland, M., Calat, G., and Schendler, C. "Projections of National

Health Expenditures 1980, 1985, and 1990." *Health Care Financing Review*, 1980, *1*, 9.

Frey, F., Engebretsen, B., Olson, W., and Carmichael, L. "Resident Participation in Residency Programs." *Journal of Medical Education*, 1975, *50*, 765–772.

Frey, J., Demick, J., and Bilbar, R. "Variation in Physician's Feelings of Control During a Family Practice Residency." *Journal of Medical Education*, 1981, *56*, 50–56.

Friedman, E. "Changing the Course of Things: Costs Enter Medical Education." *Hospitals, Journal of the American Hospital Association*, 1979, *53*, 82–85.

Fuchs, V. "What Is CBA/CBE and Why Are They Doing This to U.S.?" *New England Journal of Medicine*, 1980, *303*, 937–938.

Galen, R. S., and Gambino, S. R. *Beyond Normality: The Predictive Value and Efficiency of Medical Diagnoses.* New York: Wiley, 1975.

Garg, M. L., Gliebe, W. A., and Elkhatib, M. B. "Diagnostic Testing as a Cost Factor in Teaching Hospitals." *Hospitals, Journal of the American Hospital Association*, 1978a, *52* (14), 97–100.

Garg, M. L., Gliebe, W. A., and Elkhatib, M. B. "The Extent of Defensive Medicine: Some Empirical Evidence." *Legal Aspects of Medical Practice*, 1978b, *6*, (2), 25–29.

Garg, M. L., Gliebe, W. A., and Kleinberg, W. M. "Quality in Medical Practice: A Student Program." *Journal of Medical Education*, 1977, *52*, 514–516.

Garg, M. L., Kleinberg, W. M., and Gliebe, W. A. "A Course on Cost and Quality." *Quality Review Bulletin*, 1978, *4* (3), 22–26.

Garg, M. L., Louis, D. Z., Gliebe, W. A., Spirka, C. S., Skipper, J. K., and Parekh, R. R. "Evaluating Inpatient Costs: The Staging Mechanism." *Medical Care, 1978, 16*, 191–201.

Garg, M. L., Mulligan, J. L., McNamara, M., Skipper, J. K., and Parekh, R. R. "Teaching Students the Relationship Between Quality and Costs in Medical Care." *Journal of Medical Education*, 1975, *50*, 1085–1091.

Garland, C. H. "The Problem of Observer Error." *Bulletin of the New York Academy of Medicine*, 1960, *36*, 570–584.

Garland, M. J., McCally, M., Osterud, H. T., and Rose, B. K. *Program Descriptions. University of Oregon Health Sciences Center School of Medicine.* Portland: Department of Public Health and Preventive Medicine, University of Oregon Health Sciences Center School of Medicine, 1979.

Gibson, R. M., and Fisher, C. R. "National Health Expenditures, Fiscal 1977." *Social Security Bulletin*, 1978, *41*, 3–20.

Gifford, R. H., and Feinstein, A. R. "A Critique of Methodology in Studies of Anti-Coagulant Therapy for Acute Myocardial Infarction." *New England Journal of Medicine*, 1969, *280*, 351–357.

Ginzberg, E. "The Competitive Solution: Two Views. Competition and Cost Containment." *New England Journal of Medicine*, 1980, *303*, 1112–1115.

Gonnella, J. S., Cattani, J. A., Louis, D. Z., and others. "Use of Outcome Measures in Ambulatory Care Evaluation." In G. A. Giebink, N. H. White, and E. S. Short (Eds.), *Ambulatory Medical Care Quality Assurance*. La Jolla, Calif.: La Jolla Health Science Publications, 1977.

Gonnella, J. S., and Goran, M. S. "Quality of Patient Care. A Measurement of Change: The Staging Concept." *Medical Care*, 1975, *13*, 467–473.

Gonnella, J. S., Goran, M. S., Williamson, J. W., and Cotsonas, W. J. "Evaluation of Patient Care: An Approach." *Journal of the American Medical Association*, 1970, *214*, 2040–2043.

Gonnella, J. S., Louis, D. Z., and McCord, J. J. "The Staging Concept: An Approach to the Assessment of Outcomes of Ambulatory Care." *Medical Care*, 1976, *14*, 13.

Goodlad, J. I. *School Curriculum and the Individual*. Waltham, Mass.: Blaisdell, 1966.

Goran, M. J. "The Evolution of the PSRO Hospital Review System." *Medical Care*, 1979, *17* (5), Supplement.

Goran, M. J., Roberts, J. S., Kellogg, M., Fielding J., and Jessee, W. "The PSRO Hospital Review System." *Medical Care*, 1975, *13* (4), Supplement.

Greenbaum, D., and Hoban, J. "Teaching Peer Review at Michigan State University." *Journal of Medical Education*, 1976, *51*, 392–394.

Greene, R. *Assuring Quality in Medical Care: The State of the Art*. Cambridge, Mass.: Ballinger, 1976.

Greenspan, N., and Vogel, R. "Taxation and Its Effect upon Public and Private Health Insurance and Medical Demand." *Health Care Financing Review*, Spring 1980, 39–44.

Haefner, D. P., and Kirscht, J. P. "Motivational and Behavioral

Effects of Modifying Health Beliefs." *Public Health Report,* 1970, *85,* 478–484.

Haggerty, R. J. "Family Medicine: A Teaching Program for Medical Students and Pediatric Health Officers." *Journal of Medical Education,* 1962, *37,* 331–580.

Harrow, A. J. *A Taxonomy of the Psychomotor Domain: A Guide for Developing Behavioral Objectives.* New York: McKay, 1972.

Helfer, R. "Peer Evaluation: Its Potential Usefulness in Medical Education." *British Journal of Medical Education,* 1972, *6,* 224–231.

Hiatt, H. "Protecting the Medical Commons: Who Is Responsible?" *New England Journal of Medicine,* 1975, *293,* 235–241.

Hochbaum, G. M. *Public Participation in Medical Screening Programs: A Socio-Psychological Study.* PHS Publ No. 572. Washington, D.C.: U.S. Government Printing Office, 1958.

Horn, S. D. "Goodness-of-Fit Tests for Discrete Data: A Review and an Application to a Health Impairment Scale." *Biometrics,* 1977, *33,* 237–248.

Hsiao, W., and Stason, W. "Toward Developing a Relative Value Scale for Medical and Surgical Services." *Health Care Financing Review,* 1979, *1* (2), 23–38.

Hu, T., and Sandifer, F. H. *Synthesis of Cost of Illness Methodology.* Prepared for National Center for Health Services Research, Office of the Assistant Secretary for Health, Public Health Service, Department of Health and Human Services (Contract No. 233-79-3010), 1981.

Hubbard, W. N., Gronvall, J. A., and DeMuth, G. R. (Eds.). *The Medical School Curriculum.* Part 2: *Medical Education.* Washington, D.C.: Association of American Medical Colleges, 1970.

Huebner, L., Royner, J., and Moore, J. "The Assessment and Remediation of Dysfunctional Stress in Medical School." *Journal of Medical Education,* 1981, *56,* 547–558.

Institute of Medicine. *Advancing the Quality of Health Care: Key Issues and Fundamental Principles. A Policy Statement by a Committee of the Institute of Medicine.* Washington, D.C.: National Academy of Sciences, 1974.

Institute of Medicine. *Assessing Quality of Health Care: An Evaluation.* Washington, D.C.: National Academy of Sciences, 1976.

Inui, T. S., Yourtee, E. L., and Williamson, J. W. "Improved Outcomes in Hypertension After Physician Tutorials: A Controlled

Trial." *Annals of Internal Medicine,* 1976, *84,* 646–651.

Jessee, W. F. "Quality Assurance Systems: Why Aren't There Any?" *Quality Review Bulletin,* 1977a, *3* (11), 16–18.

Jessee, W. F. "Physician Competence and Compulsory Continuing Education: Are They Compatible?" *Journal of Community Health,* 1977b, *2,* 291–295.

Jessee, W. F., and Goran, M. J. "The Role of the Academic Medical Center in the PSRO Program." *Journal of Medical Education,* 1976, *55,* 365–369.

Joint Commission on Accreditation of Hospitals. *The PEP Primer.* Chicago: Joint Commission on Accreditation of Hospitals, 1974.

Joint Commission on Accreditation of Hospitals. *Program on Hospital Accreditation Standards.* (1st ed.) Chicago: Joint Commission on Accreditation of Hospitals, 1976.

Joint Commission on Accreditation of Hospitals. "New Quality Assurance Standard of the JCAH." *Quality Review Bulletin,* 1979, *5,* 4–5.

Joint Commission on Accreditation of Hospitals. *The QA Guide: A Resource for Hospital Quality Assurance.* Chicago: Joint Commission on Accreditation of Hospitals, 1980.

Kane, R. L. Personal communication, 1973a.

Kane, R. L. *Report on the Development of a Curriculum for Teaching Medical Care Appraisal in Medical Schools.* Salt Lake City: University of Utah Medical Center, 1973b.

Kane, R. L., and Hogben, M. "Teaching Quality of Care Evaluation to Medical Students." *Journal of Medical Education,* 1974, *49,* 778–780.

Kaplan, S. H., and Greenfield, S. "Criteria Mapping: Using Logic in Evaluation of Processes of Care." *Quality Review Bulletin,* 1978, *4,* 3–9.

Kegeles, S. S. "A Field Experiment to Change Beliefs and Behavior of Women in an Urban Ghetto." *Journal of Health and Social Behavior,* 1969, *10,* 115–124.

Keniston, K. "The Medical Student." *Yale Journal of Biology and Medicine,* 1967, *39,* 346–358.

Kessner, D. M., Kalk, C. E., and Singer, J. "Assessing Health Quality: The Case for Tracers." *New England Journal of Medicine,* 1973, *288,* 189–194.

Kinast-Porter, S., Barr, D. M., and Wollstadt, L. J. "The Effect of a Quality Assurance Curriculum on Medical Student Activities." Paper presented at annual meeting of North American Primary Care Research Group, Toronto, 1978.

Kleinberg, W. M., Garg, M. L., and Gliebe, W. A. "Cost Effective Medical Practices: A Curriculum at Medical College of Ohio." *Ohio State Medical Journal*, 1979, *75*, 298–300.

Knox, A. B. "Adult Learning." In *Adult Development and Learning: A Handbook on Individual Growth and Competence in the Adult Years for Education and the Helping Professions.* San Francisco: Jossey-Bass, 1977.

Krathwohl, D.R., Bloom, B. S., and Masia, E. B. *Taxonomy of Educational Objectives: Classification of Educational Goals.* Vol. 2: *Affective Domain.* New York: McKay, 1964.

Lawler, K., Manigold, D., Reuben, G., Silva, G., Skallerup, J., Taylor, J., Van Dam, J., Barr, D. M., Wollstadt, L. J., and Campobello, P. L. *Ambulatory Care Audit Program of the Primary Care Audit Program of the Primary Care Experience: Annual Report 1977-78.* Rockford, Ill.: Rockford School of Medicine, 1978.

Lawrence, P. R., and Lorsch, J. W. *Organization and Environment.* Homewood, Ill.: Irwin, 1969.

Lawrence, P. R., Weisbord, M. R., and Charms, M. P. "The Organization and Management of Academic Medical Centers: A Sumary of Findings." Unpublished paper, Organization Research and Development, division of Block, Petrella and Associates, 1974.

Laxdal, D. E., Jennett, P. A., Wilson, T. W., and Salisbury, G. M. "Improving Physician Performance by Continuing Medical Education." *Canadian Medical Association Journal*, 1978, *118*, 1051-1058.

Lesserman, J. "Changes in the Professional Orientation of Medical Students: A Follow-up." *Journal of Medical Education*, 1980, *55*, 415-422.

Lewis, L. A. Personal communication, 1979.

Lilienfeld, A. M. *Foundations of Epidemiology.* New York: Oxford University Press, 1976.

Lindstone, H. A., and Turoff, M. (Eds.) *The Delphi Method—Tech-*

*niques and Applications.* Reading, Mass.: Addison-Wesley, 1975.

Longmire, W., and Mellinkoff, S. "Regionalization of Operations." *New England Journal of Medicine,* 1979, *301,* 1393–1394.

Louis, D. Z., DeDiemar, N. L., Edison, S. M., Heineccius, L., and Spirka, C. S. *Application of the Staging Methodology to the Analysis and Evaluation of PHDDS Hospital Utilization Data. Final Report.* Santa Barbara, Calif.: Systemetrics, 1979.

Louis, D. Z., and Spirka, C. S. *Staging Analysis of Hospital Discharges, 1976–1978.* Santa Barbara, Calif.: Systemetrics, 1979.

Lowe, J. A. "PASport." *Quality Review Bulletin,* 1977a, *3,* 20–24.

Lowe, J. A. "The Quality Assurance Monitor and MCE Studies." Paper presented at a workshop on Alternative Approaches to MCE Studies, Chicago, 1977b.

Luft, H. "How Do Health Maintenance Organizations Achieve Their 'Savings'?" *New England Journal of Medicine,* 1978, *298,* 1336.

Luft, H., Bunker, J., and Enthoven, A. "Should Operations Be Regionalized? The Empirical Relation Between Surgical Volume and Mortality." *New England Journal of Medicine,* 1979, *301,* 1364–1369.

McCarthy, E. G., and Finkel, M. *Fundamentals of Second-Opinion Programs for Elective Surgery.* Brookfield, Wis.: International Foundation of Employee Benefit Plans, 1979.

McCarthy, E. G., and Finkel, M. "Surgical Utilization in the U.S.A." *Medical Care,* 1980, *18,* 883–892.

McCarthy, E. G., and Widmer, G. W. "Effects of Screening by Consultants on Recommended Elective Surgical Procedures." *New England Journal of Medicine,* 1974, *291,* 1331–1335.

MacDonald, C. J. "Protocol-Based Computer Reminders, the Quality of Care and the Non-perfectibility of Man." *New England Journal of Medicine,* 1975, *295,* 1351–1355.

MacMahon, B., and Pugh, T. F. *Epidemiology: Principles and Methods.* Boston: Little, Brown, 1970.

McNerney, W. "Control of Health Care Costs in the 1980's." *New England Journal of Medicine,* 1980, *303,* 1088–1095.

Mager, R. W. *Preparing Instructional Objectives.* (2nd ed.) Belmont, Calif.: Fearon, 1975.

Mather, H. G., Morgan, D. C., Pearson, N. G., Read, K. L. Q.,

Shaw, D. B., Steed, G. R., Thorne, M. G., Lawrence, C. J., and Riley, I. S. "Myocardial Infarction: A Comparison Between Home and Hospital Care for Patients." *British Journal of Medical Education,* 1976, *1,* 925–929.

Matthews, J. S. Personal communication, 1979.

Meads, S., and McLemore, T. "National Ambulatory Medical Care Survey: Symptom Classification, United States." *Vital and Health Statistics,* Series 2, No. 63. DHEW Pub. No. (HRA)74-1337. Washington, D.C.: U.S. Government Printing Office, 1974.

Meyer, G. *Tenderness and Technique: Nursing Values in Transition.* Los Angeles: Institute of Industrial Relations, University of California at Los Angeles, 1960.

Mills, D. H. "Report on the California Medical Insurance Feasibility Study." Unpublished paper, California Medical Association/ California Hospital Association, 1977.

Mills, R., Fetter, R. B., Riedel, D. C., and Averill, R. "AUTOGRP: An Interactive Computer System for the Analysis of Health Care Data." *Medical Care,* 1976, *14,* 603–615.

Mishan, E. J. "Evaluation of Life and Limb: A Theoretical Approach." *Journal of Political Economy,* 1971, *79,* 687–705.

Moloney, T., and Rogers, D. "Medical Technology—a Different View of the Contentious Debate over Costs." *New England Journal of Medicine,* 1979, *301,*1413–1419.

Monson, R. A. *An Ambulatory Care Information System for Evaluating Clinical Performance of Medicine Residents.* Little Rock: Department of Medicine, University of Arkansas for Medical Sciences, 1979.

Mooney, G. "Cost-Benefit Analysis and Medical Ethics." *Journal of Medical Ethics,* 1980, *6,* 177–179.

Muir Gray, J. "Choosing Priorities." *Journal of Medical Ethics,* 1979, *5,* 73–75.

Mulhearn, J., and Eurenius, K. "A Veterans Administration Initiative in Health Care Cost Control." *Journal of the American Medical Association,* 1979, *242,* 1285–1287.

Mulley, A. B., Thibault, G. E., Hughes, R. A., Barnett, G. O., Reder, V. A., and Sherman, E. L. "The Course of Patients with Suspected Myocardial Infarction." *New England Journal of Medicine,* 1980, *302,* 943–948.

Mulligan, J. L. Personal communication, University of Missouri School of Medicine, 1979.

Mulligan, J., Garg, M., Skipper, J., and McNamara, M. "Quality Assurance in Undergraduate Medical Education at the Medical College of Ohio." *Journal of Medical Education,* 1976, *51,* 378–385.

Mushkin, S. J., and d'A. Collings, F. "Economic Costs of Disease and Injury." *Public Health Reports,* 1959, *74,* 795–809.

Mushkin, S. J., Smelke, M., Wyss, D., Vehorn, C. L., and others. "Cost of Disease and Illness in the United States in the Year 2000." *Public Health Reports,* 1978, *494.*

Mushlin, A. I. "An Experimental Mechanism for Quality Assurance in a Pre-Paid Group Practice." In Group Health Association of America, *Proceedings of the Group Health Institute.* Washington, D.C.: Group Health Association of America, 1974.

Mushlin, A. I., and Appel, P. A. *Final Report of the Johns Hopkins University Experimental Medical Care Review Organization (EMCRO) Project at the Columbia Medical Plan.* PHS Grant No. HS01310. Baltimore, Md.: Johns Hopkins University, 1977.

Mushlin, A. I., and Appel, P. A. "Quality Assurance in Primary Care: A Strategy Based on Outcome Assessment." *Journal of Community Health,* 1978, *3,* 292–305.

Mushlin, A. I., and Appel, P. A. "Testing an Outcome Based Quality Assurance Strategy in Primary Care." *Medical Care* (Supplement), 1980, 18 (5), part 2.

Naeye, R. L. "Causes of the Excessive Rates of Perinatal Mortality and Prematurity in Pregnancies Complicated by Maternal Urinary Tract Infections." *New England Journal of Medicine,* 1979, *300,* 819–823.

National Center for Health Statistics. "National Ambulatory Medical Care Survey: Symptom Classification, United States." In *Vital and Health Statistics.* Series 2, No. 63. DHEW Pub. No. (HRA) 74-1337. Washington, D.C.: U.S. Government Printing Office, 1974.

National Center for Health Statistics. *International Classification of Diseases, Adapted for Use in the United States.* (8th revision.) DHEW Pub. No. (PHS) 1693. Washington, D.C.: U.S. Government Printing Office, 1977.

National Center for Health Statistics. "National Ambulatory Medical Care Survey: 1975 Summary. United States, January–December 1975." In *Vital and Health Statistics.* Series 13, No. 33. DHEW Pub. No. (PHS) 78-1784. Washington, D.C.: U.S. Government Printing Office, 1978a.

National Center for Health Statistics. "Inpatient Utilization of Short-Stay Hospitals by Diagnosis: 1975. United States, January–December, 1975." In *Vital and Health Statistics.* Series 13, No. 35. DHEW Pub. No. (PHS) 78-1786. Washington, D.C.: U.S. Government Printing Office, 1978b.

National Center for Health Statistics. *Health, United States.* DHEW Pub. No. (PHS) 78-1232. Hyattsville, Md.: National Center for Health Services Research, 1978c.

National Center for Health Statistics, Division of Health Resources Utilization Statistics. *National Ambulatory Medical Care Survey.* Special Communication. Washington, D.C.: U.S. Government Printing Office, 1979a.

National Center for Health Statistics. "A Reason for Visit Classification for Ambulatory Care." In *Vital and Health Statistics.* Series 2, No. 78. DHEW Pub. No. (PHS) 79-1352. Washington, D.C.: U.S. Government Printing Office. 1979b.

Nobrega, F. I., Morrow, J. W., Smoldt, R. K., and Offord, K. P. "Quality Assessment in Hypertension: Analysis of Process and Outcome Methods." *New England Journal of Medicine,* 1977, *296,* 145–148.

Noren, J., and Detmer, D. "Quality of Health Care: Evaluation and Assurance." In University of Wisconsin Medical School (Madison), *Preventive Medicine 703: Course Catalog.* Madison: University of Wisconsin Medical School, 1979.

Office of Research, Demonstration and Statistics. *Professional Standards Review Organizations, 1978. Program Evaluations.* DHEW Pub. No. (HCFA) 0300. Washington, D.C.: Health Care Financing Administration, 1979.

Office of Research, Demonstration and Statistics. *Health Care Financing Research Report: Professional Standards Review Organization 1979 Program Evaluation.* DHHS Pub. No. (HCFA) 03041. Washington, D.C.: Health Care Administration, 1980.

Office of Technology Assessment. *Assessing the Efficacy and Safety of Medical Technologies.* No. 052-003-00593-0. Washington, D.C.: U.S. Government Printing Office, 1978.

Office of Technology Assessment. *The Implications of Cost-Effectiveness Analysis of Medical Technology.* Washington, D.C.: U.S. Government Printing Office, 1980a.

Office of Technology Assessment. *The Implications of Cost-Effectiveness Analysis in Medical Technology; Background Paper: Methodological Issues and Literature Review.* Washington, D.C.: U.S. Government Printing Office, 1980b.

Ogilvie, R., and Ruedy, J. "An Educational Program in Digitalis Therapy." *Journal of the American Medical Association,* 1972, *222,* 50–55.

Osborne, C. E. "Relationship Between Medical Audit Results and the Planning of Continuing Medical Education Programs." *Medical Care,* 1980, *18,* 994–1000.

Paringer, L. C., and Berk, A. *Costs of Illness and Disease, Fiscal Year 1975.* Pub. No. PB 280-298. Springfield, Va.: Department of Commerce, National Technical Information Service, 1977.

Parker, J. L., and Rubin, L. J. *Process as Content: Curriculum Design and the Application of Knowledge.* Chicago: Rand McNally, 1960.

Parsons, V., and Lock, P. "Focus: Current Issues in Medical Ethics. Triage and the Patient with Renal Failure." *Journal of Medical Ethics,* 1980, *6,* 173–176.

Pauker, S., and Kassirer, J. "Therapeutic Decision Making: A Cost-Benefit Analysis." *New England Journal of Medicine,* 1975, *293,* 229–234.

Payne, B. C., and Lyons, T. F. *Methods of Evaluating and Improving Personal Medical Care Quality: Episode of Illness Study.* Ann Arbor: University of Michigan School of Medicine, 1972.

Peterson, P. "Teaching Peer Review." *Journal of the American Medical Association,* 1973, *224,* 884–885.

Piper, D. "Decision-Making: Decisions Made by Individuals vs. Those Made by Group Consensus or Group Participation." *Education Administration Quarterly,* 1974, *10,* 82–95.

Pliskin, N., and Taylor, A. "General Principles: Cost-Benefit and Decision Analysis." In J. Bunker and others (Eds.), *Costs, Risks, and Benefits of Surgery.* New York: Oxford University Press, 1977.

Posner, G. J., and Rudnitsky, A. N. *Course Design: A Guide to Curriculum Development for Teachers.* New York: Longmans, 1978.

Rafferty, J., and Hornbrook, M. "On Being Wrong About the Hospital: The Role of Utilization Measures." Paper presented at Public Health Conference on Records and Statistics. DHEW Pub. (PHS) 79-1214. 1979.

Reiser, D. "Struggling to Stay Human in Medicine: One Student's Reflections on Becoming a Doctor." *New Physician,* 1973, *22,* 295–299.

Relman, A. "Technology Costs and Evaluation." *New England Journal of Medicine,* 1979, *301,* 1444–1445.

Relman, A. "The Allocation of Medical Resources by Physicians." *Journal of Medical Education,* 1980, *55,* 99–104.

Renner. J. H., Miragia, M., Davis, J., and McNeil, D. "Quality Assessment and Assurance and Medical Records." In University of Wisconsin Medical School (Madison), *Fourth Year Electives Catalog.* Madison: University of Wisconsin Medical School, 1979.

Renner, J. H., and Piernot, R. W. "A Revised Symptom Code List for Ambulatory Medical Record Data." Paper prepared for Family Practice Program. Madison: University of Wisconsin, 1972.

Rice, D. P. *Estimating the Cost of Illness.* Health Economics Series No. 6. DHEW Pub. No. (PHS) 947-6. Washington, D.C.: U.S. Government Printing Office, 1966.

Rice, D. P., Feldman, J. J., and White, K. L. "The Current Burden of Illness in the United States." Occasional paper presented at annual meeting of Institute of Medicine, Washington, D.C., October 1976.

Rice, D. P., and Hodgson, T. A. "Social and Economic Implications of Cancer in the United States." Paper presented to the Expert Committee on Cancer Statistics of the World Health Organization and International Agency for Research on Cancer, Madrid, Spain, June 1978. Hyattsville, Md.: National Center for Health Statistics.

Riedel, R. L., and Riedel, D. C. *Practice and Performance: An Assessment of Ambulatory Care.* Ann Arbor, Mich.: Health Administration Press, 1979.

Rosenberg, P. "Students' Perceptions and Concerns During Their First Year in Medical School." *Journal of Medical Education,* 1971, *46,* 211–218.

Rosser, R. M., and Watts, V. "A Clinical Classification of Disability and Distress and Its Application to the Awards Made by the Courts in Personal Injury Cases." *New Law Journal,* 1975, *125,* 323.

Rubenstein, E., and others. "CME Before Audit." *Medical Care,* 1979, *17,* 1048–1053.

Rubin, L., and Kellogg, M. A. "The Comprehensive Quality Assurance System." In G. A. Giebink, N. H. White, and E. S. Short (Eds.), *Ambulatory Medical Care Quality Assurance.* La Jolla, Calif.: La Jolla Health Sciences Publications, 1977.

Rutstein, D., Berenberg, W., and Chalmers, T. C. "Measuring the Quality of Medical Care." *New England Journal of Medicine,* 1976, *294,* 582–588.

Sackett, D. L., and Haynes, R. B. *Compliance with Therapeutic Regimens.* Baltimore, Md.: Johns Hopkins University Press, 1976.

Sanazaro, P. J., and Worth, R. M. "Concurrent Quality Assurance in Hospital Care: Report of a Study by Private Initiative in PSRO." *New England Journal of Medicine,* 1978, *198,* 1171–1177.

Saylor, J. G., and Alexander, W. M. *Planning Curriculum for the Schools.* New York: Holt, Rinehart and Winston, 1974.

Schein, E. H. *Process Consultation: Its Role in Organization Development.* Reading, Mass.: Addison-Wesley, 1969.

Schein, E. H. *Organizational Psychology.* (2nd ed.) Englewood Cliffs, N.J.: Prentice-Hall, 1970.

Schein, E. H. *Professional Education: Some New Directions.* Tenth of a series of profiles sponsored by the Carnegie Commission on Higher Education. Berkeley, Calif.: McGraw-Hill, 1972.

Schelling, T. C. "The Life You Save May Be Your Own." Paper presented at the Second Conference on Government Expenditures, Brookings Institution, Washington, D.C., 1968. Cambridge, Mass.: Department of Economics, Harvard University.

Schneider, D., and Appleton, L. "Reason for Visit Classification System for Patient Records in an Ambulatory Care System." *Quality Review Bulletin,* 1977, *3,* 20–26.

Schroeder, S. A., Showstack, J. A., and Roberts, H. E. "Frequency and Clinical Description of High Cost Patients in 17 Acute-Care Hospitals." *New England Journal of Medicine,* 1979, *300,* 1306–1309.

Scitovsky, A. A., and McCall, N. *Changes in the Costs of Treatment of Selected Illnesses: 1951–1964–1971.* DHEW Pub. No. (HRA) 77-3161. Hyattsville, Md.: National Center for Health Services Research, 1977.

Senior, J. "Towards the Measurement of Competence in Medicine." *Quarterly Review Bulletin,* 1977, *3,* 19–21.

Sheber, J. "Quality Assurance Concurrent Review Assures Quick Response to Faculty Care." *Hospitals, Journal of the American Hospital Association,* 1980, *54,* 55–57.

Showstack, J. A., Blumberg, B., Schwartz, J., and Schroeder, S. "Fee-for-Service Physician Payment: Analysis of Current Methods and Their Development." *Inquiry,* 1979, *16,* 230–246.

Silva, G. Personal communication, Rockford School of Medicine, 1979.

Sivertsen, S., Meyer, T., Hassan, R., and Schoenenberger, A. "Individual Physician Profile: Continuing Education Evaluation Related to Medical Practice." *Journal of Medical Education,* 1973, *48,* 1006–1012.

Skipper, J., Mulligan, J., and Garg, M. "The Use of Peer Group Review in a Community and Family Medical Clerkship." *Journal of Medical Education,* 1974, *49,* 991–993.

Smith, W. M. "Treatment of Mild Hypertension: Results of a Ten-Year Intervention Trial." *Circulation Research,* 1977, *40* (Supplement 1), 98–105.

Smith, W. M. "Hypertension: Effectiveness of Early Treatment in Preventing Sequelae." Paper presented at a seminar on preventive interventions in the practice of medicine, Rancho Mirage, Calif., March 1979.

Solomon, N., and Cohen, H. "Hospital Cost Control in Maryland." *Health Care Financing Administration Forum,* 1978, *2,* 12–19.

Somers, A., and Somers, H. "A Proposed Framework for Health and Health Care Policies." *Inquiry,* 1977, *14,* 115–120.

Starfield, B. H. "Achieving Coordination in Primary Care." Paper presented at the Ambulatory Pediatric Association meeting, New York, April 1978.

Starr, C., and Whipple, C. "Risks of Risk Decisions." *Science,* 1980, *208,* 1114–1119.

Steel, K., Gertman, P., Crescenzi, C., and Anderson, J. "Iatrogenic Illness on a General Medical Service at a University Hospital." *New England Journal of Medicine,* 1981, *304,* 638–642.

Suter, E., Green, J. S., Lawrence, K. and Walthhall, D. B., III. "Continuing Education of Health Professionals: Proposal for a Definition of Quality." *Journal of Medical Education,* 1981, *56* (Supplement), 687–707.

Thaler, R., and Rosen, S. "The Value of Saving a Life: Evidence from the Labor Market." *Household Production Consumption, Studies in Income and Wealth* (New York: National Bureau of Economic Research), 1976, *40,* 265–294.

Thibault, G. E., Mulley, A. B., Barnett, G. O., Goldstein, R. L., Reder,, V. A., Sherman, E. L., and Skinner, E. R. "Medical Intensive Care: Indications, Interventions, and Outcomes." *New England Journal of Medicine,* 1980, *302,* 938–942.

Thompson, J. D., Averill, R. F., and Fetter, R. B. "Planning, Budgeting, and Controlling—One Look at the Future: Case Mix Cost Accounting." *Health Services Research,* 1979, *14,* 111–125.

Thompson, J. D., Fetter, R. B., and Mross, C. D. "Case Mix and Resource Use." *Inquiry,* 1975, *17,* 300–312.

Thompson, J. D., Fetter, R. B., and Shin, Y. "One Strategy for Controlling Costs in University Teaching Hospitals." *Journal of Medical Evaluation,* 1978, *53,* 167–175.

Tufo, H. M., Bouchard, R. E., Rubin, A. S., Twitchell, J. C., Van Buren, H. C., Weed, L. B., and Rothwell, M. "Problem-Oriented Approach to Practice." *Journal of the American Medical Association,* 1979, *238,* 414–417; 502; 505.

Tyler, R. "Specific Approaches to Curriculum Development." In J. Schaffarzick and D. H. Hampson (Eds.), *Strategies for Curriculum Development,* Berkeley, Calif.: McCutchan, 1975.

U.S. Congress, House of Representatives, Committee on Interstate and Foreign Commerce, Subcommittee on Oversight and Investigations. *Background Report on PSRO's: Report of a Yale University Study Group.* No. 95-16. Washington, D.C.: U.S. Government Printing Office, 1977.

Veterans Administration Cooperative Study Group on Antihypertensive Agents. "Effects of Treatment on Morbidity in Hypertension. Results in Patients with Diastolic Blood Pressure Averaging 115 Through 129 mm Hg." *Journal of the American Medical Association,* 1967, *202,* 1028–1034.

Veterans Administration Cooperative Study Group on Antihypertensive Agents. "Effects of Treatment on Morbidity in Hypertension. Part 2: Results in Patients with Diastolic Blood Pressure Averaging 90 Through 114 mm Hg." *Journal of the American Medical Association,* 1970, *213,* 1143–1152.

Veterans Administration Cooperative Study Group on Antihypertensive Agents. "Effects of Treatment on Morbidity in Hypertension. Part 3: Influence of Age, Diastolic Pressure, and Prior Cardiovascular Disease; Further Analysis of Side Effects." *Circulation,* 1972, *45,* 991–1004.

Ware, J., Davies-Avery, A., and Stewart A. "The Measurement and Meaning of Patient Satisfaction." *Health and Medical Services Review,* 1978, *1,* 1–15.

Weinstein, M., Fineberg, H., Elskin, A., Frazier, H., Neuhauser, D., Neutra, R., and McNeil, B. *Clinical Decision Analysis.* Philadelphia: Saunders, 1980.

Weisbord, M. R. "A Mixed Model for Medical Centers: Changing Structure and Behavior." In J. Adams (Ed.), *Theory and Method in Organization Development: An Evolutionary Process.* Arlington, Va.: National Institute for Applied Behavioral Science, 1974.

Weisbord, M. R. "Why Organization Development Hasn't Worked (So Far) in Medical Centers." *Health Care Management Review,* 1976, *1,* 18–31.

Williams, K. N., and Brook, R. H. "Quality Measurement and Assurance: A Literature Review." *Health and Medical Care Services Review,* 1978, *1* (3), 1.

Williamson, J. W. *Improving Medical Practice in Health Care: A Bibliographic Guide to Information Management in Quality Assurance and Continuing Medical Education.* Cambridge, Mass.: Ballinger, 1977.

Williamson, J. W. *Assessing and Improving Health Care Outcomes: The Health Accounting Approach to Quality Assurance.* Cambridge, Mass.: Ballinger, 1978.

Williamson, J. W., Alexander, M., and Miller, G. E. "Continuing Education in Patient Care Research: Physician Response to

Screening Test Results." *Journal of the American Medical Association,* 1967, *201,* 938–942.

Williamson, J. W., Alexander, M., and Miller, G. E. "Priority in Patient Care Research and Continuing Medical Education." *Journal of the American Medical Association,* 1968, *204,* 93.

Williamson, J. W., Aronovitch, S., Simonson, L., Ramirez, C., and Kelly, D. "Health Accounting, an Outcome-Based System of Quality Assurance: Illustrative Application to Hypertension." *Bulletin of the New York Academy of Medicine,* 1975, *51,* 727–738.

Williamson, J. W., Goldschmidt, P., and Jilson, I. *Medical Practice Information Demonstration Project.* Baltimore, Md.: Policy Research, 1979.

World Health Organization. *Manual of the International Statistical Classification of Diseases, Injuries, and Causes of Death.* (9th revision.) Geneva: World Health Organization, 1977.

Young, W. W. *Measuring the Cost of Care Using Generalized Patient Management Paths.* Pittsburgh: Health Research Department, Blue Cross of Western Pennsylvania, 1979.

Young, W. W., Swinkola, R. B., and Hutton, M. D. "Assessment of the AUTOGRP Patient Care Classification System." *Medical Care,* 1980, *18,* 228.

Zeleznik, C. Personal communication, Jefferson Medical College, 1979.

Zeleznik, C., and Gonnella, J. S. "The Student Model Utilization Review Committee of Jefferson Medical College." *Journal of Medical Education,* 1979, *54,* 848–851.

Zook, C. J., and Moore, F. D. "High-Cost Users of Medical Care." *New England Journal of Medicine,* 1980, *302,* 996–1002.

# Index

## A

Abt, C. C., 85, 312
Academic medical centers: curriculum integration in, 23–30; and curriculum rationale, 4–5; teaching of quality assurance and cost containment in, 231–257
Achievable benefit not achieved (ABNA), ratings of, 148
Ackerman, F., 262, 312
Acton, J. P., 83, 85, 312
Adams, R. D., 51
Affelt, J., 263, 313
Aldridge, M. G., 205, 319
Alexander, M., 143, 165, 169, 335–336
Alexander, W. M., 6, 332
Alliance for Engineering in Medicine and Biology, 128, 129
Ambulatory care: classification scheme for, 59, 62–63; evaluation in, 36; national data on, 89–94
American Academy of Pediatrics, 128, 264
American Association for Labor Legislation, Committee on Social Insurance of, 288–289
American Association of Foundations of Medical Care, 293
American Association of Professional Standards Review Organizations, 293
American Board of Medical Specialties, 190
American College of Cardiology, 127
American College of Physicians, 127, 128, 151
American College of Surgeons, 128, 151
American Federation of Labor, 289
American Heart Association, 127, 299
American Hospital Association, 57, 59, 151, 289, 313
American Hospital Supply Corporation, 69$n$
American Medical Association, 313; classification by, 89; and consensus teams, 127; criteria of, 64, 128, 129, 192, 234; and curriculum, 20; and history, 283, 285, 286, 287, 290; and Joint Commission on Accreditation of Hospitals, 151; and Peer Review Organizations, 293
American Nurses Association, 190

**337**

Hampton, J., 305, 308
Harris, J., 306, 315–316
Harrow, A. J., 9, 323
Hartley, L. H., 300, 302, 308
Hass, W. K., 52
Haynes, R. B., 225, 332
Health Accounting, for effectiveness and efficiency, 148, 155
Health care: achieving improvement in, 164–181; costs of, 260–272; effectiveness and efficiency of, 136–163; efficacy documentation of, 111–135; expenditures for, 70, 101
Health Care Cost Restraint Act of 1979 (H.R. 5740), 272
Health care facilities, inpatient days in, by disease categories, 104–105
Health Care Financing Administration, 64, 108; Office of Policy, Planning, and Research of, 156
Health Incentive Reform Act of 1979 (S. 1968), 262
Health insurance: changes in, and costs, 263–264; history of, 282–283, 288–290
Health loss: from care, cost of, 86–87; concept of, 70; health problem importance and, 71; local data on, 108; national data on, 98–101; quantifying, 79–81
Health Maintenance Organization Act of 1973, 293
Health maintenance organizations: and costs, 265; and quality assurance, 293
Health Outcomes Commission, 293
Health problems: classification systems for, 57–63; and coding systems in quality assurance studies, 63–67; direct costs of, 83–84; and efficacy, 116; implications of, 55–57; indirect costs of, 84–85; local data on, developing, 64–67; and local use of national data, 63–64; as organizing framework, 54–68; patient categories and, 55–56, 59, 62–63; provider categories and,

56, 57–61; societal importance of, 69–110; and topic selection, 185; unmeasured costs of, 85–86
Health problems importance: analysis of, 69–110; and curriculum integration, 24; and economic costs, 71–72; economic framework for, 81, 82–83; frequency of, 71; and health loss, 71; illustrations of, 72–79; implications of, 70–72; local data on, 103, 107–109; medical framework for, 80–81; national data on, 88–105; projects suggested on, 109–110; quantifying determinants of, 79–88; and topic selection, 185–186
Health Standards and Quality Bureau, 126, 127–128
Heller, S. S., 308
Herman, M. V., 308
Hiatt, H., 137–138, 261, 265, 323
Hill-Burton program, 290–291
Hirschfeld, D., 295
Hoban, J., 236–238, 322
Hochbaum, G. M., 171, 323
Hodgson, T. A., 73, 84, 331
Hoff, J. T., 52
Hogben, M., 231–232, 324
Hohman, J., 174, 318–319
Hood, W. B., 301, 310
Horn, H., 301, 310
Horn, S. D., 216, 323
Hornbrook, M., 260, 331
Hospital-centered program, evaluation in, 37
Hospital costs, and insurance, 76
Hospital of the University of Pennsylvania, and teaching program, 243–244
Hospital stays, changes in number of, 76, 78
Hospital Survey and Construction Act of 1946, 290–291
Hospitals, short-stay, national data from, 94–98
Hsiao, W., 84, 263, 323
Hu, T., 82, 83, 323
Hubbard, W. N., 19, 323